The Opioid Epidemic and Infectious Diseases

The Opioid Epidemic and Infectious Diseases

Edited by

Brianna L. Norton, MD

Division of General Internal Medicine and Infectious Diseases
Bronx, NY, United States

ELSEVIER

Elsevier
Radarweg 29, PO Box 211, 1000 AE Amsterdam, Netherlands
The Boulevard, Langford Lane, Kidlington, Oxford OX5 1GB, United Kingdom
50 Hampshire Street, 5th Floor, Cambridge, MA 02139, United States

Notices

Knowledge and best practice in this field are constantly changing. As new research and
experience broaden our understanding, changes in research methods, professional
practices, or medical treatment may become necessary.

Practitioners and researchers must always rely on their own experience and knowledge in
evaluating and using any information, methods, compounds, or experiments described
herein. In using such information or methods they should be mindful of their own safety
and the safety of others, including parties for whom they have a professional
responsibility.

To the fullest extent of the law, neither the Publisher nor the authors, contributors, or
editors, assume any liability for any injury and/or damage to persons or property as a
matter of products liability, negligence or otherwise, or from any use or operation of any
methods, products, instructions, or ideas contained in the material herein.

Library of Congress Cataloging-in-Publication Data
A catalog record for this book is available from the Library of Congress

British Library Cataloguing-in-Publication Data
A catalogue record for this book is available from the British Library

ISBN: 978-0-323-68328-9

For information on all Elsevier publications visit our website at
https://www.elsevier.com/books-and-journals

Publisher: Elsevier
Acquisitions Editor: Charlotta Kryhl
Editorial Project Manager: Sam W. Young
Production Project Manager: Sreejith Viswanathan
Cover Designer: Alan Studholme

Typeset by TNQ Technologies

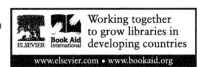

Contents

CHAPTER 6   Opioid use disorder and HCV (hepatitis C virus) 77
Irene Pericot-Valverde, PhD, Divya Ahuja, MD,
Brianna L. Norton, MD and Alain H. Litwin, MD MPH

**CHAPTER 10 Inpatient opioid use disorder treatment
for the infectious disease physician 189**
*Nikhil Seval, MD, Ellen Eaton, MD, MSPH and
Sandra A. Springer, MD*

CHAPTER 11 HIV pre-exposure prophylaxis for people who inject drugs...................................... 223

Roman Shrestha, PhD, Benjamin McCoy-Redd, BS and Jaimie P. Meyer, MD, MS, FACP

Contributors

Divya Ahuja, MD
Department of Medicine, University of South Carolina School of Medicine, Columbia, SC, United States

Wajiha Z. Akhtar, PhD, MPH
Associate Scientist, Department of Medicine, University of Wisconsin—Madison, Madison, WI, United States

Frederick L. Altice
Center for Interdisciplinary Research on AIDS (CIRA), Yale University, New Haven, CT, United States; Academic Icon Professor of Medicine, University of Malaya, Kuala Lumpur, Malaysia; Visiting Professor of Medicine, Sichuan University, Chengdu, China

Hayley Berg
College of Global Public Health, New York University, New York, NY, United States

Annick Bórquez, PhD, MSc
Assistant Professor, Division of Infectious Diseases and Global Public Health, University of California San Diego, La Jolla, CA, United States

John Cafardi, MD
The Christ Hospital, Cincinnati, OH, United States

Javier A. Cepeda, PhD, MPH
Assistant Professor, Division of Infectious Diseases and Global Public Health, University of California San Diego, La Jolla, CA, United States

Daniel Ciccarone, MD, MPH
Professor, Department of Family and Community Medicine, University of California San Francisco, San Francisco, CA, United States

Don C. Des Jarlais, PhD
Professor of Epidemiology, Social and Behavioral Sciences, College of Global Public Health, New York University, New York, NY, United States

Ellen Eaton, MD, MSPH
Assistant Professor, Department of Medicine, Division of Infectious Disease, University of Alabama at Birmingham, Birmingham, AL, United States

Jonathan Feelemyer
College of Global Public Health, New York University, New York, NY, United States

Judith Feinberg, MD
Professor, Department of Behavioral Medicine and Psychiatry and Professor, Department of Medicine, Section of Infectious Diseases, West Virginia University School of Medicine, Morgantown, WV, United States

Audrey Li, MD
Clinical Fellow in Medicine, Beth Israel Deaconess Medical Center, Boston, MA, United States

Alain H. Litwin, MD MPH
Department of Medicine, University of South Carolina School of Medicine, Greenville, SC, United States; Department of Medicine, Prisma Health, Greenville, SC, United States; Clemson University, School of Health Research, Clemson, SC, United States

Gregory M. Lucas, MD, PhD
Professor, Medicine, Johns Hopkins University, Baltimore, MD, United States

Lynn M. Madden
Department of Medicine, Section of Infectious Diseases, Yale School of Medicine, New Haven, CT, United States; Department of Epidemiology of Microbial Diseases, Yale School of Public Health, New Haven, CT, United States

Natasha K. Martin, DPhil
Associate Professor, Division of Infectious Diseases and Global Public Health, University of California San Diego, La Jolla, CA, United States

Benjamin McCoy-Redd, BS
Predoctoral Fellow, Yale School of Medicine, Section of Infectious Disease, AIDS Program, New Haven, CT, United States

Jaimie P. Meyer, MD, MS, FACP
Associate Professor of Medicine, Yale School of Medicine, Section of Infectious Disease, AIDS Program, New Haven, CT, United States

Dharushana Muthulingam
Department of Medicine, Section of Infectious Diseases, Yale School of Medicine, New Haven, CT, United States

Brianna L. Norton, MD
Division of General Internal Medicine and Infectious Diseases, Bronx, NY, United States

Irene Pericot-Valverde, PhD
Clemson University, School of Health Research, Clemson, SC, United States

David C. Perlman, MD
Professor of Medicine, Icahn School of Medicine at Mount Sinai Chief, Infectious Diseases, Mount Sinai Beth Israel New York, NY, United States

Jody Rich, MD, MPH
Professor of Medicine and Epidemiology at The Warren Alpert Medical School of
Brown University, Providence, RI, United States; Center for Prisoner Health and
Human Rights at The Miriam Hospital, Providence, RI, United States

Christopher F. Rowley, MD, MPH
Assistant Professor Medicine, Beth Israel Deaconess Medical Center, Boston,
MA, United States

Radha Sadacharan, MD, MPH
Clinical Instructor in the Department Family Medicine, The Warren Alpert
Medical School of Brown University, Providence, RI, United States; Center for
Prisoner Health and Human Rights at The Miriam Hospital, Providence, RI,
United States

Nikhil Seval, MD
Instructor of Medicine, Department of Internal Medicine, Section of Infectious
Diseases, AIDS Program, Yale School of Medicine, New Haven, CT, United States

Roman Shrestha, PhD
Associate Research Scientist, Yale School of Medicine, Section of Infectious
Disease, AIDS Program, New Haven, CT, United States

Sandra A. Springer, MD
Attending Physician, Internal Medicine, Infectious Disease, Veterans
Administration Connecticut Healthcare System, West Haven, CT, United States;
Center for Interdisciplinary Research on AIDS, Yale University School of Public
Health, New Haven, CT, United States; Associate Professor of Medicine,
Department of Internal Medicine, Section of Infectious Diseases, AIDS Program,
Yale School of Medicine, New Haven, CT, United States

Norah Terrault, MD, MPH
Professor, Division of Gastrointestinal and Liver Diseases, Keck School of
Medicine, University of Southern California, Los Angeles, CA, United States

Kali Zhou, MD, MAS
Assistant Professor, Division of Gastrointestinal and Liver Diseases, Keck School
of Medicine of University of Southern California, Los Angeles, CA, United States

The epidemiology of the opioid overdose epidemic in the United States

Daniel Ciccarone, MD, MPH

Professor, Department of Family and Community Medicine, University of California San Francisco, San Francisco, CA, United States

Introduction

The opioid overdose epidemic is the latest phase of a multidecade exponential increase in drug-related mortality in the United States [1]. The severity of the current crisis has driven up the overall US mortality rate 3 years in a row from 2014 to 2017 [2–4]. Correspondingly, life expectancy at birth has declined; the first triple-year decline since World War I and the devastating influenza pandemic 100 years ago [5]. Most of the top 10 causes of death are declining year over year; however, the third leading cause of death, unintentional injuries, has climbed in rate and rank since 2014 [3]. Driving this increase are deaths due to drug poisoning, which exceeded 70,000 in 2017 [6]. Annual deaths due to drug overdoses now exceed those caused by motor vehicle accidents, gun violence, and even HIV infection at the height of the 1990s HIV epidemic [7].

The focus of this chapter is on the epidemiology of the US opioid overdose epidemic. National trends and demographics will be presented first. Then, using the framework of the "triple wave," each phase of the opioid crisis will be discussed separately in terms of regional distribution, demographics, and supply and demand drivers. It is critical to discuss the drivers of each wave to best inform policy and intervention responses.

National trends and demographics

The annual number of drug overdose deaths (all classes) grew from 16,849 in 1999 to 70,237 in 2017; corresponding to an increase in rate from 6.1 per 100,000 population in 1999 to 21.7 in 2016 [6]. This rate more than tripled overall with an accelerated increase from 2014 to 2016 of 18% per year.

The class of drugs leading the escalation in drug poisoning, as well as the overall US mortality, is the opioids. In 2017, two-thirds of drug overdose deaths involved opioids (47,600) [8]. There were 8050 opioid overdose deaths in 1999, with a rate

The Opioid Epidemic and Infectious Diseases. https://doi.org/10.1016/B978-0-323-68328-9.00001-1

of 2.9 per 100,000; this rate increased fivefold to 14.9 in 2017 [6]. Since 1999, over 400,000 deaths have been attributed to the opioid crisis thus far.

Since 1999, overdose death rates for men were approximately twice that of women, with the rate for men tripling from 8.2 in 1999 to 29.1 in 2017. Rates increased fastest for age groups 25–34 years and 45–54 years, both achieving rates of 38 per 100,000 in 2017 [6].

The triple-wave epidemic: opioid pills, heroin, and synthetic opioids

The triple wave epidemic of overdose deaths stems from three classes of opioids: prescription opioid pills ("semisynthetic opioids" in Fig. 1.1), heroin, and synthetic opioids other than methadone [9]. Fig. 1.1 shows three waves of opioid mortality, each wave cresting on top of the one before it. In the first wave, overdoses related to opioid pills started rising in the year 2000 and have steadily grown through 2016. The second wave saw overdose deaths due to heroin, which started increasing clearly in 2007, surpassing the number of deaths due to opioid pills in 2015. The third wave mortality has arisen from fentanyl, fentanyl analogues, and other synthetic opioids of illicit supply; it has climbed slowly at first but dramatically after 2013. Data from 2017 show synthetic opioid deaths continuing to rise, reaching a

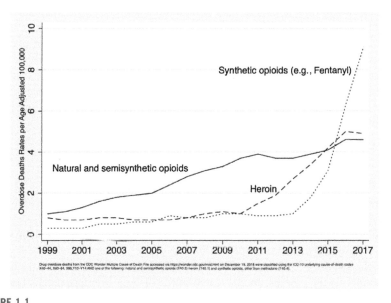

FIGURE 1.1

Opioid overdose deaths by the type of opioid.

peak of over 28,000, whereas opioid pill and heroin overdose deaths leveled off, albeit at very high levels of approximately 15,000 deaths in each category [6].

Wave 1: prescription opioid pills

The rate of prescription opioid overdose mortality increased fourfold from 1.0/ 100,000 in 1999 to 4.4 in 2016 and 2017 [6]. Men have a 50% higher rate (6.1) than women (4.2). The highest rate is among those aged 45−54 years (10.0) [8]. Rates are higher in whites (6.9) than in African Americans (3.5) or Hispanics (2.2). By level of urbanization (e.g., metro, fringe metro, nonmetro), rates are equivalent.

The supply-side drivers underlying the first wave of prescription opioid overdose have been extensively discussed [10,11]. Wave 1 is widely considered to have been driven iatrogenically with a tripling of opioid prescriptions starting in the 1990s and peaking around 2011 [12]. Increases in prescribing have been attributed to the changing medical culture and assertive marketing by pharmaceutical companies [13]. The upsurge in prescriptions has been correlated to the rising adverse consequences, particularly opioid overdose [14]. The introduction of extended-release long-acting (ERLA) opioid formulations supports both supply-side and demand-side pressure. ERLA formulations are a source of opioids in a novel form with a technologic advance that allowed higher, longer lasting doses in a single capsule. However, the ease with which their delayed-release mechanisms could be bypassed and the whole dose discharged at once, for instance, by crushing and insufflating (nasal snorting) or injecting, led to a wave of misuse [15,16].

A demand-side argument has been introduced examining the structural factors that might be driving the epidemic [17]. The "diseases of despair" analyses highlight the extraordinary rise in death rates, among middle-aged whites without a college degree, in three related categories: drug poisoning, alcohol-related disease, and suicide [18]. The most compelling structural determinants include an aging population with rises in reported pain and disability, economic distress, declining social cohesion, and rising psychologic malaise that may have led an at-risk population to seek opioids in the first place [17]. In this line of reasoning, increased opioid prescribing is a "vector" of the opioid overdose epidemic, with more proximal root causes being worsening structural forces accompanied by generational hopelessness and despair [19].

Wave 2: heroin

Heroin-related overdose mortality rates were stable from 1999 to 2007. Starting in 2008, heroin overdose rates increased fivefold from 1.0 per 100,000 (3041 deaths) to 4.9 in 2017 (15,482 deaths) [6].

Coincident with rising heroin-related deaths, the number of heroin users [20], especially young heroin users, has been increasing since the mid-2000s [21]. The first two overdose waves, from opioid pills and heroin, have been termed "intertwined epidemics" [22]. Young and new heroin users have described the reason for transitioning from opioid pills to heroin as their growing dependence that required larger and more consistent pill supplies than they could obtain either by prescription or on the street. The more ready availability of high-purity, low-cost heroin made the switch to heroin economically logical and difficult to resist [15].

Drug treatment data show that in successive cohorts from the 1960s through the 2000s, patients admitted to treatment with heroin use disorder increasingly reported starting their opioid use disorder with opioid pills [23]. However, this has begun to change as an increasing proportion of patients with heroin use disorder entering treatment report heroin as their first experience of an opioid [24]. Overdoses due to heroin began to accelerate in 2011. In late 2010, OxyContin, a brand-name ERLA formulation of oxycodone, was reformulated to be abuse-deterrent. The reformulation of this popular diverted opioid pill may have had the unintended consequence of driving a small proportion of the at-risk population to heroin use [16]. In sum, we have seen elements of demand-side drive in wave 2, with rising numbers of heroin users transitioning from opioid pill dependency followed more recently by younger persons initiating first with heroin.

Although "intertwined," the first and second opioid overdose waves show some contrasts in age and regional distribution. Examining the years 2012–14, the age distribution of patients hospitalized for opioid pill overdose had its largest peaks in the 50- to 64-year-old group. Meanwhile, the peak age group for heroin overdose admissions was 20- to 34-year-old people. In this data, we see possible evidence of population-level transitions from opioid pills to heroin use as the rates for overdose among 20- to 34-year-old people declined for opioid pills but, in the same period, increased for heroin [25]. Heroin overdose mortality is three times higher among men (7.3/100,000) than women (2.5). Although whites have higher rates (6.1) than African Americans (4.9), rates are increasing in the recent years among the latter [8].

Geographic disparities are also evident—in contrast to the national spread of opioid pill overdose, heroin-related overdose is much higher in the US Northeast and Midwest regions, along with higher rates of increase [25]. Some of this regional disparity may be endemic, stemming from the 1970s, but there are also significant new supply-side forces shaping it. A dramatic transformation in the US heroin supply, including changes in its country of origin, has occurred in the past 10 years. Prior to 2000, heroin was imported from four source regions/countries in the world, including Southeast Asia, Southwest Asia, Mexico, and South America (Colombia). The 2000s began an era in which most US heroin was transshipped by transnational criminal organizations (TCOs) from two countries: Colombia and Mexico [26]. Regional heroin distribution became starkly divided with Colombia sourced heroin predominant in the eastern United States while "black tar" heroin from Mexico being the major source-form in the western United States [27,28]. Accelerating this trend from oligopoly to monopoly, Mexican TCOs have increasingly dominated the US heroin market, with their market share increasing from 50% in 2005 to 90% in 2016 [29].

Mexico-sourced heroin is also becoming more refined. From 2005 to 2012, a growing and substantial proportion of the analyzed heroin samples obtained in the eastern US cities by the US Drug Enforcement Administration (DEA) for its Heroin Domestic Monitor Program were from an unknown source and of unknown quality. Subsequent DEA analyses have led to the conclusion that a more refined heroin has emerged from Mexican sources. This so-called "Mexican White" is a mimic of high-quality Colombia-sourced powder heroin, replacing it in its traditional retail outlets of the Northeast and Midwest [30].

Wave 3: synthetic opioids

Synthetic opioids in the heroin supply, chiefly illicitly produced fentanyl, are responsible for the third wave of overdose mortality [9,31]. Mortality due to fentanyls, including chemical analogues, has increased dramatically, with a doubling in number and rate between 2013 and 2016 (2016: 5800 deaths; 5.9/100,000) [32]. By 2016, fentanyl overdose rates are almost three times higher in men (8.6) than those in women (3.1). The age group with the highest numbers of deaths (5976) and rate (13.4/100,000) is 25- to 34-year-old people. Whites have higher rates of fentanyl mortality (7.74) than African Americans (5.55); however, the recent rate of increase is much higher in the latter, i.e., 140.6% average annual increase in 2011−16. Regional disparities are also evident, with the Northeast, Midwest, and mid-Atlantic regions most impacted.

"Heroin," particularly in the Northeast and Midwest, the regions with the greatest increases in wave 2 overdose, currently exists as fentanyl-adulterated and/or fentanyl-substituted heroin (FASH) [33]. Illicitly manufactured fentanyl is integrated into the illicit drug supply and sold as "heroin" in powder form, or as counterfeit opioid or benzodiazepine pills [34].

Fentanyl is the main chemical in a growing family of chemical analogues. These analogues come in a range of morphine-equivalent potencies, with some such as butyryl-fentanyl being less potent than fentanyl by weight while others have much greater potency [35]. In addition, there are other novel synthetic opioids in circulation, including U47700 and U48800. The greatest concern arises from a branch of the fentanyl family that includes some exceedingly potent opioids such as carfentanil, sufentanil, and remifentanil. It is unclear whether these extremely potent fentanyls will become established elements in the opioid marketplace or if they are just accidents or experiments in the rapidly evolving illicit opioid supply.

According to the US DEA, the current main source of illicitly manufactured fentanyls is China. Fentanyls sourced from China take a number of routes on their way into the United States, including internet purchases, routing through Canada (typically pill form), or through Mexico in powder or pill form [36]. Perhaps the most revealing aspect of the supply that fuels the US fentanyl epidemic is its regional discreetness. Comparing drug seizure data with overdose death data, one finds a remarkable geographic correlation between fentanyl seizures and synthetic opioid overdoses [34]. These fentanyl events overlap in the same regions as wave 2 heroin overdose: the Northeast, mid-Atlantic, and Midwest. The reasons for this regional disparity are unclear. One possibility is that fentanyl distribution is regionally orchestrated by a branch of the Sinaloa TCO [29]. Another hypothesis is that source forms of powder heroin, predominant in the Northeast and Midwest, are more easily adulterated with powder fentanyls than solid "black tar" heroin, which predominates in the western United States [9,37]. Such stark regional disparities support the notion that the third wave is a supply-side event [38]. A demand-driven or culturally driven event, such as through entrepreneurial or individual internet purchases, would more likely have led to a more even geographic spread of fentanyl-related overdose or one that reflected similar social conditions in separate geographic locations.

The "Iron Law of Prohibition" suggests that highly potent-by-volume drugs such as fentanyl are *expected* due to the honing effects of interdiction [39]. Following this is the concern that constraining the mother chemical, fentanyl, too robustly and too rapidly will foster the supply of fentanyl analogues. The number of known fentanyl analogues exceeds 200; the number of potential fentanyl analogues could exceed several hundred more. Care must be taken not to foster the ingenuity and creativity of illicit drug manufacturers to push in even more dangerous directions. Based on this concern, the DEA has imposed a first-ever class restriction on the family of fentanyls, the utility of which is uncertain.

Ethnographic research with persons who use heroin confirms that the introduction of FASH has been unexpected and unsettling, that fentanyl was not a demand-driven phenomenon, and that there is a range of desirability for FASH from abhorrence and avoidance through acceptance to enthusiasm [33,40]. Those who favor fentanyl are nevertheless hampered from choosing it in the marketplace by its concealed identity as "heroin" or counterfeit brand-name pills [33,37,40]. Importantly, cultural idioms for fentanyl have been slow to emerge despite 4 years of steady supply; slang terms have arisen for most desired illicit drugs and their absence, in this case, is evidence for a lack of strong demand. Consequentially, emergence of slang can be seen as a marker for the growing acceptance of fentanyl.

In addition to the dangerous potency of fentanyl, ethnographic observations support the notion of a possibly greater danger: rapid changes in potency and purity, as well as varying mixtures of heroin, fentanyl, and its analogues [9,33,40]. Australian research on heroin overdose has shown that fluctuations within a wider range of street heroin purity, particularly when around a higher mean purity level, are an independent predictor of a fatal overdose [41]. Vicissitudes in the potency/purity/mixture of FASH in the street market may be discovered to have profound effects on the overdose rate in a given location.

Conclusion

The triple-wave opioid overdose epidemic is an intertwined, three drug subclass epidemic. All three waves have impressive supply-side drivers including excessive prescribing of medication, a new form of highly refined Mexico-sourced heroin, and a new illicit source of synthetic opioids adulterating heroin and counterfeit pills. Demand for opioid pills partially drove demand for heroin while demand for heroin unsuspectingly feeds demand for synthetics-as-substitute. Increases in opioid mortality are now driven by deaths due to FASH. The second and third waves are regional, with the Northeast (including mid-Atlantic) and Midwest (including Appalachia) being the most affected regions.

Positive supply shocks are historically correlated with upswings in drug use and consequences and the same can be seen in the current opioid crisis. Fentanyl, in particular, comes as a positive supply shock leading to disastrous consequences. It is thus tempting to focus efforts on controlling supply. There is evidence that supply-side interventions can work if part of a comprehensive program also includes demand reduction [42]. Unipolar supply-side interventions, however, may cause paradoxical unwanted results (for example, see Ciccarone et al. 2009 [28]). These phenomena may be occurring within the current crisis. Downward pressure on opioid prescribing may be driving a portion of the at-risk population from opioid pill misuse to heroin, thus exposing them to the even more dangerous family of fentanyls. Another driver of unintended consequences may have been the reformulation of ERLA opioids to abuse-deterrent formulations, examples of which include OxyContin and Opana, with misuse of the latter implicated in the Scott County Indiana HIV outbreak [43]. The goals of curtailing excessive prescribing practices or creating abuse-deterrent formulations may be reasonable, but the untoward consequences must be recognized, monitored, and responded to accordingly.

Considering the inadequate and paradoxical effects of current opioid supply interventions, supply-side policies must be combined with sufficient investments in and expansion of effective prevention, substance use treatment, and harm reduction services [44]. Opioid use disorder has a number of medical treatment options that have been shown to be medically efficacious as well as cost-effective [45]. Improving access to medical treatment for opioid use disorder is vital; for this, efforts must be placed on workforce expansion, improving medical education, expanding insurance coverage, and reducing regulatory barriers [46,47]. In particular, reducing the regulatory burdens on prescribing buprenorphine and providing performance-based metrics and incentives for its use should greatly enhance access to this evidence-based treatment [47,48]. The US Surgeon General has called for greater distribution of naloxone, the opioid antagonist used to treat an opioid pill, heroin, or fentanyl overdose [49]. Achieving a wider distribution of naloxone into the community is an essential strategy in the current epidemic [50,51]. Sterile syringe provision must be greatly expanded to meet the increasing population at risk. Drug surveillance and drug checking can be utilized as a harm reduction strategy [9,52–55]. Supervised consumption spaces can aid in the prevention of overdose and can reduce HIV and HCV transmission risks [56–58]. These services can act as a safety net or hub for persons at risk and provide them with necessary resources and referrals to services [59].

Acknowledgments

I gratefully acknowledge research funding from the US National Institutes of Health, National Institute of Drug Abuse Grant DA037820. I thank Dr. Sarah Mars for extensive feedback and Dr. Jay Unick for creating Fig. 1.1.

References

[1] Jalal H, et al. Changing dynamics of the drug overdose epidemic in the United States from 1979 through 2016. Science 2018;361(6408):eaau1184.

[2] National Center for Health Statistics. Mortality multiple cause-of-death public use data file documentation. National Vital Statistics System, US Centers for Disease Control and Prevention; 2017.

[3] Murphy SL, et al. Mortality in the United States, 2015. In: NCHS data brief. US Department of Health and Human Services, Centers for Disease Control and Prevention; 2016.

[4] Murphy SL, et al. Mortality in the United States, 2017. In: NCHS data brief. US Department of Health and Human Services, Centers for Disease Control and Prevention; 2018.

[5] Tejada VB, et al. Mortality trends in the United States, 1900—2015. National Center for Health Statistics; 2017.

[6] Hedegaard H, Miniño AM, Warner M. Drug overdose deaths in the United States, 1999—2017. In: NCHS data brief no 329. Hyattsville, MD: National Center for Health Statistics; 2018.

[7] Katz J. Drug deaths in America are rising faster than ever. N Y Times June 5, 2017. Accessed at: https://www.nytimes.com/interactive/2017/06/05/upshot/opioid-epidemic-drug-overdose-deaths-are-rising-faster-than-ever.html.

[8] Scholl L, et al. Drug and opioid-involved overdose deaths — United States, 2013—2017. Morb Mortal Wkly Rep 2019;67:1419—27.

[9] Ciccarone D. Fentanyl in the US heroin supply: a rapidly changing risk environment. Int J Drug Pol 2017;46:107—11.

[10] Madras BK. The surge of opioid use, addiction, and overdoses: responsibility and response of the US health care system. JAMA Psychiatr 2017;74(5):441—2.

[11] Van Zee A. The promotion and marketing of OxyContin: commercial triumph, public health tragedy. Am J Publ Health 2009;99(2):221—7.

[12] Kolodny A, et al. The prescription opioid and heroin crisis: a public health approach to an epidemic of addiction. Annu Rev Publ Health 2015;36:559—74.

[13] Humphreys K. Avoiding globalisation of the prescription opioid epidemic. Lancet 2017;390(10093):437—9.

[14] Centers for Disease Control and Prevention. Vital signs: overdoses of prescription opioid pain relievers — United States, 1999—2008. Morb Mortal Wkly Rep 2011;60:1487—92.

[15] Mars SG, et al. "Every 'never' I ever said came true": transitions from opioid pills to heroin injecting. Int J Drug Pol 2014;25(2):257—66.

[16] Cicero TJ, Ellis MS, Surratt HL. Effect of abuse-deterrent formulation of OxyContin. N Engl J Med 2012;367(2):187—9.

[17] Dasgupta N, Beletsky L, Ciccarone D. Opioid crisis: No easy fix to its social and economic determinants. Am J Publ Health 2018;108(2):182—6.

[18] Stein EM, et al. The epidemic of despair among white Americans: trends in the leading causes of premature death, 1999−2015. Am J Publ Health 2017;107(10):1541−7.

[19] National Academies of Sciences, Engineering, and Medicine. Pain Management and the opioid epidemic: balancing societal and individual benefits and risks of prescription opioid use. Washington, DC: National Academies Press; 2017.

[20] What America's users spend on illegal drugs: 2000−2010. 2014, Office Of National Drug Control Policy. Washington, D.C.: Executive Office of the President.

[21] Center for Behavioral Health Statistics and Quality. Results from the 2016 national Survey on drug use and Health: detailed tables prevalence estimates, standard errors, P values, and sample sizes. Rockville, MD: Substance Abuse and Mental Health Services Administration; 2017.

[22] Unick GJ, et al. Intertwined epidemics: national demographic trends in hospitalizations for heroin- and opioid-related overdoses, 1993−2009. PloS One 2013;8(2):e54496.

[23] Cicero TJ, et al. The changing face of heroin use in the United States: a retrospective analysis of the past 50 years. JAMA Psychiatr 2014;71(7):821−6.

[24] Cicero TJ, Kasper ZA, Ellis MS. Increased use of heroin as an initiating opioid of abuse: further considerations and policy implications. Addict Behav 2018;87:267−71.

[25] Unick GJ, Ciccarone D. US regional and demographic differences in prescription opioid and heroin-related overdose hospitalizations. Int J Drug Pol 2017;46:112−9.

[26] US Drug Enforcement Administration, Update: Heroin Signature Program. Reported in the 2015 national drug threat assessment summary. 2015.

[27] Ciccarone D. Heroin in brown, black and white: structural factors and medical consequences in the US heroin market. Int J Drug Pol 2009;20(3):277−82.

[28] Ciccarone D, Unick GJ, Kraus A. Impact of South American heroin on the US heroin market 1993−2004. Int J Drug Pol 2009;20(5):392−401.

[29] US Drug Enforcement Administration, National drug threat assessment. 2017.

[30] US Drug Enforcement Administration, Domestic monitoring program. Reported in the 2015 national drug threat assessment summary. 2015.

[31] NIDA. Overdose death rates. January 2017. Available from: https://www.drugabuse.gov/related-topics/trends-statistics/overdose-death-rates.

[32] Spencer MR, et al. National Vital Statistics Reports. Drug overdose deaths involving fentanyl, 2011−2016, vol. 68 (3). Hyattsville, MD: National Center for Health Statistics; 2019.

[33] Ciccarone D, Ondocsin J, Mars SG. Heroin uncertainties: exploring users' perceptions of fentanyl-adulterated and -substituted 'heroin'. Int J Drug Pol 2017;46:146−55.

[34] Gladden RM, Martinez P, Seth P. Fentanyl Law enforcement submissions and increases in synthetic opioid-involved overdose deaths − 27 States, 2013−2014. Morb Mortal Wkly Rep 2016;65(33):837−43.

[35] Suzuki J, El-Haddad S. A review: fentanyl and non-pharmaceutical fentanyls. Drug Alcohol Depend 2017;171:107−16.

[36] US Drug Enforcement Administration, National drug threat assessment. 2016.

[37] Carroll JJ, et al. Exposure to fentanyl-contaminated heroin and overdose risk among illicit opioid users in Rhode Island: a mixed methods study. Int J Drug Pol 2017;46:136−45.

[38] Mars SG, Rosenblum D, Ciccarone D. Illicit fentanyls in the opioid street market: desired or imposed? Addiction 2018;114(5).

[39] Beletsky L, Davis CS. Today's fentanyl crisis: prohibition's Iron Law, revisited. Int J Drug Pol 2017;46:156−9.

[40] Mars SG, Ondocsin J, Ciccarone D. Sold as heroin: perceptions and use of an evolving drug in Baltimore, MD. J Psychoact Drugs 2018;50(2):167–76.

[41] Darke S, et al. Fluctuations in heroin purity and the incidence of fatal heroin overdose. Drug Alcohol Depend 1999;54(2):155–61.

[42] Caulkins JP, et al. How goes the "war on drugs"? An assessment of U.S. drug problems and policy. Santa Monica, CA: RAND; 2005. 1–49, i–ix.

[43] Broz D, et al. Multiple injections per injection episode: high-risk injection practice among people who injected pills during the 2015 HIV outbreak in Indiana. Int J Drug Pol 2018;52:97–101.

[44] Pacula RL, Powell D. A supply-side perspective on the opioid crisis. J Pol Anal Manag 2018;37(2):438–46.

[45] Volkow ND, et al. Medication-assisted therapies — tackling the opioid-overdose epidemic. N Engl J Med 2014;370(22):2063–6.

[46] Thomas CP. Addressing workforce needs for medication treatment of opioid use disorder. J Addiction Med 2019;13(1):1–2.

[47] Medications for Opioid Use Disorder Save Lives. National academies of sciences, engineering and medicine. Washington, DC: The National Academies Press; 2019.

[48] Fiscella K, Wakeman SE, Beletsky L. Buprenorphine deregulation and mainstreaming treatment for opioid use disorder: X the X Waiver. JAMA Psychiatr 2019;76(3):229–30.

[49] US Surgeon General. Surgeon general's advisory on naloxone and opioid overdose. 2018.

[50] Fairbairn N, Coffin PO, Walley AY. Naloxone for heroin, prescription opioid, and illicitly made fentanyl overdoses: challenges and innovations responding to a dynamic epidemic. Int J Drug Pol 2017;46:172–9.

[51] Wheeler E, et al. Opioid overdose prevention programs providing naloxone to laypersons-United States, 2014. Morb Mortal Wkly Rep 2015;64(23):631–5.

[52] Peiper NC, Clarke SD, Vincent LB, Ciccarone D, Kral AH, Zibbell JE. Fentanyl test strips as an opioid overdose prevention strategy: findings from a syringe services program in the Southeastern United States. Int J Drug Pol 2019;63:122–8.

[53] Butterfield RJ, et al. Drug checking to improve monitoring of new psychoactive substances in Australia. Med J Aust 2016;204(4):144–5.

[54] Barratt MJ, et al. Pill testing or drug checking in Australia: acceptability of service design features. Drug Alcohol Rev 2018;37(2):226–36.

[55] Rosenblum D, Unick J, Ciccarone D. The rapidly changing US illicit drug market and the potential for an improved early warning system: evidence from Ohio drug crime labs. Drug Alcohol Depend 2020;208:107779. https://doi.org/10.1016/j.drugalcdep.2019.107779.

[56] Potier C, et al. Supervised injection services: what has been demonstrated? A systematic literature review. Drug Alcohol Depend 2014;145:48–68.

[57] Marshall BD, et al. Reduction in overdose mortality after the opening of North America's first medically supervised safer injecting facility: a retrospective population-based study. Lancet 2011;377(9775):1429–37.

[58] Dolan K, Kimber J, Fry C, McDonald D, Fitzgerald J, Trautmann F. Drug consumption facilities in Europe and the establishment of supervised injecting centres in Australia. Drug Alcohol Rev 2000;19(3):337–46.

[59] Kerr T, et al. A micro-environmental intervention to reduce the harms associated with drug-related overdose: evidence from the evaluation of Vancouver's safer injection facility. Int J Drug Pol 2007;18(1):37–45.

The case of Scott County: injection drug use and the HIV and hepatitis C virus outbreak

John Cafardi, MD [1], Judith Feinberg, MD [2]

[1]*The Christ Hospital, Cincinnati, OH, United States;* [2]*Professor, Department of Behavioral Medicine and Psychiatry and Professor, Department of Medicine, Section of Infectious Diseases, West Virginia University School of Medicine, Morgantown, WV, United States*

Background

The syndemic of injection drug use (IDU) and HIV infection has been well recognized since the origin of the HIV epidemic. Although transmission in persons who inject drugs (PWID) was documented in 1977 [1], phylogenetic analysis suggests that the HIV infection was circulating in this population as early as 1970 [2]. Following rapid spread in this population, it is estimated that at least 100,000 PWID were infected when AIDS was first recognized in 1981, with estimates of HIV infection in PWID ranging from 900,000 to 4.8 million worldwide. At that time, HIV seroprevalence was estimated at 50% in the IDU population in New York City [3]. Since then, it has been established that IDU is one of the most efficient methods of HIV transmission, behind only blood transfusion and unprotected receptive anal intercourse [4]. Once introduced, HIV spreads rapidly through a population of PWID, with little genetic variation [5,6]. Incidence rates of up to 10 to 31/100 person-years have been observed in Bangkok [7], Vancouver [8], and Tallinn [9], while other communities have seen HIV prevalence increase up to 50% within 6—24 months, including Kathmandu [10], Manipur [11], Kiev [12], and Rio de Janeiro [13]. While these outbreaks have occurred in urban and not rural areas, they serve as an example of how rapidly HIV infection can disseminate in these at-risk populations.

Factors that have been associated with the rapid spread of HIV in communities include limited knowledge of risk, limited access to sterile injection equipment, and large, frequently changing networks of injection partners [14]. While not all factors must be present for an HIV outbreak to occur in PWID, a number of these (frequently modifiable) factors are typically present [3].

Outbreak

In December 2014, a physician in Austin, Indiana, identified two new diagnoses of HIV infection, shortly followed by a third case. These were quickly followed by 8 others and by the end of March 2015, 68 new cases of HIV infection had been identified [15]. By November 1, 2015, 181 cases had been diagnosed [16], with 205 cases by September 2016 [17] and 215 by March 2, 2017 [18] (Fig. 2.1).

Subsequent phylogenetic analysis revealed a sequence homology of over 99.5%, confirming a single common source of the outbreak while laboratory and clinical evaluation of most newly diagnosed patients was consistent with infection within 2–6 months of diagnosis [16]. Further phylodynamic analysis indicated an initial introduction into a tight network of PWID via high-risk sexual contact at some point

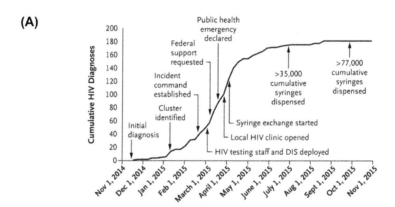

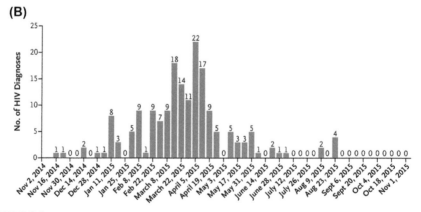

FIGURE 2.1

Outbreak of HIV infection in southeastern Indiana. (A) Cumulative HIV diagnoses and public health response. (B) HIV diagnoses according to the week of testing.

Reproduced from P.J. Peters, P. Pontones, K.W. Hoover, M.R. Patel, R.R. Galang, J. Shields, et al., HIV infection linked to injection use of oxymorphone in Indiana, 2014–2015, N Engl J Med 375 (3), 2016, 229–239.

in 2011 and rapid expansion in mid-2014, with most transmission events having occurred by early 2015 before the declaration of a public health emergency on March 26, 2015 [17] (Fig. 2.2).

The nature of the opioid itself and the associated injection practices contributed significantly to the rapid spread of HIV. In Austin, a sustained-release formulation of oxymorphone (Opana ER) was used. Oxymorphone is a semisynthetic μ-opioid agonist first approved in the United States in 1959. It was initially available only in injectable and rectal forms but was subsequently made available in both immediate- and extended-release oral formulations [19,20]. The injectable formulation has an onset of action within 5 min, has a half-life of 3−6 h, and is approximately 30-fold more potent than oral morphine [21,22]. The extended-release formulation utilized a novel proprietary drug matrix (TIMERx) that provided a different pharmacokinetic profile than either the injectable or the immediate-release oral formulation. This matrix consisted of a xanthan and locust bean gum−derived hydrophilic polymer that resulted in the gradual degradation of the matrix and release of the active medication [23]. This formulation was marketed as "abuse deterrent" and was intended to prevent immediate release of all active drugs following crushing and insufflation [21]. Owing to community perceptions of this medication being "safer" (i.e., a pharmaceutical product manufactured under sterile conditions without adulteration), it rapidly became the preferred agent for nonprescription use in this community [24]. This required complex processing of the extended-release tablets to obtain oxymorphone for injection, consisting of "browning" or slow heating of the tablet, followed by solubilization with water and finally, injection. As the resulting solution was poorly soluble in water, the total volume required multiple "takes" (drawing up and injecting) per episode. Frequently, users described using two to three "flushes" to obtain all the drug present in a single quarter tablet. Furthermore, owing to the high cost of the drug, a single delayed-release tablet was shared among multiple—frequently between two and four—injection partners [25], and given the high potency and short half-life of the injected oxymorphone, withdrawal symptoms were faster and more severe, requiring between three and seven injection episodes per day. This combination of multiple users sharing a single tablet, multiple injections required per episode, short high and rapid, intense withdrawal combined to provide an ideal situation that promoted frequent nonsterile injection practices associated with the transmission of hepatitis C virus (HCV) and HIV infections [25]. HIV subsequently spread rapidly in this population and was further amplified among those who participated in transactional sexual activity (up to 25% of the HIV-infected women in this outbreak) [16,17]. This finding of high levels of transactional sexual activity and IDU has also occurred in other populations with high incident rates of HIV and HCV infection [26]. This level of transactional sexual activity, combined with the frequent injections and close network of PWID mentioned earlier, further enhanced the spread of HIV infection in this community.

An outbreak similar to Scott County occurred in London, Ontario. This outbreak was strongly associated with the illicit injection of sustained-release hydromorphone, with the microcrystalline cellulose present in the sustained-release tablets

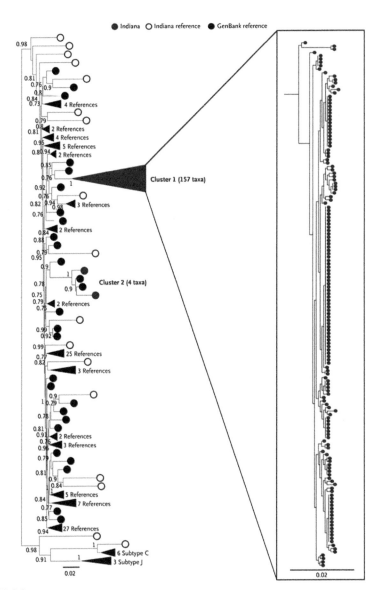

FIGURE 2.2

Maximum likelihood phylogenetic tree of HIV-1 polymerase sequences—southeastern Indiana, November 18, 2014 to November 1, 2015.

Reproduced from P.J. Peters, P. Pontones, K.W. Hoover, M.R. Patel, R.R. Galang, J. Shields, et al., HIV infection linked to injection use of oxymorphone in Indiana, 2014–2015, N Engl J Med 375 (3), 2016, 229–239.

serving to prolong the viability of HIV present [27]. As in the Scott County experience, the sustained-release hydromorphone preparation was poorly soluble in aqueous solution, so the preparation for injection also required multiple steps, in this case including crushing, heating, suspending in water, and passing through a cotton filter to remove particulate matter, and owing to the high volume required for solubilization, multiple injections were frequently shared [28,29].

Burden of injection drug use throughout the United States and the world, and association of injection drug use with HIV and hepatitis C virus infections

An accurate assessment of the burden of IDU is difficult for many reasons, including social stigma, lack of access to healthcare, poor economic status, and potential legal challenges. Evaluation of this population is, however, increasingly important, given not only their need for medical care but also the potential for this group of people to function as a reservoir for transmission of infectious diseases to both IDU and non-IDU populations. It is estimated that 2.6% of the US population has ever injected drugs, with 0.3% having done so within the past 12 months [30]. The current global prevalence of IDU is estimated at 15.6 million, with 17.8% infected with HIV, 52.3% infected with HCV, and 9% chronically infected with hepatitis B virus [31].

Acute hepatitis C virus infection and injection drug use in areas at risk for HIV outbreaks

As acute HCV infection is one of the more common sequelae of nonsterile injections, it serves as a surrogate marker for both IDU and areas at high risk for HIV infection. The Scott County outbreak ultimately resulted from the introduction of HIV into a closely related, preexisting network of PWID with extensive circulation of HCV, with 1.7% of Scott County residents using injection drugs and 92% of the new HIV cases coinfected with HCV [32]. This is consistent with findings from other high-risk rural counties, such as Cabell County, West Virginia, with 2.4% of the population reporting IDU and half of them reporting such use within the past 6 months [33]. In prior studies the illicit use of prescription opioids has been identified as an independent risk factor for the acquisition of HCV, with the use conferring an absolute risk increase of 36% during a recent outbreak in New York state; notably, the risk of using prescription opioids was significantly higher than with the use of methamphetamine, cocaine, or heroin [34]. Among prescription opioids associated with HCV infection, sustained-release oxymorphone was most commonly used, as was seen in Scott County [34].

In the United States, rates of acute HCV infection had fallen through 2005, but beginning in 2006, acute HCV infection rates have dramatically increased predominantly among individuals aged 20—29 years, although significant increases in individuals aged 30—39 years have also been noted. It is estimated that 70% of incident HCV infection in the United States since 2006 is due to IDU [35,36] and that 43% of HCV infections between 2018 and 2030 will also be due to IDU, with the impact greater in moderate- to high-income countries (79%) than in low-income countries (38%) [37].

In the United States, these increases have been most dramatic in predominantly non-urban areas in the eastern states with historically low rates of HIV infection, including Indiana, Kentucky, Tennessee, Virginia, and West Virginia. Following the Scott County outbreak, a Centers for Disease Control and Prevention (CDC) analysis was undertaken to determine whether other counties are at risk for future similar outbreaks. To date, 220 rural counties in 26 states have been identified as "high risk" for an HIV and/or HCV outbreak. Over 50% of these rural counties are in central Appalachia, including 28 of 55 counties (51%) in West Virginia, 54 of 120 counties (45%) in Kentucky, and 41 of 95 counties (43%) in Tennessee [38].

The Scott County outbreak is a clear illustration of the changing demographics of HIV infection in PWID, centered in a rural town (the population of Austin is approximately 4200) with 10% unemployment, 19% living below the poverty threshold, and low levels of educational attainment with over 20% not finishing high school [15]. Additional barriers in rural counties include significant distances between social service programs and those in need exacerbated by poor access to transportation, and limited infrastructure for HIV testing, diagnosis, and care.

Management of HIV outbreaks, methods for amelioration of existing outbreaks, and prevention of future outbreaks

The core of the initial management of outbreaks is community engagement, with access to treatment for opioid use disorder (including medication-assisted treatment [MAT] and syringe services programs [SSPs]). This is particularly challenging in rural settings, with significantly limited availability of SSPs and difficulty accessing the few that do exist, and poor coverage of MAT. At the time of the Austin outbreak, there was no available SSP in the entire state of Indiana and possession of syringes was a felony, so they were frequently reused. Governmental action to establish an SSP was taken in response to the outbreak, although it was delayed and uncoordinated, and impaired by conflicts with local law enforcement. These difficulties were ameliorated in part following changes in law as well as declaration of a public health emergency, although SSP implementation continued to face challenges from local law enforcement. Unfortunately, SSP implementation did not occur until the tail end of the outbreak, following the majority of the transmission events.

As it has been suggested that earlier implementation of SSP or the presence of a preexisting SSP would have prevented or ameliorated the outbreak, multiple modeling studies have been performed to evaluate the outcome at various earlier

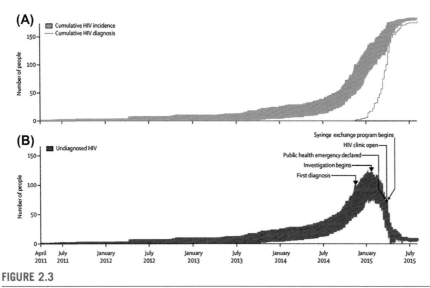

FIGURE 2.3

(A,B) Raw and reconstructed data from the HIV outbreak in Scott County, IN, USA, from April 2011 to August 2015.

Reproduced from G.S. Gonsalves and F.W. Crawford, Dynamics of the HIV outbreak and response in Scott County, IN, USA, 2011-15: a modelling study, Lancet HIV 5 (10), 2018, e569–e577.

possible timepoints of SSP implementation. If the SSP were implemented in 2013, the outbreak would likely have been reduced to 56 cases or fewer, while if it had been implemented in 2011, it would have likely reduced the total number of cases to less than 10 [18] (Figs. 2.3 and 2.4).

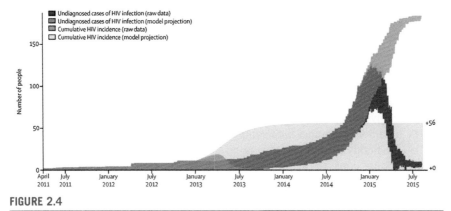

FIGURE 2.4

Evaluation of projected outbreak dynamics under the counterfactual intervention date of January 1, 2013.

Reproduced from G.S. Gonsalves and F.W. Crawford, Dynamics of the HIV outbreak and response in Scott County, IN, USA, 2011-15: a modelling study, Lancet HIV 5 (10), 2018, e569–e577.

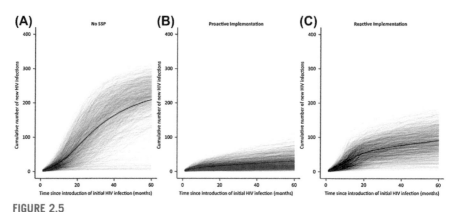

FIGURE 2.5

Cumulative HIV infections over 5 years following a single infection (A) when a syringe services program (SSP) was never implemented, (B) in the presence of an established SSP, and (C) when an SSP was implemented after 10 incident HIV infections.

Reproduced from W.C.Goedel, M.R.F.King, M.N.Lurie, S.Galea, J.P.Townsend, A.P.Galvani, Implementation of syringe services programs to prevent rapid human immunodeficiency virus transmission in rural counties in the United States: a modeling studyClin Infect Dis 70 (6), 2019, 1096–1102.

It has also been suggested that urban models of SSPs would not be applicable in rural areas, so further modeling studies evaluating various models of response to outbreaks in rural areas have been performed. These compared predicted outbreaks in the setting of no SSP, proactive SSP implementation (immediately upon recognition of an outbreak), or reactive SSP implementation (implementation following recognition of an outbreak). This modeling was based on the Scott County outbreak, which is considered to be representative of at-risk rural counties, with a 1.7% prevalence of IDU. At baseline, it was estimated that such a county without an SSP would experience 176 HIV infections over a 5-year period, an incidence of 12.1/ 100 person-years. A proactive implementation policy would reduce incident infections to 22 over the same period, which is a 90% reduction. A reactive policy, defined as implementation of SSP 10 months after the incident infection, would decrease the incident infections over this period to 69, which is a 61% reduction. Furthermore, reduction in HIV transmission in the non-PWID population would also occur, given the decreased community prevalence [39] (Fig. 2.5).

HIV treatment is another core component of prevention ("treatment as prevention") and is highly effective in preventing sexual transmission, with no genetically linked transmissions to the uninfected partner in either HPTN 052 or the PARTNER study [40,41]. When the index partner has an undetectable viral load, no sexual transmissions occurred despite >70,000 condomless sex acts, leading to the formulation that "undetectable is untransmittable" ("U = U") [42–44]. There is considerably less data regarding the effect of HIV treatment on the incidence in IDU populations, although a beneficial, albeit limited, effect has been seen to date [45].

Pre-exposure prophylaxis (PrEP) has also been shown to significantly decrease the incidence of sexually acquired HIV [46], while data in PWID are limited to the Bangkok Tenofovir Study [47]. The concept of PrEP in PWID has been investigated in dynamic compartmental modeling (PrEP alone, PrEP with intensive screening, and PrEP with intensive screening and immediate combination antiretroviral therapy [cART]). The model of PrEP + intensive screening + immediate cART is predicted to significantly reduce the burden of HIV infection among PWID, although at a significant cost ($253,000 per quality-adjusted life-year) [48]. Work is in progress to better understand the factors needed for optimal usage of PrEP in PWID.

Opioid substitution programs utilizing methadone, buprenorphine-based MAT, and syringe exchange programs have also been shown to reduce the risk of HIV transmission in PWID, with a 64% relative risk reduction achieved via opiate substitution treatment/MAT [49] and a 56% relative risk reduction achieved via SSPs [50]. A direct link between the degree of restrictive policies employed by SSPs (such as limits on the number of syringes that can be exchanged per visit) and the facilitation of safe injection practices has been identified, with efficacy ranging from 61% with no restrictions to 26% with multiple restrictions such as 1:1 exchange, no supply for exigent circumstances, and a limit on the total number of syringes exchanged. In follow-up studies, elimination of the 1:1 policy reduced unsafe injection practices by approximately 50% [51]. These programs have been highly successful over the past 30 years in preventing transmission of HIV among PWID, with the incidence in the United States falling from 13/100 person-years in 1981 to 0.1/100 person-years in 2011. This is due to multiple interventions, including education on the importance of sterile injection equipment and not sharing injection equipment, the implementation of SSPs [52,53], and the widespread use of cART [54] and opiate substitution program/MAT [55−57].

Other recent outbreaks

Recent IDU-associated outbreaks of HIV in the United States have been reported, including rural West Virginia, Seattle, Portland, and Massachusetts. In West Virginia, 57 cases in 15 rural counties were identified in 2015−17 that included some PWID [58], and a current, ongoing active cluster in Huntington, Cabell County has so far identified 61 cases, all among PWID [59]. In Seattle, 14 cases have been identified primarily in homeless PWID [60]. Outbreaks in 2019 in Portland, Oregon [61] and two communities in Massachusetts, namely, Lowell and Lawrence, have also been described [62]. This trend has also been observed globally with outbreaks throughout North America and Western Europe, including Canada, Greece, Romania, Ireland, Scotland, and Luxembourg, ranging in size from under 100 to over 1100 affected persons. There are several common themes in these outbreaks, including involvement of socioeconomically disadvantaged persons and lack of availability of SSPs. Despite the initiation of public health measures and overall

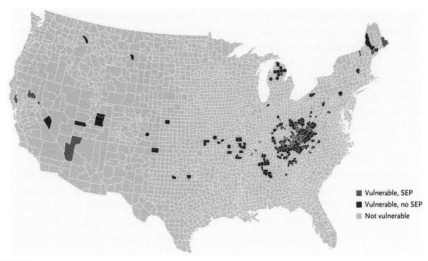

FIGURE 2.6

Vulnerability of US counties to HIV and hepatitis C virus outbreaks and their syringe exchange program (SEP) status.

Reproduced from S. Kishore, M. Hayden, J. Rich, Lessons from Scott County — Progress or Paralysis on Harm Reduction?, N Engl J Med 380(21), 2019, 1988-1990. https://doi.org/10.1056/NEJMp1901276.

control of these outbreaks, HIV incidence has not returned to baseline in any of these regions [63] (Fig. 2.6).

Scott County may be the harbinger of things to come

Cities such as Amsterdam [64,65], Vancouver [66], and New York [67] have seen a significant fall in the incidence and prevalence of HIV infection in PWID. The introduction of syringe services, the use of opioid substitution and MAT for opioid use disorder, and cART and PrEP have all contributed to reducing the risk of HIV infection among PWID. However, HIV outbreaks among PWID will continue where the political will to use these tools is lacking. We hope that Scott County can serve both as a cautionary tale and as a road map of how to prevent and interrupt future outbreaks.

References

[1] Des Jarlais DC, Friedman SR, Novick DM, Sotheran JL, Thomas P, Yancovitz SR, et al. HIV-1 infection among intravenous drug users in Manhattan, New York City, from 1977 through 1987. J Am Med Assoc 1989;261(7):1008−12.

[2]   Worobey M, Watts TD, McKay RA, Suchard MA, Granade T, Teuwen DE, et al. 1970s and 'Patient 0' HIV-1 genomes illuminate early HIV/AIDS history in North America. Nature 2016;539(7627):98−101.

[3]   Des Jarlais DC, Carrieri P. HIV infection among persons who inject drugs: ending old epidemics and addressing new outbreaks: authors' reply. AIDS 2016;30(11):1858−9.

[4]   Patel P, Borkowf CB, Brooks JT, Lasry A, Lansky A, Mermin J. Estimating per-act HIV transmission risk: a systematic review. AIDS 2014;28(10):1509−19.

[5]   Liitsola K, Tashkinova I, Laukkanen T, Korovina G, Smolskaja T, Momot O, et al. HIV-1 genetic subtype A/B recombinant strain causing an explosive epidemic in injecting drug users in Kaliningrad. AIDS 1998;12(14):1907−19.

[6]   Roudinskii NI, Sukhanova AL, Kazennova EV, Weber JN, Pokrovsky VV, Mikhailovich VM, et al. Diversity of human immunodeficiency virus type 1 subtype A and CRF03_AB protease in Eastern Europe: selection of the V77I variant and its rapid spread in injecting drug user populations. J Virol 2004;78(20):11276−87.

[7]   Vanichseni S, Kitayaporn D, Mastro TD, Mock PA, Raktham S, Des Jarlais DC, et al. Continued high HIV-1 incidence in a vaccine trial preparatory cohort of injection drug users in Bangkok, Thailand. AIDS 2001;15(3):397−405.

[8]   Strathdee SA, Patrick DM, Currie SL, Cornelisse PG, Rekart ML, Montaner JS, et al. Needle exchange is not enough: lessons from the vancouver injecting drug use study. AIDS 1997;11(8):F59−65.

[9]   Uuskula A, Kals M, Rajaleid K, Abel K, Talu A, Ruutel K, et al. High-prevalence and high-estimated incidence of HIV infection among new injecting drug users in Estonia: need for large scale prevention programs. J Public Health 2008;30(2):119−25.

[10] Oelrichs RB, Shrestha IL, Anderson DA, Deacon NJ. The explosive human immunodeficiency virus type 1 epidemic among injecting drug users of Kathmandu, Nepal, is caused by a subtype C virus of restricted genetic diversity. J Virol 2000;74(3):1149−57.

[11] Sarkar S, Das N, Panda S, Naik TN, Sarkar K, Singh BC, et al. Rapid spread of HIV among injecting drug users in north-eastern states of India. Bull Narc 1993;45(1):91−105.

[12] Booth RE, Kwiatkowski CF, Brewster JT, Sinitsyna L, Dvoryak S. Predictors of HIV sero-status among drug injectors at three Ukraine sites. AIDS 2006;20(17):2217−23.

[13] Lima ES, Bastos FI, Telles PR, Friedman SR. HIV infection and AIDS among drug injectors at Rio de Janeiro: perspectives and unanswered questions. Bull Narc 1993;45(1):107−15.

[14] Des Jarlais DC, Friedman SR. HIV infection among intravenous drug users: epidemiology and risk reduction. AIDS 1987;1(2):67−76.

[15] Janowicz DM. HIV transmission and injection drug use: lessons from the Indiana outbreak. Top Antivir Med 2016;24(2):90−2.

[16] Peters PJ, Pontones P, Hoover KW, Patel MR, Galang RR, Shields J, et al. HIV infection linked to injection use of oxymorphone in Indiana, 2014−2015. N Engl J Med 2016;375(3):229−39.

[17] Campbell EM, Jia H, Shankar A, Hanson D, Luo W, Masciotra S, et al. Detailed transmission network analysis of a large opiate-driven outbreak of HIV infection in the United States. J Infect Dis 2017;216(9):1053−62.

[18] Gonsalves GS, Crawford FW. Dynamics of the HIV outbreak and response in Scott County, IN, USA, 2011-15: a modelling study. Lancet HIV 2018;5(10):e569−77.

[19] FDA. OPANA (oxymorphone hydrochloride) tablets. CII; July 2012.

[20] FDA. OPANA® ER (oxymorphone hydrochloride) extended-release tablets, for oral use. CII; July 2012.

[21] Smith HS. Clinical pharmacology of oxymorphone. Pain Med 2009;10:3−10.

[22] Prommer E. Oxymorphone: a review. Support Care Cancer 2006;14(2):109−15.

[23] Adams MP, Ahdieh H. Pharmacokinetics and dose-proportionality of oxymorphone extended release and its metabolites: results of a randomized crossover study. Pharmacotherapy 2004;24(4):468−76.

[24] Brooks JT. In: Joint Meeting of the Drug Safety and Risk Management Advisory Committee, Committee at Anesthetic and Analgesic Drug Products Advisory, editor. CDC outbreak investigations involving OPANA® ER. Food and Drug Administration; 2017.

[25] Broz D, Zibbell J, Foote C, Roseberry JC, Patel MR, Conrad C, et al. Multiple injections per injection episode: high-risk injection practice among people who injected pills during the 2015 HIV outbreak in Indiana. Int J Drug Pol 2018;52:97−101.

[26] Ousley J, Nesbitt R, Kyaw NTT, Bermudez E, Soe KP, Anicete R, et al. Increased hepatitis C virus co-infection and injection drug use in HIV-infected fishermen in Myanmar. BMC Infect Dis 2018;18(1):657.

[27] Ball LJ, Venner C, Tirona RG, Arts E, Gupta K, Wiener JC, et al. Heating injection drug preparation equipment used for opioid injection may reduce HIV transmission associated with sharing equipment. J Acquir Immune Defic Syndr 2019;81(4):e127−34.

[28] Roy E, Arruda N, Bourgois P. The growing popularity of prescription opioid injection in downtown Montreal: new challenges for harm reduction. Subst Use Misuse 2011;46(9):1142−50.

[29] Roy E, Arruda N, Bertrand K, Dufour M, Laverdiere E, Jutras-Aswad D, et al. Prevalence and correlates of prescription opioid residue injection. Drug Alcohol Depend 2016;166:69−74.

[30] Lansky A, Finlayson T, Johnson C, Holtzman D, Wejnert C, Mitsch A, et al. Estimating the number of persons who inject drugs in the United States by meta-analysis to calculate national rates of HIV and hepatitis C virus infections. PloS One 2014;9(5):e97596.

[31] Degenhardt L, Peacock A, Colledge S, Leung J, Grebely J, Vickerman P, et al. Global prevalence of injecting drug use and sociodemographic characteristics and prevalence of HIV, HBV, and HCV in people who inject drugs: a multistage systematic review. Lancet Glob Health 2017;5(12):e1192−207.

[32] Ramachandran S, Thai H, Forbi JC, Galang RR, Dimitrova Z, Xia GL, et al. A large HCV transmission network enabled a fast-growing HIV outbreak in rural Indiana, 2015. EBioMedicine 2018;37:374−81.

[33] Allen ST, O'Rourke A, White RH, Schneider KE, Kilkenny M, Sherman SG. Estimating the number of people who inject drugs in a rural county in Appalachia. Am J Publ Health 2019;109(3):445−50.

[34] Zibbell JE, Hart-Malloy R, Barry J, Fan L, Flanigan C. Risk factors for HCV infection among young adults in rural New York who inject prescription opioid analgesics. Am J Publ Health 2014;104(11):2226−32.

[35] Zibbell JE, Iqbal K, Patel RC, Suryaprasad A, Sanders KJ, Moore-Moravian L, et al. Increases in hepatitis C virus infection related to injection drug use among persons aged </=30 years − Kentucky, Tennessee, Virginia, and West Virginia, 2006−2012. Morb Mortal Wkly Rep 2015;64(17):453−8.

[36] Suryaprasad AG, White JZ, Xu F, Eichler BA, Hamilton J, Patel A, et al. Emerging epidemic of hepatitis C virus infections among young nonurban persons who inject drugs in the United States, 2006−2012. Clin Infect Dis 2014;59(10):1411−9.

[37] Trickey A, Fraser H, Lim AG, Peacock A, Colledge S, Walker JG, et al. The contribution of injection drug use to hepatitis C virus transmission globally, regionally, and at country level: a modelling study. Lancet Gastroenterol Hepatol 2019;4(6):435−44.

[38] Van Handel MM, Rose CE, Hallisey EJ, Kolling JL, Zibbell JE, Lewis B, et al. County-level vulnerability assessment for rapid dissemination of HIV or HCV infections among persons who inject drugs, United States. J Acquir Immune Defic Syndr 2016;73(3): 323−31.

[39] Goedel WC, King MRF, Lurie MN, Galea S, Townsend JP, Galvani AP, et al. Implementation of syringe services programs to prevent rapid human immunodeficiency virus transmission in rural counties in the United States: a modeling study. Clin Infect Dis 2019;70(6):1096−102.

[40] Cohen MS, Chen YQ, McCauley M, Gamble T, Hosseinipour MC, Kumarasamy N, et al. Antiretroviral therapy for the prevention of HIV-1 transmission. N Engl J Med 2016;375(9):830−9.

[41] Rodger AJ, Cambiano V, Bruun T, Vernazza P, Collins S, van Lunzen J, et al. Sexual activity without condoms and risk of HIV transmission in serodifferent couples when the HIV-positive partner is using suppressive antiretroviral therapy. J Am Med Assoc 2016;316(2):171−81.

[42] Eisinger RW, Dieffenbach CW, Fauci AS. HIV viral load and transmissibility of HIV infection: undetectable equals untransmittable. J Am Med Assoc 2019;321(5): 451−2.

[43] Rodger AJ, Cambiano V, Bruun T, Vernazza P, Collins S, Degen O, et al. Risk of HIV transmission through condomless sex in serodifferent gay couples with the HIV-positive partner taking suppressive antiretroviral therapy (PARTNER): final results of a multi-centre, prospective, observational study. Lancet 2019;393(10189):2428−38.

[44] York A. Undetectable equals untransmittable. Nat Rev Microbiol 2019;17(7):399.

[45] Fraser H, Mukandavire C, Martin NK, Hickman M, Cohen MS, Miller WC, et al. HIV treatment as prevention among people who inject drugs − a re-evaluation of the evidence. Int J Epidemiol 2017;46(2):466−78.

[46] Riddell J, Amico KR, Mayer KH. HIV preexposure prophylaxis: a review. J Am Med Assoc 2018;319(12):1261−8.

[47] Choopanya K, Martin M, Suntharasamai P, Sangkum U, Mock PA, Leethochawalit M, et al. Antiretroviral prophylaxis for HIV infection in injecting drug users in Bangkok, Thailand (The Bangkok Tenofovir Study): a randomised, double-blind, placebo-controlled phase 3 trial. Lancet 2013;381(9883):2083−90.

[48] Bernard CL, Brandeau ML, Humphreys K, Bendavid E, Holodniy M, Weyant C, et al. Cost-effectiveness of HIV preexposure prophylaxis for people who inject drugs in the United States. Ann Intern Med 2016;165:10−9. https://doi.org/10.7326/M15-2634.

[49] MacArthur GJ, Minozzi S, Martin N, Vickerman P, Deren S, Bruneau J, et al. Opiate substitution treatment and HIV transmission in people who inject drugs: systematic review and meta-analysis. BMJ 2012;345:e5945.

[50] Aspinall EJ, Nambiar D, Goldberg DJ, Hickman M, Weir A, Van Velzen E, et al. Are needle and syringe programmes associated with a reduction in HIV transmission among people who inject drugs: a systematic review and meta-analysis. Int J Epidemiol 2014; 43(1):235−48.

[51] Kerr T, Small W, Buchner C, Zhang R, Li K, Montaner J, et al. Syringe sharing and HIV incidence among injection drug users and increased access to sterile syringes. Am J Publ Health 2010;100(8):1449−53.

[52] Abdul-Quader AS, Feelemyer J, Modi S, Stein ES, Briceno A, Semaan S, et al. Effectiveness of structural-level needle/syringe programs to reduce HCV and HIV infection among people who inject drugs: a systematic review. AIDS Behav 2013;17(9): 2878–92.

[53] Des Jarlais DC, Feelemyer JP, Modi SN, Abdul-Quader A, Hagan H. High coverage needle/syringe programs for people who inject drugs in low and middle income countries: a systematic review. BMC Publ Health 2013;13:53.

[54] Wood E, Milloy MJ, Montaner JS. HIV treatment as prevention among injection drug users. Curr Opin HIV AIDS 2012;7(2):151–6.

[55] Mattick RP, Breen C, Kimber J, Davoli M. Methadone maintenance therapy versus no opioid replacement therapy for opioid dependence. Cochrane Database Syst Rev 2009; (3):CD002209.

[56] Woody GE, Bruce D, Korthuis PT, Chhatre S, Poole S, Hillhouse M, et al. HIV risk reduction with buprenorphine-naloxone or methadone: findings from a randomized trial. J Acquir Immune Defic Syndr 2014;66(3):288–93.

[57] Vlahov D, Robertson AM, Strathdee SA. Prevention of HIV infection among injection drug users in resource-limited settings. Clin Infect Dis 2010;50(Suppl. 3):S114–21.

[58] Evans ME, Labuda SM, Hogan V, Agnew-Brune C, Armstrong J, Periasamy Karuppiah AB, et al. Notes from the field: HIV infection investigation in a rural area – West Virginia, 2017. Morb Mortal Wkly Rep 2018;67(8):257–8.

[59] Health WVBfP. Health advisory #155: increase in new HIV infections among persons who inject drugs. 2019.

[60] Golden MR, Lechtenberg R, Glick SN, Dombrowski J, Duchin J, Reuer JR, et al. Outbreak of human immunodeficiency virus infection among heterosexual persons who are living homeless and inject drugs – Seattle, Washington, 2018. Morb Mortal Wkly Rep 2019;68(15):344–9.

[61] Health officials alert public to increase in HIV infections among people who use drugs. Multnomah County Health Department; 2019.

[62] Cranston K, Alpren C, John B, Dawson E, Roosevelt K, Burrage A, et al. Notes from the field: HIV diagnoses among persons who inject drugs – Northeastern Massachusetts, 2015–2018. Morb Mortal Wkly Rep 2019;68(10):253–4.

[63] Des Jarlais VS D, Wiessing L, Abagiu A-O, Arendt V, Broz D, Devaux C, Duwve JM, Ferbineaunu C, Fitzgerald M, Goldberg DJ, Hatzakis A, Igoe D, McAuley A, editors. Complacency is the new problem: comparative analysis of recent outbreaks of HIV among persons who inject drugs in Europe and North America. AIDS2018. Amsterdam: International AIDS Society; 2018.

[64] Van Den Berg C, Smit C, Van Brussel G, Coutinho R, Prins M, Amsterdam C. Full participation in harm reduction programmes is associated with decreased risk for human immunodeficiency virus and hepatitis C virus: evidence from the Amsterdam Cohort Studies among drug users. Addiction 2007;102(9):1454–62.

[65] van der Knaap N, Grady BP, Schim van der Loeff MF, Heijman T, Speksnijder A, Geskus R, et al. Drug users in Amsterdam: are they still at risk for HIV? PloS One 2013;8(3):e59125.

[66] Hyshka E, Strathdee S, Wood E, Kerr T. Needle exchange and the HIV epidemic in Vancouver: lessons learned from 15 years of research. Int J Drug Pol 2012;23(4):261–70.

[67] Des Jarlais DC, Marmor M, Paone D, Titus S, Shi Q, Perlis T, et al. HIV incidence among injecting drug users in New York City syringe-exchange programmes. Lancet 1996;348(9033):987–91.

Opioid use disorder and rural America

3

Wajiha Z. Akhtar, PhD, MPH [1], Judith Feinberg, MD [2]

[1]*Associate Scientist, Department of Medicine, University of Wisconsin−Madison, Madison, WI, United States;* [2]*Professor, Department of Behavioral Medicine and Psychiatry and Professor, Department of Medicine, Section of Infectious Diseases, West Virginia University School of Medicine, Morgantown, WV, United States*

Opioid use disorder burden in rural communities

Although the overall prevalence of drug use in rural areas is lower than that in urban areas, the looming opioid epidemic has caused the rate of overdose deaths in rural areas to increase and surpass the rate seen in urban areas [1]. As shown in Fig. 3.1, the Centers for Disease Control and Prevention (CDC) reported a 325% increase in drug overdose deaths from 1999 to 2015 in nonmetropolitan counties of residence compared with 198% among metropolitan counties of residence [1]. In 2017, age-adjusted drug overdose rates were highest among states with large rural populations, such as West Virginia, Kentucky, Maine, and Ohio (Fig. 3.2) [2]. Additionally, several studies have reported that nonmedical prescription drug use has been mostly concentrated in nonmetropolitan areas, which is a change from the previous experience of urbanized areas [3−8].

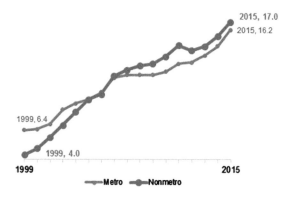

FIGURE 3.1

Age-adjusted rate per 100,000 persons for self-reported drug overdose deaths by metropolitan and nonmetropolitan counties of residence.

National Vital Statistics System, United States 1999−2015.

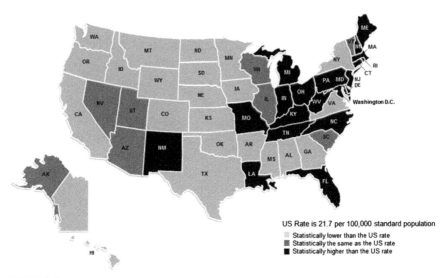

FIGURE 3.2

Age-adjusted drug overdose death rates by state: United States, 2017. Deaths were classified using the underlying cause of death codes X40-X44, X60-X64, X85, and Y10-Y14.

National Vital Statistics System, Mortality.

In a meta-analysis by Brady et al. [9], the investigators reviewed qualitative and quantitative studies in order to identify risk factors associated with prescription drug overdose death. Twenty-nine studies were assessed for six risk factors: sex, age, race, psychiatric disorders, substance use disorder, and urban/rural residence. All were associated with drug overdose deaths except for urban/rural residence. These findings are of particular interest because rural overdose death rates are exceeding those in urban areas, yet the most current meta-analysis did not find a statistical association. This could be due to the wide array of ways rurality can be assessed in studies. Studies often describe urban and rural by population density, or by grouping micropolitan and metropolitan as urban. Varying definitions of rurality may result in attenuation of the overall effect it has on overdose deaths [9,10].

Human immunodeficiency virus

Between 2008 and 2014, the overall number of new HIV diagnoses among persons who inject drugs (PWID) fell in the United States. This was driven largely by the approximate 50% decline among urban PWID of color [11]. However, transmission by injection drug use (IDU) in nonurban areas contributed to new HIV cases in greater proportion than in urban areas [12]. The HIV outbreak in Scott County, Indiana, was the first in the United States that resulted from the rural opioid epidemic.

Additional outbreaks have emerged since then. Between January and July 2017, 57 HIV cases emerged across 15 counties in the southern coalfield counties of West Virginia [13]. Although 60% of the cases reported male-to-male sexual (MSM) contact as the mode of transmission and 10% endorsed both MSM contact and IDU, 23% either could not be found or refused to speak to the CDC investigators, raising the possibility that some or all had IDU risk. From January 2018 through February 2019, 30 PWID were diagnosed with HIV in Cabell County, West Virginia, a county that had previously averaged eight new HIV cases annually based on data from 2013 to 2017 [13].

Between 2015 and 2018, 129 new HIV cases emerged in the cities of Lowell and Lawrence, Massachusetts [14]. Although Lowell and Lawrence are not rural communities, early arrival of fentanyl, homelessness, incarceration, and a decline in HIV testing were factors that played a crucial role in the spread of HIV there—the same factors that are increasingly evident in rural communities [15].

Hepatitis C, B, and A virus infections

The CDC reported a 2.9-fold increase in reported cases of acute hepatitis C virus (HCV) infections from 2010 through 2015, reflecting the increased rates of IDU, occurring mostly among young white persons living in rural communities [16,17]. Interestingly, the states with the highest rates of new HCV infections during this period—Kentucky, West Virginia, and Tennessee—were not receiving CDC funding for case finding. This reflected not only underascertainment and underreporting in these communities but also the deeper issue of limited healthcare and public health resources in rural communities with a high burden of opioid use disorder (OUD) and IDU.

Using data from the National Notifiable Diseases Surveillance System, the CDC assessed acute hepatitis B virus (HBV) infections in the same three states where HCV infections were high. Acute HBV infections also increased in Kentucky, West Virginia, and Tennessee (Fig. 3.3) among non-Hispanic whites aged 30−39 years in nonurban communities [18]. While the rate remained stable for the United States overall, the rate of HBV infections increased by 114% in 5 years in these three states [18].

In the past few years, hepatitis A virus (HAV) outbreaks have occurred among people who use drugs (PWUD), the homeless community, and men who have sex with men [19]. In 2017, the CDC received over 1000 reports of acute HAV infection from California, Kentucky, Michigan, and Utah. The majority of these cases were among IDU and non-IDU persons who use drugs and/or homeless individuals [20]. In March 2018, a cluster of HAV infections was reported by the Kanawha-Charleston Health Department in West Virginia. Testing confirmed that the outbreak, primarily among persons who use drugs and homeless persons, was caused by genotype 1B, the strain identified in ongoing HAV outbreaks in multiple states [21]. A retrospective review identified a total of 664 outbreak-associated cases

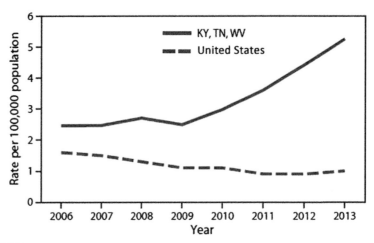

FIGURE 3.3

Incidence of acute hepatitis B virus infection, by year—United States and Kentucky (KY), Tennessee (TN), and West Virginia (WV), 2006–2013.

Reproduced from Harris AM, Iqbal K, Schillie S, et al. Increases in Acute Hepatitis B Virus Infections — Kentucky, Tennessee, and West Virginia, 2006–13. Morb Mortal Wkly Rep 2016;65:47–50.

from January 1, 2018 to August 28, 2018 that were epidemiologically linked to "… an identified outbreak case, a laboratory specimen matching the outbreak strain, or occurred in a person at high risk for infection (e.g., reported injection or noninjection drug use, experienced homelessness or unstable housing, or was recently incarcerated) …." Morbidity included hospitalization among 57% ($n = 380$) of the cases. Although mortality from HAV infection is unusual, one death has been reported in this outbreak, and deaths have been reported in San Diego and other localities with recent HAV outbreaks. This may have been exacerbated by concurrent past or current HCV infection in 314 cases (47%), past or current HBV infection in 65 cases (10%), and homelessness in 100 cases (15%). As routine surveillance data on incident cases continues to become available, the CDC expects increases in HAV infection among PWUD and/or homeless people—two characteristics that are evident in rural communities [19].

Factors that drive illicit drug use in rural communities

To explain the discrepancies evident in urban and rural illicit drug use, Keyes et al. [22] developed hypotheses regarding the disparity and shift in burden. First, there is an increase in the availability of opioids among states with large rural populations shown by high dispensing rates of prescription opioids. Rural communities, especially in central Appalachia, were exposed to aggressive marketing by prescription opioid producers such as Purdue Pharma, the maker of OxyContin

[22]. The aggressive marketing can be due in part to the higher rates of older persons who may be susceptible to chronic pain and to the drug use culture in Appalachian communities where prescription opioids are often used by mine and other heavy occupation workers [23–26]. Keyes et al. theorized that the high density of opioids available in rural communities can create opportunities for illegal markets to arise.

Second, rural communities have experienced an out-migration of young adults resulting in an aged workforce and an unstable economic infrastructure [22]. The vulnerability caused by economically deprived communities may increase the risk of substance use disorders [22]. In one qualitative study, four groups of key informants in Appalachian Kentucky described opioid misuse as an escape from hopelessness and lack of opportunity [26].

Third, large rural social and kinship network connections may contribute to the spread of opioid misuse. Unstable economic infrastructures described earlier, coupled with wider kinship networks in rural communities, can generate strain on that broader social network, thus increasing the risk of opioid misuse across a community [22]. Additionally, prescription opioids that were legitimately filled by parents, relatives, and friends were the main initial source of drug use in rural communities. This was evident in the Scott County HIV outbreak, where the size of the PWID network and the amount of syringe sharing were large for a sparsely populated area [27].

Finally, rural communities have faced industry and labor shifts. These shifts led to high rates of unemployment and fewer opportunities for upward mobility [22]. Such stressors can also increase the risk of substance use and misuse. Keyes theories gave the public health community context for the complexity of the rural opioid epidemic in order to begin understanding what is needed for treatment and care.

In response to the Scott County HIV outbreak, the CDC and the public health community raised concerns about the vulnerability of similar HIV outbreaks occurring in rural areas affected by the opioid epidemic. The socioeconomic characteristics of Scott County are not unique; other rural areas also face high unemployment, poverty, and low educational attainment. Identifying these communities became vital in order to guide public health efforts. Van Handel et al. [28] utilized a multistep analysis to identify factors that are highly associated with IDU and then identified 220 rural counties in 26 states that are most vulnerable to an HIV outbreak similar to that in Scott County by using confirmed cases of acute HCV infection from 2012 to 2013 as a proxy for IDU and 15 county-level indicators that were available nationally (Fig. 3.4). The authors found six indicators associated with acute HCV infection: drug overdose deaths, prescription opioid sales, per capita income, white non-Hispanic race/ethnicity, unemployment, and the number of buprenorphine providers per 10,000 population. The greatest proportion of counties identified were largely rural with the majority in central Appalachia—Kentucky, West Virginia, and Tennessee. Scott County ranked 32nd in their analysis.

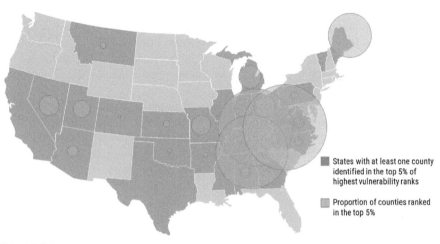

FIGURE 3.4

Identification of highest vulnerable counties in 26 states.

Reproduced from Supplement of Van Handel MM, Rose CE, Hallisey EJ, et al. County-level vulnerability
assessment for rapid dissemination of HIV or HCV infections among persons who inject drugs, United States.
J Acquir Immune Defic Syndr. 2016;73(3):323–331.

Barriers to care in rural communities

Coupled with the findings from the studies by Brady, Keyes, and Van Handel, it is imperative to understand barriers that patients, providers, and communities face in accessing and providing essential prevention and treatment services in rural areas. The first major factor rural communities face is the lack of specialty medical services, especially mental health and addiction treatment and infectious disease specialists to manage the serious sequelae of IDU. It is estimated that 80% of rural counties have no psychiatrists, 61% are without psychologists, and 91% are without psychiatric nurse practitioners (NPs) [29]. In a survey conducted by Andrilla et al. [30], 60% of rural counties lack a physician with a Drug Enforcement Administration (DEA) waiver to prescribe buprenorphine and among rural providers who had a waiver, 40% were not currently prescribing, prescribed formerly, or were not accepting new patients. It is unclear how many infectious disease specialists practice in rural communities. However, as infectious disease mortality decreases in the United States, the mortality rate in many rural communities continues to increase [31]. This suggests that lack of access to early diagnosis of life-threatening infectious diseases, case management, and care in rural communities contribute to rise in mortality.

A multitude of logistic barriers exist in rural communities. For providers who are willing to offer medication-assisted treatment (MAT) for OUD, the number of potential patients may not justify the start-up costs, office space, time, and resources needed to start an MAT program [32]. State regulations, such as those in West

Virginia, require a range of resources that may not be available in rural communities, such as availability of psychosocial counseling. Additionally, if services are available, rural communities lack public transportation options that will allow patients, who already are economically burdened, to travel to appointments. In mountainous central Appalachia, short distances can require long travel times because of the terrain and road conditions. Longer travel time for treatment may increase the risk of jeopardizing a patient's employment status and adherence to treatment [32]. Lastly, in states that have not implemented the Affordable Care Act, poverty and low employment rates preclude the option of buying private health insurance that covers care for OUD.

Developing and training the rural healthcare workforce

In lieu of specialists, rural communities depend on primary care providers (PCPs) to treat patients with OUD and the infectious consequences associated with IDU. Primary care may be practiced in a variety of settings and facilities in rural communities, including family physicians and internists in private practice, rural community health clinics, and federally qualified health centers that play an important role in serving rural residents. Rural residents of federally recognized tribes rely on the Indian Health Service that provides care to Native Americans and Alaskan Natives.

Among all buprenorphine prescribers, rural providers most frequently reported concerns about diversion or medication misuse, time constraints, and lack of available mental health or psychosocial support services as barriers to provide buprenorphine treatment [30]. In another survey by Andrilla et al. [33], nonprescribers were more likely to report time constraints, lack of patient need, resistance from practice partners, lack of specialty backup for complex problems, lack of confidence in their ability to manage OUDs, concerns about DEA intrusion on their practice, and attraction of PWUD to their practice more often than current prescribers. In a survey conducted among Wisconsin family medicine nonwaivered physicians, providers reported that they were more likely to incorporate office-based opioid treatment if patients had access to addiction counseling, had colleagues on-site who were knowledgeable about buprenorphine, and had access to a teleconsultation program [34]. Moreover, widespread stigma against MAT that is seen as substituting "a drug for a drug" is yet another obstacle to the effective treatment of OUD even when it is available in rural settings. The sentiment against MAT is persistent among even the highest federal health officials. In 2017, Tom Price, the former Health and Human Services Secretary for the United States, was quoted saying, "If we're just substituting one opioid for another, we're not moving the dial much," when he was on a listening tour in West Virginia [35].

PCPs in rural communities are also tasked with the responsibility of either independently managing their patients living with HIV infection and/or chronic viral hepatitis (HCV and HBV infections) or referring them to a specialty provider, where patients may have to travel long distances and wait many months for an appointment.

An overwhelmingly majority of PCPs still refer patients with HIV and HCV infections to specialists, even though advances in antiretroviral therapy and the development of curative, direct-acting antivirals (DAAs) for hepatitis C has made treatment simpler, safer, and highly efficacious in a primary care setting. Regardless of background and training, clinical outcomes among people living with HIV (PLWH) infection are associated with the provider's experience in managing HIV infection [36]. Because of the population size in rural communities, PCPs may not able to garner enough PLWH infection to develop the needed experience [37]. Nonetheless, data still suggests that both PCPs and NPs have comparable HIV and HCV treatment outcomes, such that infectious disease providers should collaborate with rurally practicing PCPs and NPs to expand treatment in hard-to-reach areas and to bridge gaps in the continuum of care for patients living with HCV and/or HIV infection [38–40].

Attitudes toward the use of DAAs among PWID in some communities may present continued barriers to treatment, mainly because of concerns of HCV reinfection and perceived nonadherence. The stigma around IDU in rural areas may exacerbate these concerns. However, a number of studies in PWID have shown that they can achieve the same sustained viral response at 12 weeks after the completion of therapy (SVR12, or cure) as other populations [41]. In the SIMPLIFY study, an open-label phase 4 study using the pan-genotypic combination of sofosbuvir-velpatasvir (Epclusa) for 12 weeks among 103 individuals who had injected drugs during the prior 6 months, the SVR rate was 94% (95% confidence interval, 88–98) and there were no virologic failures [42]. Available data show comparable cure rates in PWID as in the non-drug-using population and low but tolerable reinfection rates [43–46].

Community stigma, support, and policy

Although Keyes' theories revealed that large kinship circles in rural communities may allow for the spread of drug use and that the overall culture of miners and heavy machinery workers chronically taking opioids had normalized prescription opioid use, the stigma surrounding OUD poses a significant barrier that may discourage people from seeking prevention and treatment services. Studies have shown that patients with OUD are less likely to seek treatment out of fear that it would affect their employment and social relationships with friends, family, and neighbors [47]. The conservative climate, religiosity, and concerns about confidentiality are added barriers to effective HIV and HCV infection prevention and care in rural communities [37]. In order to achieve community buy-in, education on the effectiveness of MAT and routine HIV/HCV testing and treatment is warranted.

A few strategies to build support for MAT in rural communities were presented as case studies by the program funded by the Robert Wood Johnson Foundation, "Advancing Recovery: State/Provider Partnerships for Quality Addiction Care." For example, in order to overcome community resistance, Advancing Recovery West Virginia shared success stories with local papers and other media outlets

[48]. Advancing Recovery Maine worked to build statewide support for MAT by creating a recovery community called Maine Alliance for Addiction Recovery. The alliance worked to identify beliefs and attitudes toward the use of MAT, along with challenges that providers and patients may face in implementing MAT [48]. The results were then used to provide training events statewide. Patients with OUD and/or IDU frequently interact with a network of community members, including law enforcement, drug courts, probation officers, child protective services, local healthcare providers, and other community members. Efforts from local agencies with an informed approach on the disease of addiction, rather than the widespread belief that it is a character flaw or lack of willpower, and the commitment to the possibility of recovery and social reintegration, need to be integrated into the overarching community.

Local, state, and federal policies play a role in the successful prevention and treatment of HIV/HCV infection and OUD in rural communities. However, implementation of these policies may vary by jurisdiction. For example, many states have enacted a "Good Samaritan Law" by which PWUD are offered immunity from prosecution for certain drug-related offenses if they call emergency personnel when another person overdoses. As the number of overdose deaths increases, some prosecutors are treating overdose deaths as homicides and charging those who may have tried to save the victim [49]. With ambiguous laws and/or ambiguous interpretations in place, PWUD may not report overdoses, thus increasing the risk of overdose death.

Another example of a policy barrier is the discriminatory practices of some state Medicaid agencies. There are a range of restrictions to access curative therapy for HCV infection and OUD. States may require that patients reach a certain stage of liver fibrosis, which increases the risk of irreversible liver disease (cirrhosis) and hepatocellular carcinoma, or may refuse treatment to a patient with a history of alcohol or substance use or require evidence of sobriety for a specific duration. Additionally, Medicaid may restrict prescribers to specialists in gastroenterology/hepatology and infectious diseases that may not be accessible to rural PWID. Although there has been a heartening trend to reverse these restrictions nationwide, often as the result of lawsuits, restrictions remain in many hard-hit states. Additionally, among states that have begun reversing Medicaid restrictions for the treatment of HCV infection, few providers are aware of the changes even a year after the policy change and stigma in treating may still remain [50]. Interestingly, as Medicaid programs continue to enroll recipients into managed care organizations (MCOs), a few states allow for their MCOs to implement more restrictive criteria than their state's fee-for-service Medicaid restrictions [51]. Jurisdictions then have inconsistent criteria to offer HCV treatment to PWID.

All states offer some form of medication for MAT that is covered by their state Medicaid program. However, some states may limit the quantity or dosing, require prior authorization, require additional psychosocial treatment, and require step therapy [52]. Although requiring prior authorization for psychiatric medication has shown to reduce medication expenditures, the requirements may prevent timely access to treatment by an unstable PWID community. Additionally, step therapy is a common requirement through Medicaid, where a certain drug may not be used unless one or more other drugs are tried and were unsuccessful in treatment. However, this can become a barrier to treatment among PWID.

Promising models for prevention and treatment in rural communities

Evidence-based models of care that offer MAT services have been discussed elsewhere [32]. These include (1) the Project ECHO model of linking academic medical centers to resource-limited areas for various medical conditions, (2) the office-based opioid treatment collaborative care model where nurse case managers take on the responsibility of complex care, and (3) the Hub and Spoke Model where emphasis is in care coordination with a "hub" program that initiates treatment and "spoke" clinic for ongoing management, such as the Vermont model [53–55]. There are also ongoing studies to understand rural IDU, opioid use, and their infectious disease consequences, along with the effectiveness of evidence-based interventions on these communities.

Current studies on rural injection drug use
Rural opioid initiative

In order to improve understanding of the intersectionality of opioid use and HIV, HCV, and comorbid conditions, the National Institute on Drug Abuse (NIDA) funded a rural opioid initiative in 2017, with collaboration from other federal co-funders: the CDC, the Substance Abuse and Mental Health Services Administration (SAMHSA), and the Appalachian Regional Commission (ARC). This initiative was designed by NIDA and its partners to conduct community assessments; to use the assessments to design plans for implementing evidence-based practices to address opioid use, IDU, overdose, HIV infection, and other infectious comorbidities; and then to evaluate implementation of these plans. The overall objective of this initiative is to identify best practices that can be disseminated to address the unique needs of rural communities Project sites are located in Ohio, North Carolina, Kentucky, West Virginia, Oregon, Illinois, Wisconsin, and a northeast rural region encompassing Massachusetts, New Hampshire, and Vermont. To date, this cooperative agreement is the largest study assessing rural opioid and IDU in the United States. Data from the core instruments will provide a unique snapshot across the eight sites and a larger picture of the rural opioid epidemic, HIV infection, and related infectious comorbidities.

The project encompasses two phases: multimethod community assessments during the first 2 years and implementation of evidence-based practices based on those assessments in the last 3 years. The intervention projects will provide not only additional information about the epidemiology of HIV and related infectious comorbidities among opioid users but also important information about how evidence-based practices can be implemented effectively, given the challenges and obstacles in rural communities.

Healing communities study: developing and testing an integrated approach to address the opioid crisis (Healing communities)

Understanding that only a small percentage of people with OUD actually receive MAT, behavioral interventions, and naloxone to reduce overdoses, NIDA has solicited grant applications to increase access to these resources with the primary goal of reducing the opioid overdose fatality rate by 40% in a 3-year period. Three research sites will be funded to test the immediate impact of implementing an integrated set of evidence-based intervention across healthcare, behavioral health, justice, and other community-based settings to prevent and treat opioid misuse and OUD among highly affected communities. Healing Communities has an emphasis on rural communities and, in addition to the primary aim of decreasing overdose fatalities, includes a number of secondary outcomes such as reducing the supply of prescription opioids, increasing the number of specialty treatment programs and buprenorphine-waivered providers, increasing the availability of naloxone to reverse overdoses, screening to identify opioid misuse, evidence-based school and community-based prevention services, and a number of formal linkages between the justice system and healthcare.

It is anticipated that these research programs will improve our understanding of the nature of the rural opioid use and IDU epidemic and will demonstrate effective approaches to limit the associated morbidity and mortality in rural communities. It cannot happen too soon.

Acknowledgements

Dr. Akhtar is supported in part by the National Institute on Drug Abuse award number 2UG3DA044826. Dr. Feinberg is supported in part by the National Institute on Drug Abuse award number 2UG3DA044825 and the National Institute of General Medical Sciences award number 5U54GM104942-04.

References

[1] Mack KA, Jones CM, Ballesteros MF. Illicit drug use, illicit drug use disorders, and drug overdose deaths in metropolitan and nonmetropolitan areas — United States. MMWR Surveill Summ 2017;66(19):1−12. https://doi.org/10.15585/mmwr.ss6619a1.

[2] Hedegaard H, Miniño AM, Warner M. Drug overdose deaths in the United States, 1999−2017. NCHS Data Brief, no 329. Hyattsville, MD: National Center for Health Statistics; 2018.

[3] Cicero TJ, Surratt H, Inciardi JA, Munoz A. Relationship between therapeutic use and abuse of opioid analgesics in rural, suburban, and urban locations in the United States. Pharmacoepidemiol Drug Saf 2007;16(8):827−40.

[4] Wunsch MJ, Nakamoto K, Nuzzo PA, Behonick G, Massello W, Walsh SL. Prescription drug fatalities among women in rural Virginia: a study of medical examiner cases. J Opioid Manag 2009;5(4):228−36.

[5] Paulozzi LJ, Kilbourne EM, Shah NG, Nolte KB, Desai HA, Landen MG, et al. A history of being prescribed controlled substances and risk of drug overdose death. Pain Med 2012;13(1):87—95.

[6] Centers for Disease Control and Prevention. Unintentional deaths from drug poisoning by urbanization of area—New Mexico, 1994—2003. Morb Mortal Wkly Rep 2005; 54(35):870—3.

[7] Havens JR, Young AM, Havens CE. Nonmedical prescription drug use in a nationally representative sample of adolescents: evidence of greater use among rural adolescents. Arch Pediatr Adolesc Med 2011b;165(3):250—5. PMID: 21041587.

[8] Wang KH, Becker WC, Fiellin DA. Prevalence and correlates for nonmedical use of prescription opioids among urban and rural residents. Drug Alcohol Depend 2013; 127(1—3):156—62.

[9] Brady JE, Giglio R, Keyes KM, et al. Risk markers for fatal and non-fatal prescription drug overdose: a meta-analysis. Epidemiology 2017;4(1):24.

[10] Stover AN, Winstanley EL, Zhang Y, Feinberg J. The impact of rural classification systems on a comparison of risky drug-related behaviors in Kentucky and Ohio counties. J Hum Behav Soc Environ 2019. https://doi.org/10.1080/10911359.2018.1516591.

[11] Wejnert C. Vital signs: trends in HIV diagnoses, risk behaviors, and prevention among persons who inject drugs—United States. Morb Mortal Wkly Rep 2016;65:1336—42.

[12] National center for HIV/AIDs, viral hepatitis, STD, and TB prevention. division of HIV/AIDs prevention. HIV Surveillance in Urban and Nonurban areas through 2016. Available from: https://www.cdc.gov/hiv/pdf/library/slidesets/cdc-hiv-urban-nonurban-2016.pdf. [Accessed 16 April 2019].

[13] Evans ME, Labuda SM, Hogan V, et al. Notes from the field: HIV infection investigation in a rural area — West Virginia, 2017. Morb Mortal Wkly Rep 2018;67:257—8.

[14] HIV outbreak in Lawrence, Lowell is bigger than officials thought — The Boston Globe. 2019. Available from: https://www.bostonglobe.com/metro/2018/07/25/hiv-outbreak-lawrence-lowell-bigger-than-officials-thought/szlLL75UDcNTPeB022NptI/story.html.

[15] Opioids have sparked an HIV outbreak in Massachusetts. 2018. Available from: https://www.huffingtonpost.com/entry/massachusetts-fentanyl-opioids-hiv_us_5b6470bfe4b0b15abaa2958c.

[16] Increases in hepatitis C virus infection related to injection drug use among persons aged ≤30 Years — Kentucky, Tennessee, Virginia, and West Virginia, 2006—2012. Morb Mortal Wkly Rep 2015;64(17):453—8.

[17] https://www.cdc.gov/hepatitis/statistics/2015surveillance/Commentary.htm.

[18] Harris AM, Iqbal K, Schillie S, et al. Increases in acute hepatitis B virus infections — Kentucky, Tennessee, and West Virginia, 2006—2013. Morb Mortal Wkly Rep 2016;65:47—50.

[19] 2015 surveillance for viral hepatitis commentary. Available from: https://www.cdc.gov/hepatitis/outbreaks/hepatitisaoutbreaks.htm. [Accessed 16 April 2019].

[20] Foster M, Ramachandran S, Myatt K, et al. Hepatitis A virus outbreaks associated with drug use and homelessness — California, Kentucky, Michigan, and Utah, 2017. Morb Mortal Wkly Rep 2018;67:1208—10.

[21] Wilson E, Hofmeister MG, McBee S, et al. Notes from the field: hepatitis A outbreak associated with drug use and homelessness — West Virginia, 2018. Morb Mortal Wkly Rep 2019;68:330—1.

[22] Keyes KM, Cerda M, Brady JE, et al. Understanding the rural-urban differences in nonmedical prescription opioid use and abuse in the United States. Am J Publ Health 2014;104(2):e52—9.

[23] Hoffman PK, Meier BP, Council JR. A comparison of chronic pain between an urban and rural population. J Community Health Nurs 2002;19(4):213−24.

[24] Leff M, Stallones L, Keefe TJ, Rosenblatt R, Reeds M. Comparison of urban and rural non-fatal injury: the results of a statewide survey. Inj Prev 2003;9(4):332−7.

[25] Coben JH, Tiesman HM, Bossarte RM, Furbee PM. Rural−urban differences in injury hospitalizations in the US, 2004. Am J Prev Med 2009;36(1):49−55.

[26] Leukefeld CG, Walker R, Havens JR, Leedham VT. What does the community say: key informant perceptions of rural prescription drug use. J Drug Issues 2007;37(3):503−24.

[27] Peters PJ, Pontones P, Hoover KW, et al. HIV infection linked to injection use of oxymorphone in Indiana, 2014−2015. N Engl J Med 2016;375:229−39.

[28] Van Handel MM, Rose CE, Hallisey EJ, et al. County-level vulnerability assessment for rapid dissemination of HIV or HCV infections among persons who inject drugs, United States. J Acquir Immune Defic Syndr 2016;73(3):323−31.

[29] Bachhuber MA, Weiner J, Mitchell J, et al. Issue brief. Primary care: on the front lines of the opioid crisis. Philadelphia, PA: Center for Health Economics of Treatment Interventions for Substance Use Disorder, HCV, and HIV; 2016. https://ldi.upenn.edu/brief/primary-carefront-lines-opioid-crisis. [Accessed 20 February 2019].

[30] Andrilla CHA, Coulthard C, Larson EH. Changes in the supply of physicians with a DEA DATA waiver to prescribe buprenorphine for opioid use disorder. Data Brief #162. Seattle, WA: WAMI Rural Health Research Center; 2017.

[31] El Bcheraoui C, Mokdad AH, Dwyer-Lindgren L, et al. Trends and patterns of differences in infectious disease mortality among US counties, 1980−2014. J Am Med Assoc 2018;319(12):1248−60.

[32] Moran GE, Snyder CM, Noftsinger RF, et al (Prepared by Westat under Contract Number HHSP 233201500026I, Task Order No. HHSP23337003T). Implementing medication-assisted treatment for opioid use disorder in rural primary care: environmental scan, vol. 1. Rockville, MD: Agency for Healthcare Research and Quality; October 2017. Publication No. 17(18)-0050-EF.

[33] Andrilla CHA, Coulthard C, Larson EH. Barriers rural physicians face prescribing buprenorphine for opioid use disorder. Ann Fam Med 2017;15(4):359−62.

[34] Akhtar WZ, Murray M, Kung V, et al. Access to office-based opioid treatment in a rural epidemic: provider shortages in counties with high overdose burden. In: Oral presentation at addition health services research, Augusta, GA; October 2018.

[35] Eyre E, Trump officials seek opioid solutions in WV. Available from: https://www.wvgazettemail.com/news/health/trump-officials-seek-opioid-solutions-in-wv/article_52c417d8-16a5-59d5-8928-13ab073bc02b.html. [Accessed 16 April 2019].

[36] Gallant JE, Adimora AA, Carmichael JK, et al. Essential components of effective HIV care: a policy paper of the HIV medicine Association of the Infectious Diseases Society of America and the Ryan white medical providers coalition. Clin Infect Dis 2011;53:1043−50.

[37] Schafer KR, Albrecht H, Dillingham R, et al. The continuum of HIV care in rural communities in the United States and Canada: what is known and future research directions. J Acquir Immune Defic Syndr 2017;75(1):35−44.

[38] Chu C, Umanski G, Blank A, et al. HIV-infected patients and treatment outcomes: an equivalence study of community-located, primary care-based HIV treatment vs. hospital-based specialty care in the Bronx, New York. AIDS Care 2010;22(12):1522−9.

[39] Arora S, Thornton K, Murata G, et al. Outcomes of treatment for hepatitis C virus infection by primary care providers. N Engl J Med 2011;364(23):2199−207.

[40] Kattakuzhy S, Gross C, Emmanuel B, et al. Expansion of treatment for hepatitis C virus infection by task shifting to community-based nonspecialist providers: a nonrandomized clinical trial. Ann Intern Med 2017;167(5):311−8.

[41] Grebely J, Hajarizadeh B, Dore GJ. Direct-acting antiviral agents for HCV infection affecting people who inject drugs. Nat Rev Gastroenterol Hepatol 2017;14(11):641−51.

[42] Grebely J, et al. Sofosbuvir and velpatasvir for hepatitis C virus infection in people with recent injection drug use (SIMPLIFY): an open-label, single-arm, phase 4, multicentre trial. Lancet Gastroenterol Hepatol 2018;3:153−61.

[43] Dore GJ, et al. Elbasvir-grazoprevir to treat hepatitis C virus infection in persons receiving opioid Agonist therapy: a randomized trial. Ann Intern Med 2016;165(9):625−34.

[44] . Dore G, et al. Hepatitis C Virus (HCV) reinfection and injecting risk behavior following Elbasvir (EBR)/Grazoprevir (GZR) treatment in participants on opiate Agonist therapy (OAT): Co-STAR Part B. 68th annual meeting of the American Association for the Study of Liver diseases, October 20−24, 2017, Washington DC, USA. Abstract 195.

[45] . Ingiliz P, et al. Conference on retroviruses and opportunistic infections (CROI). March 4−7, 2018, Boston, MA. Abstract 612.

[46] Ingiliz P, et al. NEAT study group. HCV reinfection incidence and spontaneous clearance rates in HIV-positive men who have sex with men in Western Europe. J Hepatol 2017;66(2):282−7.

[47] Botticelli M, Koh H. Changing the language of addiction. J Am Med Assoc 2016; 316(13):1361−2.

[48] Clark L, Haram E, Johnson K, et al. Getting started with medication-assisted treatment: with lessons from advancing recovery. Madison: Network for the Improvement of Addiction Treatment, University of Wisconsin; 2010. http://www.niatx.net/PDF/NIATx-MATToolkit.pdf. [Accessed 20 February 2019].

[49] Goldensohn R. They shared drugs. Someone died. Does that make them killers? N Y Times May 25, 2018. Available from: https://www.nytimes.com/2018/05/25/us/drug-overdose-prosecution-crime.html. [Accessed 27 February 2018].

[50] Kapadia SN, Johnston CD, Marks KM, et al. Strategies for improving hepatitis C treatment access in the United States: state officials address high drug prices, stigma, and building treatment capacity. J Publ Health Manag Pract 2019;25(3):245−52.

[51] 2017 National Summary Report Harvard law school center for health law and policy innovation. Hepatitis C: the state of medicaid access. 2017. Available from: https://stateofhepc.org/wp-content/uploads/2017/10/State-of-HepC_2017_FINAL.pdf. [Accessed 27 February 2019].

[52] Substance Abuse and Mental Health Services Administration. Medicaid coverage of medication-assisted treatment for alcohol and opioid use disorders and of medication for the reversal of opioid overdose. HHS Publication No. SMA-18-5093. Rockville, MD: Substance Abuse and Mental Health Services Administration; 2018.

[53] Case study: medication assisted treatment program for opioid addiction. Arlington, VA: Association of State and Territorial Health Officials and deBeaumont Foundation; 2015. Available from: http://www.astho.org/Health-Systems-Transformation/Medicaid-and-Public-HealthPartnerships/Case-Studies/Vermont-MAT-Program-for-Opioid-Addiction/. [Accessed 24 January 2019].

[54] Arora S, Geppert CM, Kalishman S, et al. Academic health center management of chronic diseases through knowledge networks: project ECHO. Acad Med 2007;82(2):1−14.

[55] LaBelle CT, Han SC, Bergeron A, et al. Office-based opioid treatment with buprenorphine (OBOT-B): statewide implementation of the Massachusetts Collaborative Care Model in community health centers. J Subst Abuse Treat 2016;60:6−13.

Opioid use disorder, infectious diseases, and the criminal justice system

4

Radha Sadacharan, MD, MPH [1,3], Jody Rich, MD, MPH [2,3]

[1]*Clinical Instructor in the Department Family Medicine, The Warren Alpert Medical School of Brown University, Providence, RI, United States;* [2]*Professor of Medicine and Epidemiology at The Warren Alpert Medical School of Brown University, Providence, RI, United States;* [3]*Center for Prisoner Health and Human Rights at The Miriam Hospital, Providence, RI, United States*

Background on criminal justice in the United States

In the United States, the rate of incarceration has skyrocketed over the last 50 years, ignited by the "Tough on Crime" as well as the "War on Drugs" political pushes of the 1970s and disproportionately affecting people of color and people with mental health illnesses. The lifetime likelihood of incarceration for black men in the United States is 1 in 3, compared 1 in 17 for white men (Bonczar, 2013). Of the 2.2 million people incarcerated in the United States at any given time, over half have been diagnosed with a substance use disorder, with or without a serious mental illness. 12% of jail inmates report using opioids regularly, more than six times higher than the general population [8,52].

The specifics of mass incarceration based on location, medical care, and jurisdiction should also be highlighted. 1.2 million sentenced individuals are incarcerated in state prisons, while approximately 600,000 people reside in local jails in the United States. Jail stays are generally shorter, tend to be a pretrial population, and are more likely to consist of time served for misdemeanors. Prisons stays, on the other hand, are longer, for sentenced individuals, and generally sentences that involve more serious crimes. In terms of jurisdiction, jails mostly are managed under local governing bodies, while prisons are managed at the state or federal level. Within federal prisons, run by the federal Bureau of Prisons or utilizing private prisons in some places, approximately 200,000 people are currently incarcerated. Drug offense charges comprise 14.8% of sentences at a state level and 47.3% at a federal level [6]. With more states interested in implementing diversion for low-level offenses like drug possession, these statistics will hopefully change, but again, in the scope of the ongoing "War on Drugs" and the opioid epidemic, there is a real concern that this could continue to worsen.

Prisoners are the only group of people in the United States who have a constitutional right to healthcare. The federal case Estelle v Gamble (1976) determined that prisoners should be guaranteed three basic rights: the right to access to care, the right

The Opioid Epidemic and Infectious Diseases. https://doi.org/10.1016/B978-0-323-68328-9.00004-7

to care that is ordered, and the right to a professional medical judgment. Any lack of these rights for prisoners constituted a violation of the 8th Amendment, "cruel and unusual punishment" [43]. Despite a federal ruling, many prisoners still have incomprehensibly poor access to healthcare, and the variability in quality of care is wide.

Bloodborne illnesses in criminal justice settings

As other chapters in this book will delve into the details of bloodborne illnesses in the setting of opioid use disorder, we will focus specifically on the criminal justice setting.

Epidemiology

It is well known that bloodborne illnesses such as HIV/AIDS, HCV, and tuberculosis are more prevalent in criminal justice settings. In terms of prevalence, in 2006, the rate of hepatitis C was 8.7 times higher among those who were incarcerated than the general population (17.4% compared with 2.0%) [58]. The incidence of HIV and HCV acquisition is also significantly affected by incarceration. Recent incarceration, when compared with nonincarceration, increases the risk of acquiring HIV by an estimated 81% and increases the risk of acquiring HCV by an estimated 62% [59]. These staggering statistics are important to highlight: individuals leaving correctional facilities are at a tremendous risk of contracting HIV and HCV after release, most commonly through IVDU and sexual exposure.

In addition to bloodborne illnesses being more prevalent in criminal justice settings, people living with HIV/AIDS and HCV are more likely to be incarcerated. In 1997, a study on the infectious disease (ID) burden within United States correctional facilities estimated between 20% and 26% of people with HIV/AIDS passed through prisons and jails, and between 29% and 32% of people with HCV [24]. Despite a large ID burden, treatment of bloodborne illnesses in correctional facilities is not standardized.

Treatment of bloodborne illnesses in criminal justice settings

The treatment of HIV in correctional settings has long been proven to result in higher rates of viral load suppression and significant increases in CD4 counts [53]. Providing antiretrovirals in the correctional setting is relatively straightforward given consistent patient access to medications and a highly controlled environment, yet it is also complicated by the difficult and critical matter of maintaining patient confidentiality in an extremely vulnerable and stigmatizing setting and by needing to obtain costly medications that may not be on an institution's formulary. HIV treatment in correctional settings was pioneered by ID specialists and has been a successful endeavor that should be continued.

Treatment of HCV with direct-acting antivirals during incarceration is currently prohibitively expensive for many facilities but wholly necessary to cure the HCV epidemic. As the population at highest risk for contracting and transmitting HCV is within the community of people who inject drugs (PWID), and PWID are disproportionately incarcerated, the correctional setting is an important if not invaluable place to initiate HCV treatment. Given the increase in HCV transmission postrelease, a plan to treat individuals prior to release is the most effective method to improve health outcomes for the individual as well as reduce continued transmission postrelease. A dynamic mathematical model that examined HCV treatment for the incarcerated in Scotland recently demonstrated not only a reduction in overall HCV burden over a time period of 15 years but projected cost savings for the country due to reduced transmissions, in spite of high costs of treatment upfront [59,65]. Moreover, in the United States, the cost of HCV treatment has the potential to be negotiated effectively, especially in the setting of a large enough purchaser. The US Department for Veterans Administration in 2016, for example, negotiated a drug price cap of $15,000 per person for a treatment course of DAA [66]. In state correctional systems, similar negotiations are possible. To our knowledge, multiple states so far are utilizing federal 340B drug pricing. Louisiana has negotiated a novel deal with Asegua Therapeutics LLC, a wholly owned subsidiary of Gilead Sciences, Inc., where for a fixed sum of money, the state will be able to purchase an unlimited amount of Asegua's authorized generic sofosbuvir/velpatasvir to treat patients within Louisiana's Medicaid and Department of Corrections populations and caps the State's medication costs for the next 5 years [14].

ID specialists may be interested in partnering with correctional facilities to deliver this care in multiple ways. ID specialists may treat patients directly: they can contact medical personnel (information generally available on Department of Corrections websites) to identify current practices in nearby correctional facilities. If an opportunity to provide ID treatment does not already exist in a correctional facility, providers practicing in outpatient settings including community health centers and federally qualified health centers have the ability to initiate a program to treat patients with HIV and/or HCV who are currently incarcerated by utilizing federal 340B drug pricing through their community clinics.

Treatment of bloodborne illnesses after release, ID specialists as referral sites

As noted in the previous section, individuals with HIV/AIDS in correctional settings do generally achieve high rates of viral suppression and significant increases in CD4 lymphocyte counts while incarcerated, but on release, these improvements are not sustained [32,33,47]. Intensive case management and provider continuity have been shown to be some of the most effective strategies to engage other vulnerable individuals in care, but no studies to our knowledge have yet demonstrated sustained improvements for justice-involved persons with HIV [11,56]. At this time, we recommend that ID specialists work with public health departments to establish themselves as referral providers for the treatment of communicable diseases of justice-involved individuals.

The duration of effective HCV treatment again should be strongly considered while individuals are serving sentences. For jail settings, however, there can be concern of release prior to HCV treatment completion due to shorter sentences. In this scenario, an ID specialist could meet a patient while incarcerated, initiate workup, and link them to the appropriate care on the outside. This direct linkage has proven to be most effective, as patients prefer continuity of providers.

Medications for addiction (opioid use disorder) treatment

Drug overdoses are now the leading cause of death for Americans under the age of 50. There is a plethora of evidence demonstrating that methadone, buprenorphine, and naltrexone are all effective treatments for opioid use disorder, with methadone and buprenorphine being superior, and will be referred to as medications for addiction treatment, or MAT, in this chapter.

Methadone is a schedule II narcotic and full opioid agonist, first introduced as a medication to treat opioid use disorder in 1974. Methadone continues to be tightly regulated at a federal level, through opioid treatment programs. Buprenorphine, a partial opioid agonist and schedule III medication, was approved by the FDA in 2002 for the treatment of opioid use disorders. The benefits of buprenorphine include its ability to be prescribed in outpatient facilities (outpatient-based opioid treatment, or OBOTs), fewer side effects as compared with methadone, and a far-lower risk of overdose when compared to other opioids. Administration of buprenorphine to a person who has recently used opioids can precipitate withdrawal given buprenorphine's high affinity for mu receptors (knocking other opioids off the receptor). As such, buprenorphine initiation necessitates that a person be in opioid withdrawal or completely off opioids, to avoid putting patients in uncomfortable and potentially dangerous situations. Naltrexone, an opioid antagonist, is most effective as a monthly intramuscular injection, but necessitates a longer abstinence from opioids than either methadone or buprenorphine.

Treatment of opioid use disorder in criminal justice settings

Per a recent release by the National Academies of Sciences, Engineering and Medicine, "Medication-based treatment is effective across all treatment settings studied to date. Withholding or failing to have available all classes of U.S. Food and Drug Administration—approved medication for the treatment of opioid use disorder in any care or criminal justice setting is denying appropriate medical treatment" [35].

This statement is backed up by a multitude of evidence, accumulated over the last few decades particularly in the criminal justice system. In the general population, both methadone and buprenorphine, opioid agonist therapies used for the treatment of opioid use disorders, have been shown to reduce opioid misuse compared with abstinence-only interventions. [39,50]. When compared with abstinence-only interventions, opioid agonist therapy among justice-involved populations has not only been associated with lower rates of opioid misuse but also with higher retention in treatment, lower illicit substance use, and in some cases lower rates of recidivism [1,30,51] (Hedrich, 2012). Rhode Island, at the time of writing this chapter, is the only state that provides comprehensive MAT services, including screening for opioid use disorder and treatment with buprenorphine, methadone, or depot naltrexone within all state correctional facilities. It accomplished this goal by utilizing 12 community-based Centers of Excellence for MAT to promote transitions and referrals of inmates during and postincarcerations. The state of Rhode Island has already demonstrated in preliminary data from the first year of comprehensive MAT services notable success in decreasing the state's rate of fatal overdose of justice-involved individuals [17].

Despite the increasing evidence of the benefits of MAT in criminal justice settings, most correctional facilities currently rely on, at best, an opioid antagonist like naltrexone, and at worst, induced opioid withdrawal, masked as "drug-free detoxification" [13]. In addition to correctional facilities historically declining provision of MAT for people with opioid use disorder (with the exception of methadone for pregnant women, a well-accepted standard of care), some drug courts, judges, parole, and probation agencies have expressed concern with regard to the need for agonist treatment, believing that buprenorphine and methadone are replacing one drug for another. This belief and stigma presents itself in referral sources for treatment. The Substance Abuse and Mental Health Services Administration (SAMHSA) compiles and manages data regarding treatment admissions in state-regulated treatment facilities within the United States, labeled the Treatment Episodes Data Set-Admissions (TEDS-A). A retrospective study looking at the TEDS-A data for sources of referral for these treatment facilities found that justice-referred individuals were significantly less likely to receive agonist medications as part of their treatment plan compared with those referred through other sources. Less than 5% of people referred to substance use treatment for opioid use disorder through the justice system received opioid agonist treatment, compared with over 40% of people referred through other sources [28].

Due in large part to the criminal justice system's historical preference for antagonist or abstinence-based therapy, many facilities that receive funding from the criminal justice system or housing must also support nonmedication-based treatments. Instead of clinically proven medical agonist treatment, medically supervised withdrawal ("detox") is used, and return-to-use rates following detox have been reported to be as high as 65% to 91%. If patients return to using opioids post incarceration, this approach also carries a high risk of overdose due to a reduced tolerance [64].

As of late, however, multiple lawsuits have been filed against correctional facilities across the country denying inmates access to treatments like methadone and buprenorphine for their opioid use disorders. These cases will likely move the dial on better access to medications for opioid use disorder during incarceration. Despite expected progress, we still are in dire need of providers to prescribe these medications.

While people with HIV and hepatitis C are incarcerated and being treated for these and other IDs, it could not be a more opportune time to discuss treatment for opioid use disorder with patients. This work can be done seamlessly by ID specialists, both within correctional facilities and through outpatient collaboration with correctional facilities to see patients upon release.

The benefits of concurrent treatment of opioid use disorder and infectious diseases in criminal justice settings

An estimated one-third of formerly incarcerated individuals living with HIV/AIDS have an opioid use disorder [10]. People who inject drugs are at increased risk of contracting bloodborne illnesses, through needle- and other drug paraphernalia-sharing, along with sexual contact, all of which are more complicated to identify and treat in a correctional setting. Drug injection is a major method of HIV transmission, such that the National Institute on Drug Abuse has identified drug treatment as its principal strategy for preventing HIV and AIDS among this population.

Patient preference has been noted for receiving treatment for opioid use disorder and IDs, particularly HIV and HCV, in one location. Reasons cited include stigma, difficulty accessing multiple sites of care, cost, and comfort with providers, among many others [19]. Thankfully, any physician can easily obtain their waiver through an 8-h training in order to prescribe buprenorphine to treat opioid use disorders. Adding this to the fact that most ID specialists already have a thorough understanding of the effects of substance use disorders on their patients' lives, an ID specialist becomes the obvious choice of provider. Patient preference is complemented by evidence that MAT and ID treatment are more effective when provided in tandem.

In a recent systematic review, 12 studies in opioid treatment settings identified improved HIV screening uptake and clinical benefits with antiretroviral therapy when provided on-site [38]. In addition to improving screening uptake, treatment of opioid use disorder with opioid agonists has been demonstrated in systematic reviews and metaanalyses to reduce an individual's risk of acquiring HIV by about 54%, as well as reducing an individual's risk of acquiring HCV by about half [15,49, 61−63]. As stated in a previous section, ID specialists can contact correctional facilities to provide this care while individuals are incarcerated, and perhaps more importantly build bridges for patients to more easily access care on release.

Transitions of care surrounding release, the role of the ID physician

Within the first 2 weeks after release from incarceration, there is greater than a 100-fold higher risk of fatal overdose for justice-involved individuals, compared with the general population [5]. The transitions of care at time of release for patients are a critical point at which outpatient ID specialists are uniquely poised to link patients to success in the community. One retrospective cohort study that followed over 2000 HIV-infected inmates in the Texas prison system demonstrated 95% of people on HIV treatment at the time of release had their treatment interrupted (i.e., did not fill a prescription for ART within 10 days), a time at which they were more likely to engage in sexual relationships and/or drug use, thus being more likely to transmit the infection [2]. In addition to an increase in risky behaviors at the time of release, individuals are obviously more likely to develop resistance to ART with missed doses [26].

Typically, patients do not only have HIV or HCV and criminal justice involvement but also often have mental illness, trauma, psychiatric conditions, and other medical issues, in addition to tremendous social and legal problems. HIV + patients on buprenorphine maintenance treatment who have been recently incarcerated are more likely to be homeless, unemployed, and previously diagnosed with mental illness, compared with those who were not recently incarcerated [42]. Given these known barriers to care and social determinants of health, the biggest challenge often is to maintain a continuity of care through release and into the community. Here exists the real opportunity to help stop people from discontinuing life-saving medications or relapsing to drug use. If there is a familiar face or any type of warm hand-off, even if it is possible to meet part of the care team (healthcare provider, case worker, nurse, telemedicine visit) prior to release, this can change the trajectory of a patient's reentry into a person's community. Coordination of care at release is imperative to achieve better health outcomes.

While the current state of fragmented healthcare for justice-involved individuals postrelease feels like an uphill battle, we do have some effective tools to engage this vulnerable population. For one, methadone initiated in prison or immediately postrelease is associated with reduced HIV and overdose risk compared with counseling in prison without methadone and passive referral to treatment at release. Significant declines in risky behaviors are also noted in association with methadone treatment during the postrelease time periods [54]. Initiation and maintenance on buprenorphine and extended-release naltrexone, like methadone for OUD, has also been shown to improve HIV outcomes [45,46]. Unlike methadone, buprenorphine and naltrexone can be prescribed by ID specialists for the treatment of OUD. ID specialists in the community have the ability, and, we believe, the moral responsibility, to treat individuals at the greatest risk of contracting and living with bloodborne illnesses.

All healthcare providers preventing and treating IDs should be assessing risk and identifying harm reduction measures. This includes asking their patients about justice involvement. An integrated delivery system is necessary to achieve goals of HIV suppression, HCV cure, reduction of overdoses, and opioid use disorder treatment. The criminal justice system provides an unparalleled opportunity for ID specialists to engage in this work.

We must also acknowledge that the discussion around incarceration should not just be about IDs, incarceration nor opioid use disorder, but also about combating the overarching discrimination in who becomes involved in the criminal justice system. Much of the risks for HIV, HCV, and opioid use disorder parallel high rates of trauma, poverty, homelessness, depression, and a whole host of other social determinants of health. The fact that one in three black men will end up involved in the criminal justice system tells us that race and the ZIP code you were born into may be more predictive of incarceration than anything else. Physicians can play a role in advocating for a fair criminal justice system, as well as for improved access to healthcare within and outside this system.

References

[1] Aronowitz SV, Laurent J. Screaming behind a door: the experiences of individuals incarcerated without medication-assisted treatment. J Correct Health Care 2016; 22(2):98−108.

[2] Baillargeon J, Giordano TP, Rich JD, et al. Accessing antiretroviral therapy following release from prison. JAMA 2009;301(8):848−57.

[3] Baillargeon J, Penn JV, Knight K, Harzke AJ, Baillargeon G, Becker EA. Risk of reincarceration among prisoners with co-occurring severe mental illness and substance use disorders. Adm Policy Ment Health 2010;37(4):367−74.

[4] Binswanger IA. Opioid use disorder and incarceration - hope for ensuring the continuity of treatment. N Engl J Med 2019;380(13):1193−5.

[5] Binswanger IA, Stern MF, Deyo RA, et al. Release from prison−a high risk of death for former inmates. N Engl J Med 2007;356(2):157−65.

[6] Bronson J, Carson EA. Prisoners in 2017 (NCJ 252156). 2019. Retrieved from U.S. Department of Justice, Bureau of Justice Statistics website:https://www.bjs.gov/index.cfm?ty=pbdetail&iid=6546.

[7] Cepeda JA, Eritsyan K, Vickerman P, et al. Potential impact of implementing and scaling up harm reduction and antiretroviral therapy on HIV prevalence and mortality and overdose deaths among people who inject drugs in two Russian cities: a modelling study. Lancet HIV 2018;5(10):e578−87.

[8] Chandler RK, Finger MS, Farabee D, et al. The SOMATICS collaborative: introduction to a National Institute on Drug Abuse cooperative study of pharmacotherapy for opioid treatment in criminal justice settings. Contemp Clin Trials 2016;48:166−72.

[9] Dasgupta N, Beletsky L, Ciccarone D. Opioid crisis: No easy fix to its social and economic determinants. Am J Public Health 2018;108(2):182−6.

[10] Di Paola A, Altice FL, Powell ML, Trestman RL, Springer SA. A comparison of psychiatric diagnoses among HIV-infected prisoners receiving combination antiretroviral therapy and transitioning to the community. Health Justice 2014;2(11).

[11] DiPrete BL, Pence BW, Golin CE, et al. Antiretroviral adherence following prison release in a randomized trial of the imPACTintervention to maintain suppression of HIV viremia. AIDS Behav 2019;23(9):2386−95. https://doi.org/10.1007/s10461-019-02488-7.

[12] Fiscella K, Beletsky L, Wakeman SE. The inmate exception and reform of correctional health care. Am J Public Health 2017;107(3):384−5.

[13] Fiscella K, Wakeman SE, Beletsky L. Implementing opioid agonist treatment in correctional facilities. JAMA Intern Med 2018;178(9):1153−4.

[14] Gilead. Louisiana launches hepatitis C innovative payment model with Asegua Therapeutics, aiming to eliminate the disease. Gilead Sciences Inc. Press Release; June 26 ,2019. Available from:https://www.gilead.com/news-and-press/press-room/press-releases/2019/6/louisiana-launches-hepatitis-c-innovative-payment-model-with-asegua-therapeutics-aiming-to-eliminate-the-disease.

[15] Gowing LR, Hickman M, Degenhardt L. Mitigating the risk of HIV infection with opioid substitution treatment. Bull World Health Organ 2013;91(2):148−9.

[16] Green TC, Bratberg J, Dauria EF, Rich JD. Responding to opioid overdose in Rhode Island: where the medical community has gone and where we need to go. R I Med J (2013) 2014;97(10):29−33.

[17] Green TC, Clarke J, Brinkley-Rubinstein L, et al. Postincarceration fatal overdoses after implementing medications for addiction treatment in a statewide correctional system. JAMA Psychiatry 2018;75(4):405−7.

[18] Green TC, McGowan SK, Yokell MA, Pouget ER, Rich JD. HIV infection and risk of overdose: a systematic review and meta-analysis. AIDS 2012;26(4):403−17.

[19] Haley DF, Golin CE, Farel CE, et al. Multilevel challenges to engagement in HIV care after prison release: a theory-informed qualitative study comparing prisoners' perspectives before and after community reentry. BMC Public Health 2014;14:1253.

[20] Hammett TM. Making the case for health interventions in correctional facilities. J Urban Health 2001;78(2):236−40.

[21] Hammett TM. HIV/AIDS and other infectious diseases among correctional inmates: transmission, burden, and an appropriate response. Am J Public Health 2006;96(6): 974−8.

[22] Hammett TM, Donahue S, LeRoy L, et al. Transitions to care in the community for prison releasees with HIV: a qualitative study of facilitators and challenges in two states. J Urban Health 2015;92(4):650−66.

[23] Hammett TM, Gaiter JL, Crawford C. Reaching seriously at-risk populations: health interventions in criminal justice settings. Health Educ Behav 1998;25(1):99−120.

[24] Hammett TM, Harmon MP, Rhodes W. The burden of infectious disease among inmates of and releasees from US correctional facilities, 1997. Am J Public Health 2002;92(11): 1789−94.

[25] Hammett TM, Trang NT, Oanh KTH, et al. The relationship between health policy and public health interventions: a case study of the DRIVE project to "end" the HIV epidemic among people who inject drugs in Haiphong, Vietnam. J Public Health Policy 2018;39(2):217−30.

[26] Hill LM, Golin CE, Gottfredson NC, et al. Drug use mediates the relationship between depressive symptoms and adherence to ART among recently incarcerated people living with HIV. AIDS Behav 2019;23(8):2037−47. https://doi.org/10.1007/s10461-018-2355-3.

[27] Kinnard EN, Philbin MM, Beletsky L. Government actions to curb the opioid epidemic. JAMA 2018;319(15):1619−20.

[28] Krawczyk N, Picher CE, Feder KA, Saloner B. Only one in twentyjustice-referred adults in specialty treatment for opioid use receive methadone or buprenorphine. Health Aff (Millwood) 2017;36(12):2046−53.

[29] Lincoln T, Kennedy S, Tuthill R, Roberts C, Conklin TJ, Hammett TM. Facilitators and barriers to continuing healthcare after jail: a community-integrated program. J Ambul Care Manage 2006;29(1):2−16.

[30] McKenzie M, Nunn A, Zaller ND, Bazazi AR, Rich JD. Overcoming obstacles to implementing methadone maintenance therapy for prisoners: implications for policy and practice. J Opioid Manag 2009;5(4):219−27.

[31] McKenzie M, Zaller N, Dickman SL, et al. A randomized trial of methadone initiation prior to release from incarceration. Subst Abus 2012;33(1):19−29.

[32] Meyer JP, Cepeda J, Springer SA, Wu J, Trestman RL, Altice FL. HIV in people rein-carcerated in Connecticut prisons and jails: an observational cohort study. Lancet HIV 2014a;1(2):e77–84.

[33] Meyer JP, Cepeda J, Wu J, Trestman RL, Altice FL, Springer SA. Optimization of human immunodeficiency virus treatment during incarceration: viral suppression at the prison gate. JAMA Intern Med 2014b;174(5):721–9.

[34] National Academies of Sciences E, and Medicine. Integrating responses at the intersection of opioid use disorder and infectious disease epidemics: proceedings of a workshop. Washington, DC: The National Academies Press; 2018.

[35] National Academies of Sciences E, and Medicine. Medications for opioid use disorder save lives. Washington, DC: The National Academies Press; 2019.

[36] Nunn A, Zaller N, Dickman S, Trimbur C, Nijhawan A, Rich JD. Methadone and buprenorphine prescribing and referral practices in US prison systems: results from a nationwide survey. Drug Alcohol Depend 2009;105(1–2):83–8.

[37] Oldfield BJ, Muñoz N, Boshnack N, et al. "No more falling through the cracks": a qualitative study to inform measurement of integration of care of HIV and opioid use disorder. J Subst Abuse Treat 2019;97:28–40.

[38] Oldfield BJ, Muñoz N, Mcgovern MP, et al. Integration of care for HIV and opioid use disorder: a systematic review of interventions in clinical and community-based settings. AIDS 2019;33(5):873–84. https://doi.org/10.1097/QAD.0000000000002125.

[39] Potter JS, Marino EN, Hillhouse MP, et al. Buprenorphine/naloxone and methadone maintenance treatment outcomes for opioid analgesic, heroin, and combined users: findings from starting treatment with agonist replacement therapies (START). J Stud Alcohol Drugs 2013;74(4):605–13.

[40] Rich JD, Green TC, McKenzie MS. Opioids and deaths. N Engl J Med 2011;364(7):686.

[41] Rich JD, Holmes L, Salas C, et al. Successful linkage of medical care and community services for HIV-positive offenders being released from prison. J Urban Health 2001;78(2):279–89.

[42] Riggins DP, Cunningham CO, Ning Y, Fox AD. Recent incarceration and buprenorphine maintenance treatment outcomes among human immunodeficiency virus-positive patients. Subst Abus 2017;38(3):297–302.

[43] Rold WJ. Thirty years after Estelle v. Gamble: alegal retrospective. J Correct Health Care 2008;14(1):11–20.

[44] Spaulding AC, Seals RM, Page MJ, Brzozowski AK, Rhodes W, Hammett TM. HIV/AIDS among inmates of and releasees from US correctional facilities, 2006: declining share of epidemic but persistent public health opportunity. PLoS One 2009;4(11):e7558.

[45] Springer SA, Chen S, Altice FL. Improved HIV and substance abuse treatment outcomes for released HIV-infected prisoners: the impact of buprenorphine treatment. J Urban Health 2010;87(4):592–602.

[46] Springer SA, Di Paola A, Barbour R, Azar MM, Altice FL. Extended-release naltrexone improves viral suppression among incarcerated persons living with HIV and alcohol use disorders transitioning to the community: results from a double-blind, placebo-controlled trial. J Acquir Immune Defic Syndr 2018;79(1):92–100.

[47] Springer SA, Pesanti E, Hodges J, Macura T, Doros G, Altice FL. Effectiveness of antiretroviral therapy among HIV-infected prisoners: reincarceration and the lack of sustained benefit after release to the community. Clin Infect Dis 2004;38(12):1754–60.

[48]   Springer SA, Qiu J, Saber-Tehrani AS, Altice FL. Retention on buprenorphine is associated with high levels of maximal viral suppression among HIV-infected opioid dependent released prisoners. PLoS One 2012;7(5):e38335.

[49]   Tsui JI, Evans JL, Lum PJ, Hahn JA, Page K. Association of opioid agonist therapy with lower incidence of hepatitis C virus infection in young adult injection drug users. JAMA Intern Med 2014;174(12):1974–81.

[50]   Volkow ND, Frieden TR, Hyde PS, Cha SS. Medication-assisted therapies—tackling the opioid-overdose epidemic. N Engl J Med 2014;370(22):2063–6.

[51]   Vorma H, Sokero P, Aaltonen M, Turtiainen S, Hughes LA, Savolainen J. Participation in opioid substitution treatment reduces the rate of criminal convictions: evidence from a community study. Addict Behav 2013;38(7):2313–6.

[52]   Wakeman SE. Why it's inappropriate not to treat incarcerated patients with opioid agonist therapy. AMA J Ethics 2017;19(9):922–30.

[53]   Wakeman SE, Rich JD. HIV treatment in US prisons. HIV Ther 2010;4(4):505–10.

[54]   Wilson ME, Kinlock TW, Gordon MS, O'Grady KE, Schwartz RP. Postprison release HIV-risk behaviors in a randomized trial of methadone treatment for prisoners. Am J Addict 2012;21(5):476–87.

[55]   Winkelman TNA, Chang VW, Binswanger IA. Health, polysubstanceuse, and criminal justice involvement among adults with varying levels of opioid use. JAMA Netw Open 2018;1(3):e180558.

[56]   Wohl DA, Golin CE, Knight K, et al. Randomized controlled trial of an intervention to maintain suppression of HIV viremiaafter prison release: the imPACT trial. J Acquir Immune Defic Syndr 2017;75(1):81–90.

[57]   Zaller N, McKenzie M, Friedmann PD, Green TC, McGowan S, Rich JD. Initiation of buprenorphine during incarceration and retention in treatment upon release. J Subst Abuse Treat 2013;45(2):222–6.

[58]   Varan AK, Mercer DW, Stein MS, Spaulding AC. Hepatitis C seroprevalence among prison inmates since 2001: still high but declining. Public Health Rep 2014;129(2): 187–95. https://doi.org/10.1177/003335491412900213.

[59]   Stone J, Fraser H, Lim AG, et al. Incarceration history and risk of HIV and hepatitis C virus acquisition among people who inject drugs: a systematic review and meta-analysis. Lancet Infect Dis 2018;18(12):1397–409. https://doi.org/10.1016/S1473-3099(18)30469-9.

[60]   Hedrich D, Alves P, Farrell M, Stöver H, Møller L, Mayet S. The effectiveness of opioid maintenance treatment in prison settings: a systematic review. Addiction 2012;107: 501–17. https://doi.org/10.1111/j.1360-0443.2011.03676.x.

[61]   Aspinall EJ, Nambiar D, Goldberg DJ, Hickman M, Weir A, Van Velzen E, Palmateer N, Doyle JS, Hellard ME, Hutchinson SJ. Are needle and syringe programmes associated with a reduction in HIV transmission among people who inject drugs: a systematic review and meta-analysis. Int J Epidemiol 2014;43(1):235–48. https://doi.org/10.1093/ije/dyt243.

[62]   Platt L, Minozzi S, Reed J, Vickerman P, Hagan H, French C, Jordan A, Degenhardt L, Hope V, Hutchinson S, Maher L, Palmateer N, Taylor A, Bruneau J, Hickman M. Needle syringe programmes and opioid substitution therapy for preventing hepatitis C transmission in people who inject drugs. Cochrane Database Syst Rev 2017;(90). https://doi.org/10.1002/14651858.CD012021.pub2. Art. No.: CD012021.

[63] MacArthur Georgie J, Minozzi Silvia, Martin Natasha, Vickerman Peter, Deren Sherry, Bruneau Julie, et al. Opiate substitution treatment and HIV transmission in people who inject drugs: systematic review and meta-analysis. BMJ 2012;345:e5945.

[64] Chutuape MA, Jasinski DR, Fingerhood MI, Stitzer ML. One-, three-, and six-month outcomes after brief inpatient opioid detoxification. Am J Drug Alcohol Abuse 2001; 27(1):19−44. https://doi.org/10.1081/ada-100103117.

[65] Martin NK, Vickerman P, Goldberg D, Hickman M. HCV treatment as prevention in prison: key issues. Hepatology 2015;61(1):402−3. https://doi.org/10.1002/hep.27194.

[66] Spaulding AC, Chhatwal J, Adee MG, Lawrence RT, Beckwith CG, von Oehsen W. Funding hepatitis C treatment in correctional facilities by using a nominal pricing mechanism. J Correct Health Care 2019;25(1):15−24. https://doi.org/10.1177/1078345818805770.

Opioid use disorder and HIV

Gregory M. Lucas, MD, PhD

Professor, Medicine, Johns Hopkins University, Baltimore, MD, United States

Injection drug use is an important HIV risk factor

Transmission among People Who Inject Drugs (PWID) early in the HIV epidemic

Soon after the identification of acquired immune deficiency syndrome (AIDS), it became clear that injection drug use was a major risk factor for the acquisition of human immunodeficiency virus (HIV). Des Jarlais and colleagues tested for HIV antibodies in stored sera from people who inject drugs (PWID) who entered opioid treatment programs in New York City and found that HIV seroprevalence increased from below 10% in 1978 to 50% in 1983, with stabilization thereafter [1]. This observation highlights the rapidity with which HIV was able to spread in an unprepared and underresourced population of PWID. However, the finding that HIV seroprevalence plateaued at 50%—60% contrasted with hepatitis B virus seroprevalence of greater than 80% in studies of PWID, suggesting that HIV was less infectious in this context than hepatitis B virus. Other studies identified HIV nucleic acids in 39%—68% of used syringes recovered by syringe service programs (SSPs) or retrieved from shooting galleries [2,3].

Analyses, using varying methods, estimate that the transmission risk for a single episode of needle sharing from an HIV-positive to an HIV-negative individual is approximately 7 per 1000 exposures, with a range from 6 to 16 per 1000 [2,4—7]. Compared with other transmission risks [7—11], needle sharing is more risky (per episode) than penile-vaginal intercourse or accidental needlesticks, but slightly less risky than unprotected receptive anal intercourse, and much less risky than the transmission risk from mother to child or from a blood transfusion from an HIV-positive source patient (Table 5.1).

Viral load in the source individual is a strong and consistent determinant of HIV transmission across all exposure categories [12—15]. Among PWID, behaviors that increase the risk of HIV acquisition include frequency of sharing, younger age, injecting in shooting galleries [16], concurrent sexual risk factors [17—19], and use of syringes with relatively high dead space [19].

Table 5.1 Comparison of HIV transmission risks associated with different exposure types.

Exposure type (references)	HIV transmission risk per 1000 exposures (estimate range)
Penile-vaginal intercourse [9,10]	1 (0.8, 1.0)
Insertive anal intercourse [7]	2 (0.6, 6.2)
Accidental percutaneous needlestick [6]	2 (0, 24)
Needle sharing during injection drug use [2,4–6]	7 (6, 16)
Receptive anal intercourse [11]	14
Maternal to child transmission [8]	226
Blood transfusion [6]	925 (270, 1000)

The (largely unheralded) success of HIV risk reduction among PWID

According to estimates from the Centers for Disease Control and Prevention (CDC), PWID accounted for over 30,000 new HIV infections annually in the late 1980s, and, briefly, had a higher rate of new infections than men who have sex with men (MSM) [20]. By the early 1990s, HIV incidence rates had fallen sharply for both MSM and PWID, but while MSM-related incidence rebounded and tracked upward through 2006, PWID-related infections continued on a downward course. In 2015, the most recent year for which the CDC has estimates [21], only 2200 HIV infections were attributed to injection drug use, 5.7% of HIV infections that year (another 1200 infections were attributed to men with same sex exposure and injection drug use). In a long-running community-based cohort study of PWID in Baltimore, the HIV incidence declined from 4.6% annually in 1988 to near 0% by 2001 [22], and a similar decline in estimated HIV incidence among PWID in New York City was reported in serial cross-sectional surveys [23]. Compared with the late 1980s peak, HIV infections attributed to injection drug use have declined over 90% nationally, an accomplishment second only to the decline in infections attributed to mother-to-child transmission [24]. Fig. 5.1 shows the numbers of adults and adolescents diagnosed with AIDS by calendar year since 1985. Although AIDS diagnoses are not necessarily an accurate reflection of new infections, this figure underscores the long-term success of reducing HIV disease attributable to injection drug use.

Factors contributing to declining HIV incidence among PWID: 1992–2015

There are several factors that likely contributed to the large decline in HIV incidence among PWID in the United States and most other higher-income countries. The

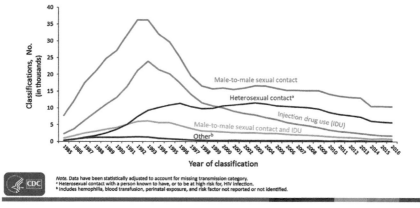

FIGURE 5.1

Stage 3 (AIDS) Classifications among Adults and Adolescents with Diagnosed HIV Infection, by Transmission Category and Year of Classification, 1985—2016. United States and six Dependent Areas. Note. Data have been statistically adjusted to account for missing transmission category. a Heterosexual contact with a person known to have, or to be at high risk for, HIV infection. b Includes hemophilia, blood transfusion, perinatal exposure, and risk factor not reported or not identified.

most important factor was reduction in needle sharing among PWID, aided, where available, by SSPs.

Reduced needle sharing and syringe service programs

Between 1991 and 1994, the estimated number of clean syringes provided in New York City increased fivefold to 1.3 million per year [23]. Among PWID recruited in New York City, receptive needle sharing in the prior 6 months declined from 42% in 1990—91 to 24% in 1996—97. In tandem with reduced injection-related risk, reported use of SSPs and HIV testing approximately doubled over this same time period [25]. Additionally, PWID who were aware of their HIV-positive status when surveyed reported 65% lower odds of unsafe sex with and 37% lower odds of distributive syringe sharing (behaviors that put others at risk), but no difference in receptive needle sharing, compared with other PWID, highlighting the importance of HIV diagnosis in supporting behavioral changes that reduce the risk of onward transmission [25]. In addition to providing access to clean needles/syringes, SSPs provide additional services to this hidden and difficult to reach population, including HIV testing, wound care, and referrals to drug treatment programs.

Although never evaluated in a randomized controlled trial, a wealth of observational data supports the benefits of SSPs in reducing HIV transmission and dispels concerns that providing clean syringes encourages drug use [26—28]. The CDC

[29], the Institute of Medicine [30], and the World Health Organization and other international health organizations [31] strongly endorse SSPs as an essential service for PWID to reduce HIV transmission.

The full potential benefits of SSPs in the United States have not been realized due to inadequate support and implementation. Political support for SSPs has been tepid and grudging at best, and outright hostile at worst. The Netherlands, the United Kingdom, and Australia began implementing robust SSPs in the 1980s when the rapidity of HIV transmission among PWID became clear. At that time in the United States, almost all states had laws criminalizing possession and distribution of drug paraphernalia, which could be invoked against SSPs. In 1988, the federal government instituted a ban on federal funding for SPPs, which has remained in effect since, with the exception of a one-year period in 2009 [32]. Consequently, legislative support and funding for SSPs has been left up to state and local governments, with substantial heterogeneity across states. In a 2014 review of state laws in 36 states with available data, there were 10 states that had not passed laws explicitly authorizing SSPs and provided no public funding for SSPs [32]. In this analysis, the authors found a correlation between an absence of state-level funding for SSPs and unfavorable trends in HIV incidence among PWID in the state. A global systematic review of PWID services conducted in 2010 [33] estimated that only 22 needle/syringes were distributed per PWID per year in the United States, a distribution rate that lagged not only Canada (46 per PWID per year) and Western Europe (59 per PWID per year) but also central Asia (92 per PWID per year), south Asia (37 per PWID per year), and east and southeast Asia (30 per PWID per year). For reference, the WHO has recommended a target distribution rate of at least 200 clean syringes per PWID per year. Revealingly, a 4-year follow-up to this report assessed the six countries with the largest numbers of PWID (China, Malaysia, Russia, Ukraine, Vietnam, and the United States) and found that only two countries had made no progress in expanding coverage of SSP, medication-assisted treatment (MAT), or antiretroviral therapy (ART) to PWID since the original report—Russia and the United States [34]. By virtue of preventing HIV infection and being relatively inexpensive per person served, expansion of SSP in the United States is highly cost-effective [35].

Transitions from injection to noninjection use of heroin

A second factor that contributed to decreased HIV transition among heroin users has been the transition from injection as the primary route of use to intranasal use (sniffing) [36,37]. For example, among treatment seeking individuals with heroin use disorder in New York City, the percentage reporting their primary administration route as intranasal increased from 25% in 1988 to 59% in 1998 [37]. Interestingly, this transition away from heroin injection (and the inherent risk of HIV transmission) was facilitated by increases in the purity of street heroin. The average purity of heroin on the street in New York City increased from less than 10% before 1988 to over

60% by the late 1990s [37]. The co-occurrence of the HIV/AIDS epidemic among PWID and increased heroin purity at the level of street sales (facilitating noninjection routes of use) seems unlikely to be coincidental. One study reported that transitioning from injection to noninjection use of heroin was associated with a lower hepatitis C seroprevalence [38].

Medication-assisted treatment

A third factor in the decades-long decline in injection drug use-related HIV transmission is the availability of effective MAT for opioid use disorder, notably methadone and later buprenorphine. Compared with being out-of-care, MAT is associated with cessation of compulsive opioid use, a two- to threefold decrease in all-cause mortality [39,40], decreased criminal activity, and improved psychosocial functioning (mood disorders, employment, relationships, etc.) [41–43]. There is strong face validity and empiric support for the proposition that MAT reduces HIV incidence [44–46]. An observational study in Philadelphia followed HIV-negative PWID in the late 1980s and early 1990s, the peak of the HIV epidemic among PWID in the United States, and found a 22% HIV incidence rate over 18 months in out-of-treatment PWID compared with a 3.5% incidence rate among those receiving methadone maintenance [46]. One randomized trial, conducted in China and Thailand, aimed to compare the incidence of HIV infection or death among HIV-negative PWID with opioid use disorder randomized to risk reduction counseling combined with either short-term (18 days) or long-term (52 weeks) buprenorphine-based MAT. Although the prevalence of opioid-negative urine drug tests was approximately twice as high in long-term than short-term MAT at 26-week follow-up, the trial was stopped early for futility, because of lower than expected HIV incidence in the study cohort overall [47]. In the United States, methadone maintenance can be provided only by heavily regulated opioid treatment programs that require patient visits multiple days a week, factors that limit rapid expansion of treatment slots.

In October of 2000, the Drug Addiction Treatment Act was passed that allowed qualified physicians, in office practice settings, to prescribe schedule III, IV, and V medications for detoxification or maintenance of patients with opioid use disorder [48]. In 2002, buprenorphine and buprenorphine/naloxone were approved by the US Food and Drug Administration for the treatment of opioid dependence. Over the subsequent years, buprenorphine-based treatment has been increasingly prescribed and provides an important, more flexible alternative to methadone maintenance. The number of physicians qualified to prescribe buprenorphine increased from approximately 5000 in 2004 to 15,662 by 2008 [49]. Yet, despite introduction of buprenorphine, overall MAT availability still remains inadequate in the United States, and substantially lower than in Western Europe [33,50]. Because MAT is associated with improvements in multiple domains, in addition to HIV prevention, it is highly cost-effective [35].

Antiretroviral therapy and "treatment as prevention"

Fourth, "treatment as prevention" may have played some role in declining HIV incidence among PWID. For sexual HIV transmission, strong and consistent data support the premise that effective treatment of HIV-positive individuals greatly reduces the risk of HIV transmission to sex partners [51−54]. In HIV Prevention Trials Network (HPTN) 052, 1763 serodiscordant couples, in which the seropositive partner was ART naïve and had a CD4 count above 350 cells/μL, were randomly assigned to either immediate ART or delayed ART until the CD4 count had declined below 250 cells/μL (which reflected standard care at the time in the countries where conducted). Of 28 genetically linked transmission observed during the trial, 27 occurred in the delayed ART arm and 1 in the immediate ART arm, translating to 96% efficacy [51]. Mathematical models indicate that a strategy of universal annual HIV testing and immediate treatment of infected persons is capable of ending the HIV epidemic in sub-Saharan Africa [55,56]. In contrast to the data for sexual transmission, there are no direct observational or experimental data from PWID showing that viral control with ART in an index HIV-positive person is associated with decreased HIV transmission risk to uninfected injecting partners. The HPTN 074 study explored the feasibility of measuring HIV seroconversion of uninfected injecting partners of HIV-positive index individuals as a primary outcome for a larger prevention trial [57]. However, the overall observed incidence was only approximately 1% among uninfected injecting partners, which the authors concluded was insufficient to support a larger trial. Although direct randomized data are lacking, ecological studies among PWID suggest a link between community viral load and the risk of new HIV infections [58,59].

It is worth noting that the impact of treatment as prevention on observed declines in PWID-associated HIV incidence has likely been modest, at least to date. First, because of very high viral loads during acute HIV infection, HIV-infected persons are most infectious in the months immediately following infection. For example, among MSM, it has been estimated that half of onward transmissions from an index individual occur in the first year of HIV infection [14] and a similar association likely applies to injection-related transmissions. Only a minority of HIV-infected individuals are diagnosed during this period of highest infectivity, which limits the impact of ART in averting transmissions. Additionally, it was not until 2015 when all major HIV treatment guidelines endorsed treating asymptomatic individuals with CD4 counts ≥ 350 cells/μL. Second, as discussed below, since the introduction of effective combination treatment for HIV in the 1990s, HIV-positive PWID have consistently lagged other groups in access to ART and achieving and maintaining viral suppression, which translates to reduced benefit of treatment as prevention.

Preexposure prophylaxis

A fifth consideration for declining HIV incidence among PWID is preexposure prophylaxis (PrEP) with oral antiretroviral drugs, which was shown to reduce HIV incidence by approximately 50% among HIV-negative PWID in Bangkok, Thailand

[60]. However, unlike MSM, where PrEP has made gains in the past 5 years [61,62], meaningful implementation or scale-up of PrEP among PWID has been extremely limited in the United States and elsewhere. For example, in a recent survey of 265 SSP clients and peers in Baltimore, Maryland, only one-quarter of participants was aware of PrEP and only two participants reported taking PrEP [63]. Additionally, modeling studies suggest that implementation of PrEP among PWID in the United States is likely not cost-effective [35,64], due to relatively low HIV incidence among PWID currently and major competing adversities (psychosocial effects of addiction, hepatitis C virus (HCV), bacterial infections, and overdose) that are not addressed by PrEP. In contrast, SSP and MAT are more cost-effective. Consequently, to this point, PrEP has played no appreciable role in the declining HIV incidence among PWID.

The current opioid epidemic threatens decades of decline in PWID-related HIV

The current US opioid epidemic and the associated rise in injection drug use seem poised to reverse the decades-long downward trend in PWID-associated HIV incidence. The dramatic HIV outbreak among PWID in a rural Indiana county in 2015 underscores the rapidity with which HIV can spread among a PWID population that lacks risk reduction services, has high rates of needle and syringe sharing, and is densely networked [65−67]. In fact, the spread of HIV among PWID in the Scott County, Indiana, outbreak was similar to the introduction of HIV among PWID in New York City in the late 1970s [1].

Compared with 2001, the estimated prevalence of persons in the United States reporting past year heroin use has increased over fourfold [68]. The opioid epidemic has been associated with sharp nationwide increases in injection drug use-associated endocarditis [69] and hepatitis C infection [70]. It seems inevitable that increases in injection drug use-related HIV transmission will follow. However, as of this writing, a clear change in course for injection drug use-related HIV transmission has not been observed through the most recent CDC HIV incidence estimates in 2015. However, harbingers of more PWID-related HIV transmission have been noted. For example, compared with the two prior years, the Philadelphia Department of Public Health noted a 48% increase in the number of individuals with newly diagnosed HIV attributed to injection drug use in the year ending August 2018 [71].

The epidemiology of the current opioid crisis is starkly different from the inner-city concentrated heroin epidemics in the second half of the 20th century, in which African Americans were overrepresented. The current epidemic involves larger percentages of white individuals living in suburban or rural areas [68,72,73]. It appears that prescription opioid abuse claimed a foothold in these areas [74], with subsequent transitions to less expensive heroin, further complicated by widespread introduction of synthetic opioids, such as fentanyl, into drug supply chains [75], a major factor in sharply rising rates of opioid overdose mortality [76]. Van Handel and colleagues from the CDC built a model to predict county-level vulnerability to rapid dissemination of HIV or HCV [77]. Strong correlates for increased HCV/HIV transmission risk in a given county included higher prescription opioid sales, higher unemployment, and higher population percentage of white non-Hispanic individuals. The study highlighted 220 counties with risk scores in the top 5% of US counties: almost all were nonurban and highly concentrated in Appalachia, the Midwest, areas of New England, and areas in the Southwest—regions that also have the highest per capita rates of drug overdose deaths [76].

The evolving epidemiology of opioid use disorder outside of major metropolitan areas is likely to further challenge an optimal public health response. After years of confronting the HIV epidemic among PWID, most large cities provide core services for PWID: SSP, MAT, and free testing for HIV and HCV. However, outside of metropolitan areas, such services are sparse to nonexistent. None of these evidence-based services was available in Scott County, Indiana, prior to the HIV outbreak among PWID there. As of March 2014, only 204 SSPs were known to be operating in the United States, and of these, only 29% served suburban or rural areas [78]. In fact, at the time this survey of SSPs was conducted in 2013, there was only a single SSP serving four states that constitute the epicenter of the opioid epidemic: Kentucky, Tennessee, Virginia, and West Virginia [78].

Treatment of HIV-positive people with opioid use disorder or who inject drugs

Stigma, barriers to retention, and limited access to ART

Since the introduction of effective combination therapy, HIV-positive PWID have faced stigma and barriers to HIV treatment [79–82]. Underuse of ART among HIV-positive PWID is likely a function of several factors. First, active drug use is strongly associated with missed clinic visits and lapses in care [83], reducing the opportunity to start ART. Second, a defining feature of addiction is the crowding out of typical concerns by the consuming need to obtain and use drugs. Third, many clinicians held negative views about people who use drugs and the utility of trying to treat them [79]. Fourth, even clinicians who were amenable to treating PWID worried that inconsistent adherence to treatment would rapidly select for drug-resistant strains of HIV that would reduce future treatment options and risk transmission of resistant virus to others [84–87]. In a community-based cohort study of 400 HIV-positive PWID conducted in Baltimore in 1997, half of the participants reported no ART use and only 14% were using combination therapy with a protease inhibitor, the optimal treatment at the time [88]. In a survey of 764 persons attending an urban HIV clinic in 1998 and 1999, 44% of persons who reported active drug use had never used combination ART, compared with 22% of inactive drug users (abstinent >6 months), and 18% of nondrug users [89]. More recent data show that delays in ART initiation persist for PWID compared with other groups [90]. Among HIV-positive patients with opioid use disorder, engagement in MAT with methadone or buprenorphine stabilizes patients, facilitates engagement in care, and likely increases medical providers' comfort in offering ART. In a cohort of PWID followed in Vancouver, Wood and colleagues reported that among 235 HIV-positive participants who had not been treated with ART at baseline, those who were receiving methadone maintenance treatment were twice as likely to initiate ART over 24-month follow-up [91].

Direct biologic effects of opioids on HIV and immune function

There has long been interest in whether opioid use per se has direct effects on the immune system or HIV itself. This question retains relevance today given that the most effective MAT for opioid use disorder is based on long-acting opioid agonists [92] and that opioid prescriptions for chronic pain are more common among HIV-infected persons than in the general population [93]. Researchers have pursued this topic with in vitro studies, animal models, and analyses of human data [94].

In vitro studies are best suited to characterizing mechanisms, but cannot account for complex system effects. Animal models have the potential to account for system effects, but may not reflect human processes accurately. In preclinical studies, opioids have been associated with decreased phagocytic function [95], increased HIV-1 replication in peripheral blood mononuclear cells [96], and abnormal lymphoproliferative index and soluble markers of immune function [97]. One study reported that opioids increased the viral replication rate in a primate model [98]. Conversely, in a study that used a different primate model, long-term opioid dependency was associated with slowed progression of simian immunodeficiency virus and increased survival [99].

Some clinical studies have reported associations that support the hypothesis that opioid use has direct biologic effects that adversely affect HIV natural history. However, clinical studies also face important limitations from confounding by socioeconomic status, psychological stress, adherence with treatment, survival bias, and PWID-associated coinfections (hepatitis C infection, tuberculosis, and bacterial infections). Additionally, opioid abuse is strongly correlated with use of other substances, including tobacco, alcohol, marijuana, and stimulants (all of which have also been proposed to have direct effects on immune function or HIV pathogenesis [100−102]). Consequently, unlike in controlled animal models, substance use by people is heterogenous and affords limited ability to ascribe observed associations to a specific drug or drug class. Despite these caveats, it is notable that several carefully conducted studies in the era prior to the availability of effective ART (which minimizes access to treatment and adherence as potential confounders) cast doubt on a major adverse biologic effect on HIV pathogenesis by opioids. Studies with long-term follow-up of HIV seroconverters found no difference in CD4 count trajectory (in the absence of treatment) in PWID and MSM [103,104]. Similarly, after accounting for sex differences and CD4 cell counts, another study found no difference in viral loads in HIV-positive PWID and MSM [105]. A Dutch study of HIV-infected participants with documented dates of seroconversion found no difference in the time from seroconversion to an AIDS-defining condition in PWID and MSM, after excluding Kaposi's sarcoma (which is much more common in MSM than PWID) and accounting for higher pre-AIDS mortality among PWID compared with MSM [106]. Finally, a Swedish study of persons with documented HIV seroconversion even found that PWID were significantly less likely than MSM to progress to a CD4 count below 200 cells/μL, an AIDS-defining condition, or death from AIDS [107]. These studies suggest that if opioids (or other abused drug classes) have direct adverse effects on immune function or HIV pathogenesis, the effect magnitude is not clinically meaningful.

HIV medication adherence and treatment outcomes

Substance use disorder is a reliable risk factor for poor HIV treatment outcomes. Early in the era of combination ART, an urban cohort study found that injection drug use as an HIV risk factor was the strongest predictor of failure to achieve viral suppression 12 months after initiating ART, with only 27% suppressed compared with 47% of non-PWID [83]. Subsequent research clarified that poorer treatment outcomes among PWID were mediated by nonretention [108,109] and low medication adherence. In a nationally representative cohort collaboration that followed over 60,000 HIV-positive patients between 2000 and 2008, those with injection drug use as an HIV risk factor had 68% higher odds (95% confidence interval: 49%, 89%) of nonretention to HIV care [109]. Wood and colleagues in British Columbia found that viral suppression rates following ART initiation among PWID lagged non-PWID by 20 percentage points. However, this difference disappeared when adjusted for adherence, calculated from medication refill data [110]. Additional studies showed that history of injection drug use was not a monolithic risk factor for poor outcomes with HIV treatment. In fact, PWID who were abstinent or in substance use disorder treatment had HIV treatment outcomes that were indistinguishable from non-PWID [89,111,112]. However, the effect of active drug use was profound. Arnsten and colleagues used electronic pill bottle monitors to quantify ART adherence in 85 current and former drug users, and found that average adherence was only 27% among active users, compared with 68% among former users [113].

A longitudinal study emphasized the cumulative impact of drug use on HIV treatment outcomes. The study—which assessed 10-year restricted mean time in each care continuum stage following enrollment in an HIV clinic—found that PWID spent 17 fewer months on ART and virally suppressed, and lost 8.9 more months of life compared with non-PWID [114]. Engagement in MAT is a mediator of improved treatment outcomes among HIV-positive persons with opioid use disorder [91,115]. A systematic review and metaanalysis found that MAT was associated with a 69% increased odds ART use, twofold increased odds of medication adherence, and 45% increased odds of viral suppression [116].

But what about HIV-positive persons with active opioid use disorder (or another substance use disorder) who are not engaged in MAT? Early in the era of combination ART, active substance use was widely considered a relative contraindication to prescribing ART [87]. However, clinical experience and observational studies show that some individuals with moderate to severe drug or alcohol use disorders do well on ART, although clinicians' ability to predict who will do well was no better than chance [117]. Moreover, a longitudinal study of HIV-positive people who use drugs (including opioids, cocaine, and methamphetamine), followed in seven HIV clinics and four clinical studies, found that abstinence, but also decreased frequency of drug use were both associated with increased likelihood of viral suppression during follow-up [118]. These data suggest that achieving reductions in drug use, even without reaching abstinence, can translate into improved HIV treatment outcomes.

However, even clinicians who were open-minded about treating individuals who were actively using *drugs* worried about the emergence of antiretroviral drug resistance and the loss of future treatment options when a patient might accept substance use disorder treatment and be more prepared to commit to HIV treatment. In this regard, the arrival of ritonavir-boosted protease inhibitor-based regimens—beginning with ritonavir-lopinavir in 2000 and later with ritonavir-boosted atazanavir and darunavir—likely led to greater willingness to prescribe ART for those with untreated substance use disorder. While reasonably well tolerated and easy to take (particularly the later drugs) the key strength of these regimens was the extremely low emergence of resistance mutations with virologic failure due to nonadherence [119,120]. Consequently, and in contrast with nonnucleoside reverse transcriptase regimens that were also first-line treatment during this time, clinicians could offer treatment with boosted protease inhibitor-based regimens with little concern that early nonadherence would burn bridges for future treatment options. Currently, some integrase strand-transfer inhibitors (in particular dolutegravir and bictegravir) appear to have similarly high genetic barriers to resistance as boosted protease inhibitors, while also having a favorable side effect profile, low pill burden, and once daily dosing [121−123].

HIV treatment gaps in PWID have slowly, but not completely, closed

Progress has been made in the past decade in reducing HIV treatment disparities among PWID compared with other risk groups. In a recurring survey of PWID in 20 US cities conducted by the CDC every 3 years, a recent report noted that current ART use among HIV-positive respondents in the survey increased from 58% in 2009 to 67% in 2012 to 71% in 2015 [124]. Similarly, in a cohort study examining trends in the HIV care continuum in a large clinical cohort in Baltimore, Lesko and coworkers reported that differences between PWID and non-PWID in retention to care, receipt of ART, and viral suppression diminished between 2001 and 2012 [125]. For example, in 2001, the estimated viral suppression rates in PWID and non-PWID were 28% and 42%, respectively. However, by 2011 substantial temporal improvements were noted in both groups and the gap between PWID and non-PWID had nearly closed, with viral suppression rates of 69% and 71%, respectively.

Interventions to improve HIV care continuum outcomes among persons with substance use disorders

Strategies to improve treatment outcomes among people with HIV and substance use disorders have been assessed in randomized controlled trials (Table 5.2). Interventions have included patient navigation, integrated (substance use and HIV) care models, incentives, and directly observed therapy (DOT) for HIV. HPTN study 074, which was conducted in Ukraine, Vietnam, and Indonesia, found that an intervention comprising systems navigation and psychosocial counseling significantly increased use of ART, viral suppression, and use of MAT, compared with the control condition [57]. Additionally, cumulative mortality was 53% lower (95% CI; 10%, 78%) in the intervention arm compared with control. In contrast, Metsch and colleagues reported that a 6-month patient navigation intervention that targeted hospitalized persons with HIV and substance use disorder was not associated with improved survival with viral suppression compared with usual care [126].

Cunningham and colleagues reported that a 24-week patient navigation intervention that overlapped with prison discharge was associated with a significantly higher viral suppression rate at 12 months compared with usual care [127]. In a smaller trial, Wohl and colleagues found that a case management intervention targeting prison discharge was not significantly associated with postrelease medical follow-up [128].

One trial compared opioid treatment with HIV clinic-based buprenorphine versus referral to an opioid treatment program in HIV-positive participants with untreated opioid use disorder [129]. Compared with the referred treatment arm, participants assigned to clinic-based buprenorphine were significantly more likely to be engaged and retained in opioid agonist treatment over 12-month follow-up, significantly less likely to have opiate or cocaine positive urine drug tests, and attended significantly more visits with their HIV provider. However, there were no differences in viral load suppression or CD4 cell counts in the two arms.

Treatment incentives (also called contingency management) have also been explored as a way to improve adherence and treatment outcomes through demand generation. Small pilot trials, targeting HIV-positive persons with substance use disorders, reported that treatment incentives produced improvements in electronically monitored medication adherence [130–132]. More recently, a study conducted in Chennai, India, found that voucher incentives were associated with significantly greater linkage to HIV care and initiation of ART among PWID compared with active control, although there were no differences in viral suppression rates in the two arms [133]. A large, multisite trial that enrolled hospitalized HIV-positive persons with substance use disorder found that the combination of patient navigation and multitarget contingency management (contingency management was not evaluated without patient navigation) was associated with a rate of survival with viral

Table 5.2 Randomized controlled trials of interventions to improve outcomes in HIV-positive people who use drugs.

Category First author (reference) Setting	N	Intervention	Control	Key findings
Navigation				
Wohl [128] US, prison discharge	104	Bridging case management 3 months prior to and 6 months after prison release	Standard prison discharge planning	65% in intervention versus 54% in control attended ≥1 postrelease medical appointment (primary; $P = .3$)
Metsch [126] US, hospitalized persons with substance use disorder	530	Up to 11 sessions of motivational interviewing, case management with patient navigator over 6 months	Treatment as usual	No difference in survival with viral suppression at 6 or 12 months (primary)
Miller [57] Ukraine, Vietnam, Indonesia, HIV clinics	502	Systems navigation and counseling to facilitate engagement and retention in HIV care	Standard of care	Participants in intervention significantly more likely to use MAT, use ART, and have suppressed viral load, compared with control
Cunningham [127] US, prison discharge	356	12-session, 24-week navigation intervention in before and after prison release	Standard prison case management	50% in intervention versus 36% in control had viral suppression at 12 months (primary; $P = .03$)
Integrated (co-located care)				
Lucas [129] US, HIV clinic	93	HIV clinic-based buprenorphine for opioid use disorder	Referral to opioid treatment program	Average participation in MAT over 12 months 74% in intervention versus 41% in control (primary; $P < .001$)
Incentives				
Rigsby [130] US, HIV clinic	55	Feedback on electronic adherence data + cash reinforcement	Nondirective inquiries about adherence	Electronically monitored adherence significantly higher in incentive than control arm (primary <0.001)
Javanbakht [131] US, HIV clinic	90	Case management + monetary reinforcement	Standard of care	• The proportion with a 1 log or greater decline in HIV RNA, 55% in intervention versus 28% ($P = .01$). • Increase in CD4 count significantly larger in intervention than control

Continued

Table 5.2 Randomized controlled trials of interventions to improve outcomes in HIV-positive people who use drugs.—*cont'd*

Category First author (reference) Setting	N	Intervention	Control	Key findings
Rosen [132] US, HIV clinic	56	Supportive counseling plus prize bowl drawings for achieving adherence benchmarks	Supportive counseling	Electronically monitored adherence significantly higher in incentive than control arm (primary; $P = .01$)
Sorensen [142] US, HIV clinic	66	Medication coaching every 2 weeks plus cash reinforcement of electronically recorded adherence	Medication coaching every 2 weeks	• Medication adherence 78% in intervention arm versus 56% in control ($P < .001$) • No differences in HIV RNA or CD4 count
Solomon [133] India	120	Vouchers earned for achieving HIV care benchmarks	Opportunity to win vouchers in prize-bowl drawing	• 45% started ART in intervention arm versus 27% in control arm (primary; $P = .04$) • No difference in viral suppression (secondary)
Metsch [126] US, hospitalized persons with substance use disorder	535	Financial incentives for achieving HIV care benchmarks plus patient navigation	Treatment as usual	• No difference in survival with viral suppression at 12 months (primary) • Survival with viral suppression significantly higher at 6 months (secondary) in incentive versus control (46% vs. 35%, $P = .04$)
Directly observed therapy				
Altice [135] US, mobile health van	141	Mobile healthcare van provided DOT 5 days per week	Self-administered ART	71% in intervention achieved viral suppression at 6 months versus 55% in control (primary; $P = .02$)
Macalino [138] US, HIV clinic	87	Outreach worker provided DOT 7 days per week	Self-administered ART	64% in intervention had viral suppression at 3 months versus 41% in control (primary; $P = .05$)
Berg [136] US, methadone clinics	77	DOT provided in conjunction with methadone maintenance	Self-administered ART	Pill-count adherence 86% in intervention versus 56% in control at 24 weeks (primary; $P < .001$)
Lucas [137] US, methadone clinics	107	DOT provided in conjunction with methadone maintenance	Self-administered ART	• Average viral suppression over 12 months 51% in intervention versus 40% in control (primary; $P = .09$) • No difference in electronically measured adherence

ART, antiretroviral therapy; MAT, medication-assisted treatment.

suppression at 6 months that was 11 percentage points higher in the intervention than usual care ($P = .04$). The 6-month time point immediately followed the intervention period and was a secondary endpoint in the trial. However, the benefit was not maintained at 12 months (6 months after the conclusion of the intervention and the primary endpoint for the trial), with survival with viral suppression 39% and 35% in the intervention and control arms, respectively. Finally, although not targeted to people with substance use disorders, a large cluster randomized trial conducted in New York City and Washington DC found that financial incentives were associated with a 3.8 percentage point increase in viral suppression rates of persons on HIV treatment at incentive clinics compared with control clinics ($P = .01$). However, incentives were not associated with increased linkage to care among persons newly diagnosed with HIV [134].

Several small trials have assessed DOT for HIV, analogous to the public health approach to tuberculosis management, with most suggesting a benefit [135−138]. However, unlike tuberculosis, HIV treatment is lifelong for the foreseeable future, which raises the logistical and resource challenges of observing all or most doses for extended periods of time. For this reason, some have proposed that DOT should be an intervention of last resort—restricted to persons with advanced HIV disease and repeated failures of maximally supported self-administered therapy [139,140]. Two trials assessed DOT in the setting of opioid treatment programs as feasible venues to deliver long-term DOT. However, this strategy is limited in rationale and scope as the intervention targets in-treatment rather than out-of-treatment persons with OUD persons (the latter being more in need of services). Additionally, HIV prevalence among persons in opioid treatment programs has declined substantially from the late 1990s and, unlike opioid treatment programs, office-based buprenorphine does not lend itself to observed dosing. However, long-acting injectable ART [141] may offer a new opportunity for DOT approaches for HIV-positive patients with major barriers to long-term adherence to oral ART.

Conclusion

Shortly after identification of AIDS in the early 1980s, it became clear that injection drug use was a major risk factor for acquisition of HIV. Studies conducted on stored sera from persons seeking treatment for opioid use disorder in New York City in the late 1970s and early 1980s showed that HIV seroprevalence increased from less than 10% to 50% in 5 years. However, since the early 1990s, the number of people acquiring HIV from injection drug use steadily declined over the ensuing 25 years, with a cumulative 90% decrease in PWID-related HIV. Large reductions in needle sharing were supported by SSPs in most large cities and effective MAT for opioid use disorder was associated with greatly reduced risks for HIV infection and mortality. However, despite the success of SSPs and MAT, these important interventions are perennially maligned, underappreciated, and underfunded. Opioid and other substance use disorders have historically been associated with large disparities in HIV treatment outcome compared with nonusers. However, data increasingly show that gaps in access to HIV treatment and treatment outcomes among PWID in the United States have closed since the early 2000s. The current opioid crisis has led to a four-fold increase nationally in the number of people reporting past year heroin use. Importantly, the opioid crisis has disproportionately affected non-Hispanic white persons living in suburban and rural communities, areas where risk reduction services are scant. This opioid crisis has already exacted an enormous toll in overdose mortality and threatens to reverse the decades-long success in reducing HIV infections attributed to injection drug use in the United States.

References

[1] Des Jarlais DC, Friedman SR, Novick DM, Sotheran JL, Thomas P, Yancovitz SR, et al. HIV-1 infection among intravenous drug users in Manhattan, New York City, from 1977 through 1987. J Am Med Assoc 1989;261(7):1008–12.

[2] Kaplan EH, Heimer R. A model-based estimate of HIV infectivity via needle sharing. J Acquir Immune Defic Syndr 1992;5(11):1116–8.

[3] Shapshak P, Fujimura RK, Page JB, Segal D, Rivers JE, Yang J, et al. HIV-1 RNA load in needles/syringes from shooting galleries in Miami: a preliminary laboratory report. Drug Alcohol Depend 2000;58(1–2):153–7.

[4] Hudgens MG, Longini Jr IM, Halloran ME, Choopanya K, Vanichseni S, Kitayaporn D, et al. Estimating the transmission probability of human immunodeficiency virus in injecting drug users in Thailand. J Roy Stat Soc C Appl Stat 2001; 50(1):1–14.

[5] Hudgens MG, Longini Jr IM, Vanichseni S, Hu DJ, Kitayaporn D, Mock PA, et al. Subtype-specific transmission probabilities for human immunodeficiency virus type 1 among injecting drug users in Bangkok, Thailand. Am J Epidemiol 2002;155(2): 159–68.

[6] Baggaley RF, Boily MC, White RG, Alary M. Risk of HIV-1 transmission for parenteral exposure and blood transfusion: a systematic review and meta-analysis. AIDS 2006;20(6):805–12.

[7] Patel P, Borkowf CB, Brooks JT, Lasry A, Lansky A, Mermin J. Estimating per-act HIV transmission risk: a systematic review. AIDS 2014;28(10):1509–19.

[8] Sperling RS, Shapiro DE, Coombs RW, Todd JA, Herman SA, McSherry GD, et al. Maternal viral load, zidovudine treatment, and the risk of transmission of human immunodeficiency virus type 1 from mother to infant. Pediatric AIDS Clinical Trials Group Protocol 076 Study Group. N Engl J Med 1996;335(22):1621–9.

[9] Gray RH, Wawer MJ, Brookmeyer R, Sewankambo NK, Serwadda D, Wabwire-Mangen F, et al. Probability of HIV-1 transmission per coital act in monogamous, heterosexual, HIV-1-discordant couples in Rakai, Uganda. Lancet 2001;357(9263): 1149–53.

[10] Boily M-C, Baggaley RF, Wang L, Masse B, White RG, Hayes RJ, et al. Heterosexual risk of HIV-1 infection per sexual act: systematic review and meta-analysis of observational studies. Lancet Infect Dis 2009;9(2):118–29.

[11] Baggaley RF, White RG, Boily MC. HIV transmission risk through anal intercourse: systematic review, meta-analysis and implications for HIV prevention. Int J Epidemiol 2010;39(4):1048–63.

[12] Quinn TC, Wawer MJ, Sewankambo N, Serwadda D, Li C, Wabwire-Mangen F, et al. Viral load and heterosexual transmission of human immunodeficiency virus type 1. Rakai Project Study Group. N Engl J Med 2000;342(13):921−9.

[13] Wawer MJ, Gray RH, Sewankambo NK, Serwadda D, Li X, Laeyendecker O, et al. Rates of HIV-1 transmission per coital act, by stage of HIV-1 infection, in Rakai, Uganda. J Infect Dis 2005;191(9):1403−9.

[14] Volz EM, Ionides E, Romero-Severson EO, Brandt MG, Mokotoff E, Koopman JS. HIV-1 transmission during early infection in men who have sex with men: aphylodynamic analysis. PLoS Med 2013;10(12):e1001568.

[15] Hollingsworth TD, Anderson RM, Fraser C. HIV-1 transmission, by stage of infection. J Infect Dis 2008;198(5):687−93.

[16] Vlahov D, Munoz A, Anthony JC, Cohn S, Celentano DD, Nelson KE. Association of drug injection patterns with antibody to human-immunodeficiency-virus type-1 among intravenous-drug-users in Baltimore, Maryland. Am J Epidemiol 1990;132(5):847−56.

[17] Solomon L, Astemborski J, Warren D, Munoz A, Cohn S, Vlahov D, et al. Differences in risk factors for human immunodeficiency virus type 1 seroconversion among male and female intravenous drug users. Am J Epidemiol 1993;137(8):892−8.

[18] Astemborski J, Vlahov D, Warren D, Solomon L, Nelson KE. The trading of sex for drugs or money and HIV seropositivity among female intravenous drug users. Am J Publ Health 1994;84(3):382−7.

[19] Zule WA, Bobashev G. High dead-space syringes and the risk of HIV and HCV infection among injecting drug users. Drug Alcohol Depend 2009;100(3):204−13.

[20] Hall HI, Song R, Rhodes P, Prejean J, An Q, Lee LM, et al. Estimation of HIV incidence in the United States. J Am Med Assoc 2008;300(5):520−9.

[21] Centers for Disease Control and Prevention. Estimated HIV incidence and prevalence in the United States, 2010−2015. HIV Surveillance Rep 2018;23(1). Available at: https://www.cdc.gov/hiv/library/reports/hiv-surveillance.html.

[22] Mehta SH, Galai N, Astemborski J, Celentano DD, Strathdee SA, Vlahov D, et al. HIV incidence among injection drug users in Baltimore, Maryland (1988−2004). J Acquir Immune Defic Syndr 2006;43(3):368−72.

[23] Des Jarlais DC, Perlis T, Arasteh K, Torian LV, Beatrice S, Milliken J, et al. HIV incidence among injection drug users in New York City, 1990 to 2002: use of serologic test algorithm to assess expansion of HIV prevention services. Am J Publ Health 2005;95(8):1439−44.

[24] Mofenson LM. Protecting the next generation−eliminating perinatal HIV-1 infection. N Engl J Med 2010;362(24):2316−8.

[25] Des Jarlais C, Perlis T, Friedman SR, Chapman T, Kwok J, Rockwell R, et al. Behavioral risk reduction in a declining HIV epidemic: injection drug users in New York City, 1990−1997. Am J Publ Health 2000;90(7):1112−6.

[26] Wodak A, Cooney A. Do needle syringe programs reduce HIV infection among injecting drug users: a comprehensive review of the international evidence. Subst Use Misuse 2006;41(6−7):777−813.

[27] Aspinall EJ, Nambiar D, Goldberg DJ, Hickman M, Weir A, Van Velzen E, et al. Are needle and syringe programmes associated with a reduction in HIV transmission among people who inject drugs: a systematic review and meta-analysis. Int J Epidemiol 2014;43(1):235−48.

[28] Degenhardt L, Mathers B, Vickerman P, Rhodes T, Latkin C, Hickman M. Prevention of HIV infection for people who inject drugs: why individual, structural, and combination approaches are needed. Lancet 2010;376(9737):285—301.

[29] Lurie P, Reingold A, Bowser B, Chen D, Foley J, Guydish J, et al. The public health impact of needle exchange programs in the United States and abroad: summary, conclusions and recommendations. 1993.

[30] Council NR. Proceedings—Workshop on needle exchange and bleach distribution programs. National Academies Press; 1994.

[31] WHO, UNODC, UNAIDS technical guide for countries to set targets for universal access to HIV prevention, treatment and care for injecting drug users — 2012 revision. Available at:http://wwwwhoint/hiv/pub/idu/targets_universal_access/en/.

[32] Bramson H, Des Jarlais DC, Arasteh K, Nugent A, Guardino V, Feelemyer J, et al. State laws, syringe exchange, and HIV among persons who inject drugs in the United States: history and effectiveness. J Publ Health Pol 2015;36(2):212—30.

[33] Mathers BM, Degenhardt L, Ali H, Wiessing L, Hickman M, Mattick RP, et al. HIV prevention, treatment, and care services for people who inject drugs: a systematic review of global, regional, and national coverage. Lancet 2010;375(9719):1014—28.

[34] Degenhardt L, Mathers BM, Wirtz AL, Wolfe D, Kamarulzaman A, Carrieri MP, et al. What has been achieved in HIV prevention, treatment and care for people who inject drugs, 2010—2012? A review of the six highest burden countries. Int J Drug Pol 2014; 25(1):53—60.

[35] Bernard CL, Owens DK, Goldhaber-Fiebert JD, Brandeau ML. Estimation of the cost-effectiveness of HIV prevention portfolios for people who inject drugs in the United States: a model-based analysis. PLoS Med 2017;14(5):e1002312.

[36] Schottenfeld RS, Omalley S, Abdulsalaam K, Oconnor PG. Decline in intravenous drug-use among treatment-seeking opiate users. J Subst Abuse Treat 1993;10(1): 5—10.

[37] Frank B. An overview of heroin trends in New York city: past, present and future. Mt Sinai J Med 2000;67(5—6):340—6.

[38] Des Jarlais DC, McKnight C, Arasteh K, Feelemyer J, Perlman DC, Hagan H, et al. Transitions from injecting to non-injecting drug use: potential protection against HCV infection. J Subst Abuse Treat 2014;46(3):325—31.

[39] Sordo L, Barrio G, Bravo MJ, Indave BI, Degenhardt L, Wiessing L, et al. Mortality risk during and after opioid substitution treatment: systematic review and meta-analysis of cohort studies. BMJ 2017;357:j1550.

[40] Degenhardt L, Bucello C, Mathers B, Briegleb C, Ali H, Hickman M, et al. Mortality among regular or dependent users of heroin and other opioids: a systematic review and meta-analysis of cohort studies. Addiction 2011;106(1):32—51.

[41] Effective medical treatment of opiate addiction. National consensus development panel on effective medical treatment of opiate addiction. J Am Med Assoc 1998; 280(22):1936—43.

[42] Joseph H, Stancliff S, Langrod J. Methadone maintenance treatment (MMT): a review of historical and clinical issues. Mt Sinai J Med 2000;67(5—6):347—64.

[43] Dole VP, Joseph H. Long-term outcome of patients treated with methadone maintenance. Ann N Y Acad Sci 1978;311:181—9.

[44] MacArthur GJ, van Velzen E, Palmateer N, Kimber J, Pharris A, Hope V, et al. Interventions to prevent HIV and Hepatitis C in people who inject drugs: a review of reviews to assess evidence of effectiveness. Int J Drug Pol 2014;25(1):34—52.

[45] Ahamad K, Hayashi K, Nguyen P, Dobrer S, Kerr T, Schutz CG, et al. Effect of low-threshold methadone maintenance therapy for people who inject drugs on HIV incidence in Vancouver, BC, Canada: an observational cohort study. Lancet HIV 2015; 2(10):e445−50.

[46] Metzger DS, Woody GE, Mclellan AT, Obrien CP, Druley P, Navaline H, et al. Human-immunodeficiency-virus seroconversion among intravenous-drug-users in-of-treatment and out-of-treatment − an 18-month prospective follow-up. J Acquir Immune Defic Syndr 1993;6(9):1049−56.

[47] Metzger DS, Donnell D, Celentano DD, Jackson JB, Shao Y, Aramrattana A, et al. Expanding substance use treatment options for HIV prevention with buprenorphine-naloxone: HIV Prevention Trials Network 058. J Acquir Immune Defic Syndr 2015; 68(5):554−61.

[48] Fiellin DA, O'Connor PG. New federal initiatives to enhance the medical treatment of opioid dependence. Ann Intern Med 2002;137(8):688−92.

[49] Arfken CL, Johanson C-E, di Menza S, Schuster CRJJ. Expanding treatment capacity for opioid dependence with office-based treatment with buprenorphine: national surveys of physicians 2010;39(2):96−104.

[50] Volkow ND, Frieden TR, Hyde PS, Cha SS. Medication-assisted therapies−tackling the opioid-overdose epidemic. N Engl J Med 2014;370(22):2063−6.

[51] Cohen MS, Chen YQ, McCauley M, Gamble T, Hosseinipour MC, Kumarasamy N, et al. Prevention of HIV-1 infection with early antiretroviral therapy. N Engl J Med 2011;365(6):493−505.

[52] Cohen MS, Chen YQ, McCauley M, Gamble T, Hosseinipour MC, Kumarasamy N, et al. Antiretroviral therapy for the prevention of HIV-1 transmission. N Engl J Med 2016;375(9):830−9.

[53] Rodger AJ, Cambiano V, Bruun T, Vernazza P, Collins S, van Lunzen J, et al. Sexual activity without condoms and risk of HIV transmission in serodifferent couples when the HIV-positive partner is using suppressive antiretroviral therapy. J Am Med Assoc 2016;316(2):171−81.

[54] Smith K, Powers KA, Kashuba AD, Cohen MS. HIV-1 treatment as prevention: the good, the bad, and the challenges. Curr Opin HIV AIDS 2011;6(4):315.

[55] Granich RM, Gilks CF, Dye C, De Cock KM, Williams BG. Universal voluntary HIV testing with immediate antiretroviral therapy as a strategy for elimination of HIV transmission: a mathematical model. Lancet 2009;373(9657):48−57.

[56] Hontelez JA, Lurie MN, Barnighausen T, Bakker R, Baltussen R, Tanser F, et al. Elimination of HIV in South Africa through expanded access to antiretroviral therapy: a model comparison study. PLoS Med 2013;10(10):e1001534.

[57] Miller WC, Hoffman IF, Hanscom BS, Ha TV, Dumchev K, Djoerban Z, et al. A scalable, integrated intervention to engage people who inject drugs in HIV care and medication-assisted treatment (HPTN 074): a randomised, controlled phase 3 feasibility and efficacy study. Lancet 2018;392(10149):747−59.

[58] Wood E, Kerr T, Marshall BD, Li K, Zhang R, Hogg RS, et al. Longitudinal community plasma HIV-1 RNA concentrations and incidence of HIV-1 among injecting drug users: prospective cohort study. BMJ 2009;338:b1649.

[59] Solomon SS, Mehta SH, McFall AM, Srikrishnan AK, Saravanan S, Laeyendecker O, et al. Community viral load, antiretroviral therapy coverage, and HIV incidence in India: a cross-sectional, comparative study. Lancet HIV 2016;3(4):e183−90.

[60] Choopanya K, Martin M, Suntharasamai P, Sangkum U, Mock PA, Leethochawalit M, et al. Antiretroviral prophylaxis for HIV infection in injecting drug users in Bangkok, Thailand (the Bangkok Tenofovir Study): a randomised, double-blind, placebo-controlled phase 3 trial. Lancet 2013;381(9883):2083—90.

[61] McCormack S, Dunn DT, Desai M, Dolling DI, Gafos M, Gilson R, et al. Pre-exposure prophylaxis to prevent the acquisition of HIV-1 infection (PROUD): effectiveness results from the pilot phase of a pragmatic open-label randomised trial. Lancet 2016; 387(10013):53—60.

[62] Siegler AJ, Mouhanna F, Giler RM, Weiss K, Pembleton E, Guest J, et al. The prevalence of pre-exposure prophylaxis use and the pre-exposure prophylaxis-to-need ratio in the fourth quarter of 2017, United States. Ann Epidemiol 2018;28(12):841—9.

[63] Sherman SG, Schneider KE, Nyeong Park J, Allen ST, Hunt D, Chaulk CP, et al. PrEP awareness, eligibility, and interest among people who inject drugs in Baltimore, Maryland. Drug Alcohol Depend 2018;195:148—55.

[64] Bernard CL, Brandeau ML, Humphreys K, Bendavid E, Holodniy M, Weyant C, et al. Cost-effectiveness of HIV preexposure prophylaxis for people who inject drugs in the United States. Ann Intern Med 2016;165(1):10—9. PMID:27110953.

[65] Peters PJ, Pontones P, Hoover KW, Patel MR, Galang RR, Shields J, et al. HIV infection linked to injection use of oxymorphone in Indiana, 2014—2015. N Engl J Med 2016;375(3):229—39.

[66] Campbell EM, Jia H, Shankar A, Hanson D, Luo W, Masciotra S, et al. Detailed transmission network analysis of a large opiate-driven outbreak of HIV infection in the United States. J Infect Dis 2017;216(9):1053—62.

[67] Broz D, Zibbell J, Foote C, Roseberry JC, Patel MR, Conrad C, et al. Multiple injections per injection episode: high-risk injection practice among people who injected pills during the 2015 HIV outbreak in Indiana. Int J Drug Pol 2018;52:97—101.

[68] Martins SS, Sarvet A, Santaella-Tenorio J, Saha T, Grant BF, Hasin DS. Changes in US lifetime heroin use and heroin use disorder: prevalence from the 2001—2002 to 2012—2013 national epidemiologic survey on alcohol and related conditions. JAMA Psychiatr 2017;74(5):445—55.

[69] Njoroge LW, Al-Kindi SG, Koromia GA, ElAmm CA, Oliveira GH. Changes in the association of rising infective endocarditis with mortality in people who inject drugs. JAMA Cardiol 2018;3(8):779—80.

[70] Zibbell JE, Asher AK, Patel RC, Kupronis B, Iqbal K, Ward JW, et al. Increases in acute hepatitis C virus infection related to a growing opioid epidemic and associated injection drug use, United States, 2004 to 2014. Am J Publ Health 2018;108(2):175—81.

[71] Philadelphia Department of Public Health. HIV spread among people who inject drugs. Chart 2018;3(4). Available at:https://www.phila.gov/departments/department-of-public-health/data/chart/.

[72] Cicero TJ, Ellis MS, Surratt HL, Kurtz SP. The changing face of heroin use in the United States: a retrospective analysis of the past 50 years. JAMA Psychiatr 2014; 71(7):821—6.

[73] Jalal H, Buchanich JM, Roberts MS, Balmert LC, Zhang K, Burke DS. Changing dynamics of the drug overdose epidemic in the United States from 1979 through 2016. Science 2018;361(6408).

[74] Saha TD, Kerridge BT, Goldstein RB, Chou SP, Zhang H, Jung J, et al. Nonmedical prescription opioid use and DSM-5 nonmedical prescription opioid use disorder in the United States. J Clin Psychiatr 2016;77(6):772—80.

[75] Gladden RM, Martinez P, Seth P. Fentanyl law enforcement submissions and increases in synthetic opioid-involved overdose deaths — 27 states, 2013—2014. Morb Mortal Wkly Rep 2016;65(33):837—43.

[76] Centers for Disease Control and Prevention. 2018 Annual surveillance report of drug-related risks and outcomes — United States Surveillance Special Report. Centers for Disease Control and Prevention, U.S. Department of Health and Human Services; August 31, 2018. Available from: https://www.cdc.gov/drugoverdose/pdf/pubs/2018-cdc-drug-surveillance-report.pdf.

[77] Van Handel MM, Rose CE, Hallisey EJ, Kolling JL, Zibbell JE, Lewis B, et al. County-level vulnerability assessment for rapid dissemination of HIV or HCV infections among persons who inject drugs, United States. J Acquir Immune Defic Syndr 2016;73(3):323—31.

[78] Des Jarlais DC, Nugent A, Solberg A, Feelemyer J, Mermin J, Holtzman D. Syringe service programs for persons who inject drugs in urban, suburban, and rural areas — United States, 2013. Morb Mortal Wkly Rep 2015;64(48):1337—41.

[79] Gerbert B, Maguire BT, Bleecker T, Coates TJ, McPhee SJ. Primary care physicians and AIDS. Attitudinal and structural barriers to care. J Am Med Assoc 1991;266(20):2837—42.

[80] Altice FL, Mostashari F, Friedland GH. Trust and the acceptance of and adherence to antiretroviral therapy. J Acquir Immune Defic Syndr 2001;28(1):47—58.

[81] O'Connor PG, Selwyn PA, Schottenfeld RS. Medical care for injection-drug users with human immunodeficiency virus infection. N Engl J Med 1994;331(7):450—9.

[82] Fairfield KM, Libman H, Davis RB, Eisenberg DM. Delays in protease inhibitor use in clinical practice. J Gen Intern Med 1999;14(7):395—401.

[83] Lucas GM, Chaisson RE, Moore RD. Highly active antiretroviral therapy in a large urban clinic: risk factors for virologic failure and adverse drug reactions. Ann Intern Med 1999;131(2):81—7.

[84] Bassetti S, Battegay M, Furrer H, Rickenbach M, Flepp M, Kaiser L, et al. Why is highly active antiretroviral therapy (HAART) not prescribed or discontinued? Swiss HIV Cohort Study. J Acquir Immune Defic Syndr Hum Retrovirol 1999;21(2):114—9.

[85] Wood E, Hogg RS, Yip B, Dong WW, Wynhoven B, Mo T, et al. Rates of antiretroviral resistance among HIV-infected patients with and without a history of injection drug use. AIDS 2005;19(11):1189—95.

[86] Sherer R. Adherence and antiretroviral therapy in injection drug users. J Am Med Assoc 1998;280(6):567—8.

[87] Bangsberg DR, Moss A. When should we delay highly active antiretroviral therapy? J Gen Intern Med 1999;14(7):446—8.

[88] Celentano DD, Vlahov D, Cohn S, Shadle VM, Obasanjo O, Moore RD. Self-reported antiretroviral therapy in injection drug users. J Am Med Assoc 1998;280(6):544—6.

[89] Lucas GM, Cheever LW, Chaisson RE, Moore RD. Detrimental effects of continued illicit drug use on the treatment of HIV-1 infection. J Acquir Immune Defic Syndr 2001;27(3):251—9.

[90] Hanna DB, Buchacz K, Gebo KA, Hessol NA, Horberg MA, Jacobson LP, et al. Trends and disparities in antiretroviral therapy initiation and virologic suppression among newly treatment-eligible HIV-infected individuals in North America, 2001—2009. Clin Infect Dis 2013;56(8):1174—82.

[91] Wood E, Hogg RS, Kerr T, Palepu A, Zhang R, Montaner JS. Impact of accessing methadone on the time to initiating HIV treatment among antiretroviral-naive HIV-infected injection drug users. AIDS 2005;19(8):837—9.

[92] Reece AS. Epidemiologic and molecular pathophysiology of chronic opioid dependence and the place of naltrexone extended-release formulations in its clinical management. Subst Abuse 2012;6:115−33.

[93] Silverberg MJ, Ray GT, Saunders K, Rutter CM, Campbell CI, Merrill JO, et al. Prescription long-term opioid use in HIV-infected patients. Clin J Pain 2012;28(1):39−46.

[94] Kapadia F, Vlahov D, Donahoe RM, Friedland G. The role of substance abuse in HIV disease progression: reconciling differences from laboratory and epidemiologic investigations. Clin Infect Dis 2005;41(7):1027−34.

[95] Peterson PK, Sharp B, Gekker G, Brummitt C, Keane WF. Opioid-mediated suppression of cultured peripheral blood mononuclear cell respiratory burst activity. J Immunol 1987;138(11):3907−12.

[96] Peterson PK, Sharp BM, Gekker G, Portoghese PS, Sannerud K, Balfour Jr HH. Morphine promotes the growth of HIV-1 in human peripheral blood mononuclear cell cocultures. AIDS 1990;4(9):869−73.

[97] Sacerdote P, Franchi S, Gerra G, Leccese V, Panerai AE, Somaini L. Buprenorphine and methadone maintenance treatment of heroin addicts preserves immune function. Brain Behav Immun 2008;22(4):606−13.

[98] Chuang RY, Suzuki S, Chuang TK, Miyagi T, Chuang LF, Doi RH. Opioids and the progression of simian AIDS. Front Biosci 2005;10:1666−77.

[99] Donahoe RM, O'Neil SP, Marsteller FA, Novembre FJ, Anderson DC, Lankford-Turner P, et al. Probable deceleration of progression of Simian AIDS affected by opiate dependency: studies with a rhesus macaque/SIVsmm9 model. J Acquir Immune Defic Syndr 2009;50(3):241−9.

[100] Baum MK, Rafie C, Lai S, Sales S, Page B, Campa A. Crack-cocaine use accelerates HIV disease progression in a cohort of HIV-positive drug users. J Acquir Immune Defic Syndr 2009;50(1):93−9.

[101] Baldwin GC, Roth MD, Tashkin DP. Acute and chronic effects of cocaine on the immune system and the possible link to AIDS. J Neuroimmunol 1998;83(1−2):133−8.

[102] Haorah J, Heilman D, Diekmann C, Osna N, Donohue Jr TM, Ghorpade A, et al. Alcohol and HIV decrease proteasome and immunoproteasome function in macrophages: implications for impaired immune function during disease. Cell Immunol 2004;229(2):139−48.

[103] Margolick JB, Munoz A, Vlahov D, Solomon L, Astemborski J, Cohn S, et al. Changes in T-lymphocyte subsets in intravenous drug users with HIV-1 infection. J Am Med Assoc 1992;267(12):1631−6.

[104] Galai N, Vlahov D, Margolick JB, Chen K, Graham NM, Munoz A. Changes in markers of disease progression in HIV-1 seroconverters: a comparison between cohorts of injecting drug users and homosexual men. J Acquir Immune Defic Syndr Hum Retrovirol 1995;8(1):66−74.

[105] Lyles CM, Vlahov D, Farzadegan H, Astemborski J, Margolick JB, Masters BA, et al. Comparison of two measures of human immunodeficiency virus (HIV) type 1 load in HIV risk groups. J Clin Microbiol 1998;36(12):3647−52.

[106] Spijkerman IJ, Langendam MW, Veugelers PJ, van Ameijden EJ, Keet IP, Geskus RB, et al. Differences in progression to AIDS between injection drug users and homosexual men with documented dates of seroconversion. Epidemiology 1996;7(6):571−7.

[107] Pehrson P, Lindback S, Lidman C, Gaines H, Giesecke J. Longer survival after HIV infection for injecting drug users than for homosexual men: implications for immunology. AIDS 1997;11(8):1007−12.

[108] Giordano TP, Gifford AL, White Jr AC, Suarez-Almazor ME, Rabeneck L, Hartman C, et al. Retention in care: a challenge to survival with HIV infection. Clin Infect Dis 2007;44(11):1493—9.

[109] Rebeiro P, Althoff KN, Buchacz K, Gill J, Horberg M, Krentz H, et al. Retention among North American HIV-infected persons in clinical care, 2000—2008. J Acquir Immune Defic Syndr 2013;62(3):356—62.

[110] Wood E, Montaner JS, Yip B, Tyndall MW, Schechter MT, O'Shaughnessy MV, et al. Adherence and plasma HIV RNA responses to highly active antiretroviral therapy among HIV-1 infected injection drug users. Can Med Assoc J 2003;169(7): 656—61.

[111] Lucas GM, Gebo KA, Chaisson RE, Moore RD. Longitudinal assessment of the effects of drug and alcohol abuse on HIV-1 treatment outcomes in an urban clinic. AIDS 2002;16(5):767—74.

[112] Lucas GM, Griswold M, Gebo KA, Keruly J, Chaisson RE, Moore RD. Illicit drug use and HIV-1 disease progression: a longitudinal study in the era of highly active antiretroviral therapy. Am J Epidemiol 2006;163(5):412—20.

[113] Arnsten JH, Demas PA, Grant RW, Gourevitch MN, Farzodegan H, Howard AA, et al. Impact of active drug use on antiretroviral therapy adherence and viral suppression in HIV-infected drug users. J Gen Intern Med 2002;17(5):377—81.

[114] Lesko CR, Edwards JK, Moore RD, Lau B. A longitudinal, HIV care continuum: 10-year restricted mean time in each care continuum stage after enrollment in care, by history of IDU. AIDS 2016;30(14):2227—34.

[115] Nosyk B, Min JE, Colley G, Lima VD, Yip B, Milloy MJ, et al. The causal effect of opioid substitution treatment on HAART medication refill adherence. AIDS 2015; 29(8):965—73.

[116] Low AJ, Mburu G, Welton NJ, May MT, Davies CF, French C, et al. Impact of opioid substitution therapy on antiretroviral therapy outcomes: asystematic review and meta-analysis. Clin Infect Dis 2016;63(8):1094—104.

[117] Bangsberg DR, Hecht FM, Clague H, Charlebois ED, Ciccarone D, Chesney M, et al. Provider assessment of adherence to HIV antiretroviral therapy. J Acquir Immune Defic Syndr 2001;26(5):435—42.

[118] Nance RM, Trejo MEP, Whitney BM, Delaney JAC, Altice F, Beckwith CG, et al. Impact of abstinence and of reducing illicit drug use without abstinence on HIV viral load. Clin Infect Dis 2019;70(5):867—74. PMID:30994900.

[119] Daar ES, Tierney C, Fischl MA, Sax PE, Mollan K, Budhathoki C, et al. Atazanavir plus ritonavir or efavirenz as part of a 3-drug regimen for initial treatment of HIV-1. Ann Intern Med 2011;154(7):445—56.

[120] Walmsley S, Bernstein B, King M, Arribas J, Beall G, Ruane P, et al. Lopinavir-ritonavir versus nelfinavir for the initial treatment of HIV infection. N Engl J Med 2002;346(26):2039—46.

[121] Sax PE, Pozniak A, Montes ML, Koenig E, DeJesus E, Stellbrink HJ, et al. Coformulated bictegravir, emtricitabine, and tenofovir alafenamide versus dolutegravir with emtricitabine and tenofovir alafenamide, for initial treatment of HIV-1 infection (GS-US-380-1490): a randomised, double-blind, multicentre, phase 3, non-inferiority trial. Lancet 2017;390(10107):2073—82.

[122] Walmsley SL, Antela A, Clumeck N, Duiculescu D, Eberhard A, Gutierrez F, et al. Dolutegravir plus abacavir-lamivudine for the treatment of HIV-1 infection. N Engl J Med 2013;369(19):1807—18.

[123] Sax PE, DeJesus E, Crofoot G, Ward D, Benson P, Dretler R, et al. Bictegravir versus dolutegravir, each with emtricitabine and tenofovir alafenamide, for initial treatment of HIV-1 infection: a randomised, double-blind, phase 2 trial. Lancet HIV 2017;4(4):e154—60.

[124] Hoots BE, Finlayson TJ, Broz D, Paz-Bailey G, Group NS. Antiretroviral therapy use among HIV-infected people who inject drugs-20 cities, United States, 2009-—2015. J Acquir Immune Defic Syndr 2017;75(Suppl. 3):S392—6.

[125] Lesko CR, Tong W, Moore RD, Lau B. Retention, antiretroviral therapy use and viral suppression by history of injection drug use among HIV-infected patients in an urban HIV clinical cohort. AIDS Behav 2017;21(4):1016—24.

[126] Metsch LR, Feaster DJ, Gooden L, Matheson T, Stitzer M, Das M, et al. Effect of patient navigation with or without financial incentives on viral suppression among hospitalized patients with HIV infection and substance use: arandomized clinical trial. J Am Med Assoc 2016;316(2):156—70.

[127] Cunningham WE, Weiss RE, Nakazono T, Malek MA, Shoptaw SJ, Ettner SL, et al. Effectiveness of a peer navigation intervention to sustain viral suppression among HIV-positive men and transgender women released from jail: the LINK LA randomized clinical trial. JAMA Intern Med 2018;178(4):542—53.

[128] Wohl DA, Scheyett A, Golin CE, White B, Matuszewski J, Bowling M, et al. Intensive case management before and after prison release is no more effective than comprehensive pre-release discharge planning in linking HIV-infected prisoners to care: a randomized trial. AIDS Behav 2011;15(2):356—64.

[129] Lucas GM, Chaudhry A, Hsu J, Woodson T, Lau B, Olsen Y, et al. Clinic-based treatment of opioid-dependent HIV-infected patients versus referral to an opioid treatment program: a randomized trial. Ann Intern Med 2010;152(11):704—11.

[130] Rigsby MO, Rosen MI, Beauvais JE, Cramer JA, Rainey PM, O'Malley SS, et al. Cue-dose training with monetary reinforcement: pilot study of an antiretroviral adherence intervention. J Gen Intern Med 2000;15(12):841—7.

[131] Javanbakht M, Prosser P, Grimes T, Weinstein M, Farthing C. Efficacy of an individualized adherence support program with contingent reinforcement among nonadherent HIV-positive patients: results from a randomized trial. J Int Assoc Phys AIDS Care 2006;5(4):143—50.

[132] Rosen MI, Dieckhaus K, McMahon TJ, Valdes B, Petry NM, Cramer J, et al. Improved adherence with contingency management. AIDS Patient Care STDS 2007;21(1):30—40.

[133] Solomon SS, Srikrishnan AK, Vasudevan CK, Anand S, Kumar MS, Balakrishnan P, et al. Voucher incentives improve linkage to and retention in care among HIV-infected drug users in Chennai, India. Clin Infect Dis 2014;59(4):589—95.

[134] El-Sadr WM, Donnell D, Beauchamp G, Hall HI, Torian LV, Zingman B, et al. Financial incentives for linkage to care and viral suppression among HIV-positive patients: arandomized clinical trial (HPTN 065). JAMA Intern Med 2017;177(8):1083—92. PMID:28628702.

[135] Altice FL, Maru DSR, Bruce RD, Springer SA, Friedland GH. Superiority of directly administered antiretroviral therapy over self-administered therapy among HIV-infected drug users: a prospective, randomized, controlled trial. Clin Infect Dis 2007;45(6):770—8.

[136] Berg KM, Litwin A, Li X, Heo M, Arnsten JH. Directly observed antiretroviral therapy improves adherence and viral load in drug users attending methadone maintenance clinics: a randomized controlled trial. Drug Alcohol Depend 2011;113(2—3):192—9.

[137] Lucas GM, Mullen BA, Galai N, Moore RD, Cook K, McCaul ME, et al. Directly administered antiretroviral therapy for HIV-infected individuals in opioid treatment programs: results from a randomized clinical trial. PloS One 2013;8(7):e68286.

[138] Macalino GE, Hogan JW, Mitty JA, Bazerman LB, DeLong AK, Loewenthal H, et al. A randomized clinical trial of community-based directly observed therapy as an adherence intervention for HAART among substance users. AIDS 2007;21(11):1473—7.

[139] Lucas GM, Flexner CW, Moore RD. Directly administered antiretroviral therapy in the treatment of HIV infection: benefit or burden? AIDS Patient Care STDS 2002;16(11): 527—35.

[140] Liechty CA, Bangsberg DR. Doubts about DOT: antiretroviral therapy for resource-poor countries. AIDS 2003;17(9):1383—7.

[141] Margolis DA, Gonzalez-Garcia J, Stellbrink HJ, Eron JJ, Yazdanpanah Y, Podzamczer D, et al. Long-acting intramuscular cabotegravir and rilpivirine in adults with HIV-1 infection (LATTE-2): 96-week results of a randomised, open-label, phase 2b, non-inferiority trial. Lancet 2017;390(10101):1499—510.

[142] Sorensen JL, Haug NA, Delucchi KL, Gruber V, Kletter E, Batki SL, et al. Voucher reinforcement improves medication adherence in HIV-positive methadone patients: a randomized trial. Drug Alcohol Depend 2007;88(1):54—63.

Opioid use disorder and HCV (hepatitis C virus)

Irene Pericot-Valverde, PhD[3], **Divya Ahuja, MD**[4], **Brianna L. Norton, MD**[5], **Alain H. Litwin, MD MPH**[1,2,3]

[3]*Clemson University, School of Health Research, Clemson, SC, United States;* [4]*Department of Medicine, University of South Carolina School of Medicine, Columbia, SC, United States;* [5]*Division of General Internal Medicine and Infectious Diseases, Bronx, NY, United States;* [1]*Department of Medicine, University of South Carolina School of Medicine, Greenville, SC, United States;* [2]*Department of Medicine, Prisma Health, Greenville, SC, United States*

Introduction

Hepatitis C virus (HCV) has a significant impact on the healthcare system in the United States and the Centers for Disease Control and Prevention (CDC) estimates that the number of deaths associated with HCV has surpassed the combined deaths from 60 other nationally notifiable infectious conditions, including HIV (human immunodeficiency virus) and tuberculosis [1]. The last 5 years however have seen a dramatic change in the HCV treatment paradigm, and with the advent of highly effective direct-acting antivirals (DAA) for HCV, we can for the first time envision the eradication of the HCV epidemic.

The rise in death and overdoses related to opioid prescription drug use observed in the United States led to national efforts on restricting the access to prescription opioids, such as opioid prescription guidelines, dose-limit laws, and prescription monitoring programs [2,3]. While these efforts began to take effect, and prescription opioids become harder to obtain, many people with opioid use disorder began to use and inject illicit heroin [4], a less expensive and accessible substitute for prescription opioids. Coinciding with this national increase in injection drug use (IDU), the number of incident HCV infections has been escalating as IDU represents the most common route of transmission [5]. The HIV and HCV outbreak in 2015 in Scott's county Indiana was a wake-up call for the nation. There were 185 HIV infections and 171 HCV infections in a period of 4 years in a county with a total population of 24,000 [6]. Similar concerning increases in HCV infection have been seen in West Virginia, Kentucky, and Tennessee [7]. HCV is predominantly concentrated in people who inject drugs (PWID), which is defined as people who report injecting an illicit drug at least once in their life. It should be noted that PWID is a broad definition that includes both people who currently inject drugs (e.g., past month, past year) and former PWID who have permanently ceased injecting drugs [8].

Epidemiology

Multiple studies have estimated the prevalence of chronic HCV at or close to 1% among the overall US population [9]. Up until 2005, in the United States, HCV primarily affected the birth cohort between years 1945—1965, also known as the baby boomer generation. This cohort had been identified as the population with the highest prevalence of HCV infection in the United States (3.3%) and was estimated to account for 75% of all HCV infections in the United States [10]. More recently, however, there has been an alarming increase in HCV infection among people in a younger age group and this is largely related to the opioid epidemic that is sweeping the nation [11]. For example, recent state surveillance data from 15 US states have shown equal or higher rates of HCV infection among young adults aged 20—39 years old as compared with baby boomers [12]. On a global scale, estimates of PWID with chronic HCV vary widely, and have relied on rates of HCV antibody positivity, extrapolating that 65%—75% of antibody-positive individuals will be viremic, with chronic HCV. A review in 2011 estimated about 10.0 million PWID may be anti-HCV positive. In the same review, estimates of PWID with hepatitis B infection (HBcAb positive) and chronic hepatitis B (HBsAg positive) were 6.4 million and 1.2 million, respectively [13]. In another systematic review, investigators estimated 6.1 million PWID living with HCV worldwide. There were wide regional variations, with the United States, Russia, Brazil, and China accounting for 51% of all infections [14]. Despite the high rates of HCV among PWID, most PWID have never been offered HCV care or treatment [15].

Natural history of HCV and mortality

Although acute HCV infection is typically asymptomatic, 15%—30% of individuals may develop acute hepatitis within 5—12 weeks of exposure. It is estimated that 65%—75% of persons who get infected with HCV will develop chronic infection, and of the remaining 25%—35% the majority will clear the infection by 6—12 months. Once chronically infected, the rate of progression from cirrhosis is extremely variable and infected individuals may not develop significant sequelae for decades after initial infection [16]. In patients with chronic HCV, serious liver disease such as cirrhosis develops in 20%—30% of patients in the third and fourth decades after initial infection. In a meta-analysis of PWID with chronic HCV, the estimated time to cirrhosis was 34 years [17].

Cirrhosis itself can lead to a wide spectrum of liver disease, but once it ensues, patients with cirrhosis have an approximately 5% annual risk of developing decompensated liver disease, which heralds a poor prognosis, repeat hospitalizations, and in the absence of HCV treatment or a liver transplant, progressive deterioration, and death [18]. In a National Health Institutes-sponsored observational study, 220 patients with HCV-related cirrhosis were followed for approximately 8 years. A primary outcome of death, hepatic decompensation, and hepatocellular carcinoma (HCC) occurred at a rate of 7.5% per year and patients with a Child Turcotte Pugh score of >7 experienced a death rate of 10% per year [19].

Mortality among PWID is significantly higher than that of the general population [20]. Causes of death are often associated with injecting drug use, including fatal overdoses and blood-borne infections. PWID are also at higher risk of dying prematurely than the general population [21,22]. Investigators used data from the Global Burden of Disease 2013 to measure the morbidity and mortality among PWID attributable to HBV, HCV, and HIV, including cirrhosis and HCC. They calculated estimates of burden of disease through years of life lost, years of life lived with disability, deaths, and disability-adjusted life-years (DALYs). Globally, in 2013, more than 10 million DALYs were estimated to be attributable to previous exposure to HIV, HBV, and HCV via IDU [23]. In the United States, HCV causes greater than 18,000 deaths annually [24], and is the leading cause in the United States of both end-stage liver disease and HCC, and is one of the most common indications for liver transplantation [25,26]. Without imminent action, mortality from HCV is projected to triple over the next decade [27,28]; HCV-related deaths have now surpassed deaths from HIV infection [29]. Because mortality in PWID with HCV is 12 times that of the general population, we need innovative interventions to screen, treat, and cure HCV among PWID [29,30].

Screening of HCV among PWID and point-of-care testing

In 2012, the CDC established HCV screening recommendations, including a one-time testing of the birth cohort 1945−1965, as well as other individuals perceived to be at increased risk [10] (Table 6.1).

Table 6.1 Groups that should be tested for hepatitis C virus (HCV).

All persons born from 1945 through 1965
Anyone who has ever injected illegal drugs
Recipients of blood transfusions or solid organ transplants before July 1992, or clotting factor concentrates made before 1987
Patients who have ever received long-term hemodialysis treatment
Persons with known exposures to HCV, such as
• Healthcare workers after needle sticks involving blood from a patient with HCV
• Recipients of blood or organs from a donor who later tested positive for HCV
People living with HIV
People with signs or symptoms of liver disease (e.g., abnormal liver enzyme tests)
Children born to mothers who have HCV

Source: https://www.hcvguidelines.org/unique-populations/pwid.

As a result of the screening recommendations and highly effective treatment regimens for chronic HCV, screening across large healthcare systems has increased [31]. Unfortunately, the proportion of HCV infections occurring outside the designated birth cohort is growing rapidly and at a minimum, annual HCV testing is recommended in PWID. In 2020, CDC developed two new recommendations [32]: (1) HCV screening at least once in a lifetime for all adults aged $\geq$18 years, except in settings where the prevalence of HCV infection is <0.1% and (2) HCV screening for all pregnant women during each pregnancy, except in settings where the prevalence of HCV infection is <0.1%.

The screening algorithm for HCV testing begins with an antibody test, which can be conducted using a rapid antibody test (e.g., OraQuick Rapid Antibody Test) or a laboratory-based assay (e.g., enzyme immunoassay, chemiluminescence immunoassay). This initial test provides a result in terms of reactive or nonreactive. A nonreactive result suggests no evidence of HCV antibody, and, consequently, no further action is required. A reactive result should be taken as evidence of presumptive HCV infection and must be followed by HCV RNA testing. If HCV RNA is not detected, the reactive antibody represents past but cleared HCV infection. If HCV RNA is detected, the diagnosis of current HCV infection is confirmed. Next steps should include providing appropriate counseling on risk avoidance, and linkage to medical care and treatment [33]. Guidelines currently recommend conducting reflex testing, which implies that the RNA test is automatically performed on all reactive HCV antibody specimens. This automatic testing facilitates a complete evaluation within one visit, thus expediting subsequent steps in staging and clinical management (Fig. 6.1)

The advent of point-of-care (POC) tests for HCV represents a remarkable advance for HCV diagnosis that have important implications in HCV care. Major advantages of the use of the POC HCV testing are (1) simplification of the testing process; (2) increase in the number of people both tested and given results in the same encounter; and (3) as such may facilitate linkage to care [34]. POC may be particularly useful for screening vulnerable populations in healthcare, such as PWID. While several POC rapid antibody tests have been developed, only the OraQuick HCV Rapid Antibody Test is approved as POC for HCV testing and CLIA [35] waived by the Food and Drug Administration. The OraQuick test uses whole blood samples obtained by finger stick or venipuncture, is >98% accurate, and provides results regarding the presence of HCV antibody, either reactive or nonreactive, within 20 min.

Staging of liver disease and HCC screening

HCV-induced hepatic fibrosis is a dynamic process in which chronic inflammation stimulates production and deposition of collagen and extracellular matrix proteins. Assessment of the stage of fibrosis provides prognostic information as well as guidance on the choice and duration of the treatment regimen. The most widely used

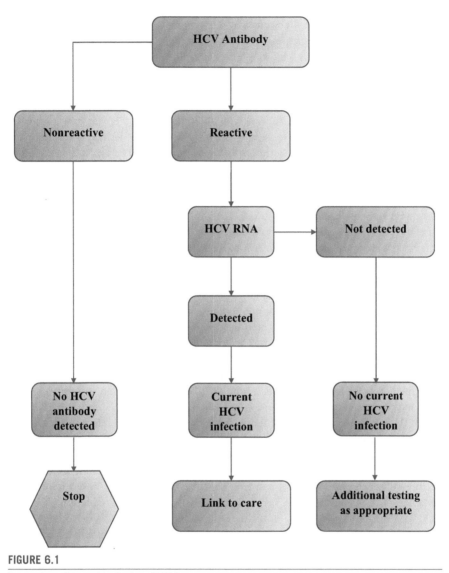

FIGURE 6.1

Screening of hepatitis C virus (HCV).

staging method is the Metavir scoring system which is used to assess the extent of inflammation and fibrosis by histopathological evaluation in a liver biopsy of patients with hepatitis C. Metavir is scored from F0 to F4, where F0 = no fibrosis and F4 = compensated cirrhosis. Liver biopsy was once considered the gold standard for assessment of liver stiffness, but is a painful, invasive, and expensive procedure with a small but not negligible risk of medical complications. Liver biopsies are rarely required anymore for staging and evaluating patients with chronic HCV [31].

The AASLD/IDSA guidelines currently recommend the use of noninvasive techniques to determine liver stiffness [10,31]. Fibrosis/liver stiffness can be assessed with noninvasive blood tests including Fibrosure/Fibrotest, AST to platelet ratio index (APRI), and FIB-4, among others. Ultrasound-based Transient elastography (TE), more commonly known by the brand name of Fibroscan (Ecosens, France), is a fast ($<$5 min), noninvasive, painless technique that can be performed in an outpatient clinic [36] and its results are available immediately. It assesses liver stiffness (fibrosis) by measuring the velocity of a shear wave as it travels through the liver. The higher the velocity, the more advanced the fibrosis. It examines an area of liver tissue 100 times larger than a liver biopsy, and results are expressed in Kilo Pascal (kPa) units. Cut-off values differ between different etiologies of hepatitis (hepatitis B, Alcohol, NASH, etc.) and in HCV values $>$ 9.5 kPa and $>$12.5 kPa are considered indicative of severe fibrosis (Metavir F3) and cirrhosis (Metavir F4), respectively. The AASLD/IDSA guidelines recommend that both Metavir F3 and Metavir F4 are treated and followed as compensated cirrhosis. Various factors may produce unreliable TE measures and these include obesity (body mass index $\geq$30 kg/m^2), steatosis, cardiac failure, high necroinflammatory activity, ascites, cholestasis, and a nonfasting state.

In general, the noninvasive staging modalities have sensitivities and specificities that range between 75% and 85%, and the combination of liver elastography and a noninvasive blood test has the best ROC (Receiver Operating Curve) for assessing liver fibrosis [37,38].

Risk factors for HCC include cirrhosis of any etiology, and patients with cirrhosis should undergo lifelong surveillance for HCC, because surveillance improves survival and increases the detection of early-stage HCC [39]. HCV-induced HCC is seen in about 1% of infected individuals after 30 years of chronic infection; however, the risk is significantly higher in cirrhotic patients and is estimated to be 3.5% per year [40]. In a Veteran Affairs cohort of 3271 persons living with HCV cases of HCC, HCC was highest in patients with cirrhosis together with HCV treatment failure, regardless of whether the treatment was interferon or DAA-based treatment. Sustained virologic response (SVR) was associated with a 71% reduction in HCC. [41] According to the AASLD guidelines, surveillance for HCC should be with a liver ultrasound (with or without an alpha-fetoprotein) every 6—9 months in patients with cirrhosis [42].

SVR outcomes in PWID

Despite barriers to receiving care, studies indicate that very high SVR rates can be achieved in the PWID population, due to the new DAA regimens, which are highly efficacious and short in duration.

Glecaprevir/pibrentasvir: In a retrospective analysis of pooled data from 7 phase III trials to evaluate the efficacy and safety of 8 or 12 weeks of glecaprevir/pibrentasvir in patients with chronic HCV infection, in persons who used drugs, SVR rates were achieved by 93% (n/N = 91/98) in people who recently used drugs and 97% (n/N = 591/610) in persons with former drug use. Patients considered as having recently used drugs were those who self-reported IDU within 12 months of screening, had a positive urine illicit drug screen result, or both. In addition, treatment adherence and completion rates were ≥96% regardless of drug use status [43].

Elbasvir/grazoprevir: In a randomized controlled trial of 301 HCV GT1, 4, 6, infected treatment naïve patients on opioid agonist therapy, the SVR rates after 12 weeks of treatment with elbasvir/grazoprevir were >90% [44]. Importantly, nearly 60% of participants had positive urine illicit drug screens at baseline, and there was no difference in SVR rates of those with or without a positive drug screen. Adherence greater than 95% (>79 doses) was reported by nearly all participants.

Sofosbuvir/velpatasvir: The coformulated formulation of sofosbuvir/velpatasvir was approved in August 2017 for the treatment of all HCV genotypes. In the SIMPLIFY trial, investigators assessed the efficacy of sofosbuvir/velpatasvir for 12 weeks in 103 participants, of whom 100% had injected drugs in the last 3 months, 74% had injected drugs in the past month, and nearly 60% were on opioid agonist therapy (OAT). The majority were GT3 (58%), 35% had GT1 and 8% participants had cirrhosis. The regimen was well tolerated with one serious adverse event (rhabdomyolysis), and SVR rate was 94% with only one reinfection in the follow-up period [45].

All DAAs: A recent meta-analysis also provides robust evidence that PWID, both on medications for opioid use disorder (MOUD) and actively injecting drugs, can indeed be successfully treated for HCV with SVR similar to non-PWID [46]. Including data from 2010 to 2018 of all oral DAA regimens, authors compared HCV outcomes (adherence, discontinuation, SVR) of controls (non-PWID) to over 1700 patients on MOUD and over 500 patients actively injecting drugs. The overall intention to treat SVR was 90% for PWID on MOUD and 88% for those PWID actively using drugs. Importantly, the majority of those who did not achieve SVR were those lost to follow-up (LTFU) rather than true virologic failures, with 43% of those LTFU having completed the full HCV treatment regimen.

Barriers to care for PWID

Despite the evidence that supports treating PWID with HCV DAAs, there is a huge gap in the care continuum and overall <10% of PWID have been initiated these life-saving treatment regimens [42,47]. Innovative methods to get more PWID on HCV treatment and achieve SVR are desperately needed. HCV treatment uptake among PWID has been limited due to multiple interrelated barriers at the level of the patient, the provider, and the health system [48]. Patient-level barriers include asymptomatic infection and lack of awareness related to HCV and its treatment, which often results in a low perceived need for engagement in care. These issues are compounded by general barriers to healthcare access (e.g., having insurance, a primary care provider (PCP)), competing comorbidities which may require more immediate attention, as well as social determinants of health which impede stability including unemployment, unstable housing, lack of transportation, incarceration, and ongoing substance use. Providers are often unwilling to prescribe HCV treatment to even former PWID because of concerns related to ongoing substance use, low adherence, and the potential risk of reinfection [49]. Some studies have suggested that physicians have suboptimal knowledge regarding HCV and its treatment which can impact screening and referral to care. Additional structural barriers include insufficient locations where HCV testing can be performed and where treatment can be delivered [50,51]. There is also a dearth of providers who feel competent to treat HCV, as well as inadequate numbers of patient navigators dedicated to linking HCV-infected PWID and others into care and treatment. Finally, HCV care has historically been delivered in specialist settings which means it is segregated from other services that PWID utilize including primary care, opiate substitution therapy, and HIV care (Fig. 6.2).

Cascade of care and Co-located models of care

The "cascade of care" model, also known as "care continuum," is frequently used when the course of a medical condition has distinct, measurable endpoints, such as diagnosis, linkage to care, and treatment [52]. Critical stages of the cascade of care for HCV may involve (1) screening for initial HCV infection, (2) HCV RNA confirmatory testing, (3) staging the degree of liver fibrosis, (4) engagement in care and HCV treatment, (5) and finally achieving a SVR (i.e., undetectable viral load 12 weeks after treatment completion) [53]. This model provides a framework for clinicians, public health officials, and stakeholders to monitor a given disease at population level, and identify gaps in the delivery of care [54].

Despite life-saving HCV medications, the HCV cascade of care remains dismal for PWID in this country. Lack of testing services, especially at alcohol and other drug centers, lack of linkage services, an inadequate number of treatment providers, and expensive HCV medications with restrictive state insurance policies have all led to limited access to HCV care for PWID, negatively impacting the care continuum [55].

Screening

The first step toward improving HCV treatment outcomes among PWID is widespread screening. To date, screening strategies have focused on either risk-factor screening and/or age-based screening of the baby boomer population (those born between 1945 and 1965). In March 2020, the United States Preventative Services Task Force updated its recommendation, which now specifies that HCV screening is recommended for all adults (ages 18–79). This recommendation is based in part on the evolving bimodal age distribution of HCV infection, including both baby boomers and younger PWID, who have transitioned from oral prescription pain killers to injection of opioids. The AASLD/IDSA HCV Guidance Panel and CDC have also endorsed one-time HCV screening for all adults in the United States [56]. Increasing

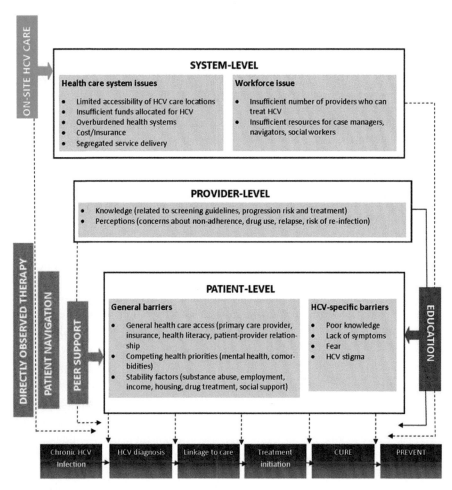

FIGURE 6.2

Barriers to care.

Published with kind permission of Dr. Shruti Metha.

incident HCV infections have paralleled the current opioid epidemic, yet many PWID continue to go unscreened. Consequently, updated guidelines are a welcome addition in order to increase screening rates.

Multiple innovative programs and models have demonstrated that co-located models of screening and care for HCV are feasible at community health centers as well as alcohol and drug treatment programs. In a community-based testing program in San Diego, HIV testing counselors were cross-trained on HCV testing and counseling, and between April 2013 and September 2013 conducted 453 rapid tests at three clinic sites and six residential alcohol and drug treatment programs. Overall, 94 (21%) of tested patients were HCV antibody positive, 67% fell within the birth cohort of 1945−1965, and 70% of patients were linked to care [57].

HCV linkage to care

Though screening must improve, linkage to HCV care for those PWID already diagnosed and aware of their infection remains a primary barrier to receiving life-saving treatment. The CHAMPS study investigated novel interventions (peer navigators and cash incentives), as compared with usual care, to increase the rate of HCV treatment initiation and cure in a population of persons with HIV/HCV coinfection who use drugs [58]. Overall, 110 of 144 (76%) of participants initiated treatment with ledipasvir/sofosbuvir. The initiation rate was higher in persons randomized to peers (83%) or cash incentives (76%) compared with usual care (67%)—however, these differences did not reach statistical significance ($P = 0.11$). Among the participants who initiated treatment, SVR rates were high, achieved by 91% of participants. Importantly, PWIDs who attended their first linkage to care appointment without rescheduling were more likely to initiate treatment and obtain cure. Those who were unemployed were more likely to benefit from peers. These data stress the importance of expedited linkage to care for PWID and interventions that are tailored to each individual's needs. Furthermore, active alcohol consumption and drug use did not lower treatment initiation rates, and SVR remained high.

For PWID outside of the healthcare system, linkage to care has been even more difficult [59–61]. Though the data are sparse, linking PWID from needle and syringe programs and from correctional settings could be beneficial and should be actively implemented and studied.

Co-located care

Co-located care models in which HCV care is provided in the same settings as substance use treatment programs may be one of the most effective approaches to deliver HCV care among PWID. Co-locating HCV treatment in other settings where PWID are already accessing services, such as primary care clinics, syringe service programs, or jails and prisons, has also been shown to be effective. Components of care in these clinical settings are varied but may include (1) HCV treatment to prevent transmission (i.e., treatment as prevention), (2) provision of MOUD to reduce risk of HCV reinfection or infection of other infectious diseases, (3) access to HIV preexposure prophylaxis (PrEP), (4) behavioral services to address psychiatric symptoms, and (5) harm reduction services (i.e., syringe service programs and naloxone).

Co-located HCV care in opioid treatment programs (OTPs)

OTPs may be an ideal setting to treat PWID with chronic HCV given that OTPs are staffed by a multidisciplinary team able to provide medical, psychiatric, and addiction treatment, adherence support, peer support, group education and support, and potentially directly observed HCV therapy (DOT).

Many real-world cohort studies have shown high SVR rates, similar to registration trials, among those treated at OTPs in the DAA era [62–64]. Many of these studies also took advantage of daily methadone distribution to offer DOT for HCV medication. The potential significance of such co-located care models is extensive given that nationwide, over 375,000 patients receive methadone or buprenorphine from approximately 1500 OTPs and conservative estimates suggest that over 60% of PWID in OTPs are infected with HCV. Understanding how best to incorporate HCV models of care within OTPs is important.

The PREVAIL study was a randomized controlled trial (RCT) conducted within three OTPs in Bronx, New York, to determine whether DOT and group treatment (GT) were more effective than self-administered individual treatment (SIT) in promoting adherence and achieving SVR among PWID receiving OAT [65]. Among 150 PWID, 65% of participants had a positive illicit urine drug screen 6 months prior to HCV treatment. Overall SVR was high at 94%; 98% in the DOT group, 94% in the GT group, and 90% in the SIT group ($P = .152$), no difference between study arms. Overall daily adherence was 78% and was greater among participants randomly assigned to DOT (86%) than those assigned to SIT (75%; $P = .001$). This study demonstrates that PWID receiving onsite HCV treatment at an OTP can achieve high SVR rates, despite ongoing drug use. Though it did not impact SVR, adherence was higher in the DOT group, indicating that leveraging the OTP infrastructure to offer DOT may be beneficial for those most at risk of nonadherence. These data support the widespread application of co-location of HCV treatment within substance use disorder treatment centers.

Co-located HCV treatment in primary care

Co-locating HCV treatment in primary care clinics is another model that can aid in expanding HCV treatment to PWID, circumventing the dearth of specialty care for many locations throughout the United States. Even in the arduous era of interferon, the ECHO study (RCT comparing SVR rates of participants treated via specialty care vs. primary care in rural clinics and prisons) proved that primary care physicians could successfully treat patients at comparable rates as specialists after telemedicine training [66]. Nationally, there are over 1200 federally qualified health centers serving over 20 million marginalized patients, many with HCV prevalence rates higher than the national average [67]. Though DAAs are highly efficacious, we will need to decentralize HCV treatment in order to increase access to care to these life-saving medications for the three to four million persons living with HCV in the United States.

The ASCEND trial evaluated the efficacy of HCV treatment managed by three provider types—nurse practitioners (NPs), primary care providers (PCPs), and specialists—set within a real-world, urban population. Patients with chronic HCV infection were assigned to receive treatment with ledipasvir and sofosbuvir from an NP (n = 150; 25%), a PCP (n = 160; 27%), or a specialist (n = 290; 48%). Overall, patients predominantly were male (69%) and black (96%); 40% had a fibrosis score 3/4, 25% had HIV coinfection, and 15% had active drug use.

There were no differences in SVR rates among the three provider types: NPs 89%; PCPs 87%; and specialists 84%. Importantly, adherence to appointments was higher among patients treated by NP and PCPs as compared with those treated by specialists, indicating that this relationship may improve engagement while on HCV treatment or after-treatment care for those that may need it most, such as PWID.

In a cohort study conducted at a primary care clinic in the Bronx, New York, SVR rates were found to be high for HCV-infected patients (n = 89) initiating DAA treatment [68]. SVR rates were 95% (n = 41/43) for those who did not use drugs and 96% (n = 44/46) for patients actively using drugs and/or receiving OAT ($P = .95$). These data support both treatment of PWID and using primary care clinics as important settings in which to engage patients who otherwise may not reach specialty care.

With the goal of HCV elimination, the United States will need to engage a larger pool of those living with HCV by task-shifting to nonspecialists, particularly for hard-to-treat populations such as PWID. Data support the reversal of state polices that prohibit nonspecialists from delivering HCV care to their patients, and treating HCV in these community-based centers will be key to the rapid scale-up of treatment and cure.

Similar models of collocated care may also be effective in increasing HCV treatment uptake in needle and syringe programs and correctional facilities, including jails and prisons, but more data are needed to support the implementation of best practices.

HCV treatment adherence

For decades, HCV treatment has been neglected for PWID due to provider's misconceptions regarding medication adherence. Of note, recent studies have demonstrated that PWID can achieve optimal adherence rates. In the SIMPLIFY study, a multicenter study involving active PWID, the average daily adherence to therapy was 94%, and 94% of PWID achieved HCV cure. In the PREVAIL study, the HCV daily adherence rate among PWID receiving OAT was lower (74%), yet SVR rates remained high (94%). Furthermore, a recent meta-analysis found that adherence rates were similar between PWID and non-PWID in the era of DAAs (adherence defined as >90%). There were no differences in SVR rates between those defined as adherent and those that were not. This may indicate that, in the era of DAAs, a 90% adherence threshold is too high to predict failure. From these studies, it is evident that most PWID can achieve high rates of DAA adherence, and that nonperfect adherence can still lead to high SVR rates. Overall, the decision to exclude PWID from HCV treatment should be avoided even if patients have poor adherence during HCV treatment, and emphasis on treatment completion should be encouraged.

HCV reinfection

HCV antibody does not provide immunity from reinfection. HCV reinfection is defined as a positive HCV RNA test after a documented SVR at least 12 weeks after the completion of HCV treatment [49], and overall estimates indicate that reinfection rates are low. A recently published study using data from the British Columbia Hepatitis Testers Cohort [69], which includes all individuals tested for HCV or HIV at the British Columbia Center for Disease Control Public Health Lab from 1990 to 2010, is one of the largest HCV cohorts reporting reinfection to date. Among 2225 individuals who achieved SVR following HCV treatment, the overall reinfection rate was (0.48/100 PY) suggesting low rates of HCV reinfection. Higher HCV reinfection rates were reported among PWID (1.14/100 PY) and persons with HIV infection (2.56/100 PY), yet reinfection rates still remained relatively low.

Now, there are increasing data available on reinfection rates for PWID in the era of DAAs, and reinfection rates continue to be low [70]. For example, the reinfection rate found in the SIMPLIFY study conducted among active PWID with recent IDU was found to be 2.6/100 PY [45]. In the PREVAIL study conducted among PWID on MOUD, the incidence of reinfection reported was even lower (1.22/100 PY) [32], which mirrors findings from earlier studies indicating that receiving MOUD reduces HCV reinfection risk among PWID [69]. Importantly, all reinfections in this study were among participants reporting ongoing IDU, thus emphasizing the need for "wrap around" harm reduction services in conjunction with HCV treatment programs in PWID.

In a meta-analysis of 35 studies which included interferon-based regimens as well as DAAs, the overall rate of HCV reinfection was 6.2/100 person-years (95% CI 4.3−9.0) among people recently injecting drugs, 5.9/100 person-years (95% CI 4.1−8.5) among people with any recent drug use (injecting or non-injecting), and lowest, 3.8/100 person-years (95% CI 2.5−5.8) among those receiving MOUD [71]. There were no significant differences in reinfection rates between people treated with interferon-based versus DAA therapy, and overall reinfection was reported to be relatively low.

Given the increasing evidence that reinfection rates remain low for PWID post SVR in the era of DAAs, concern for reinfection should not be used as a reason to withhold therapy from people who use drugs. Instead, target interventions to lower reinfection, such as MOUD and Syringe Services Programs (SSPs), should be offered in conjunction with HCV treatment; as well as regular posttreatment HCV assessment for early detection of reinfection and nonstigmatized HCV retreatment. If we are to approach HCV elimination, we must proactively treat the population most at risk for transmitting the virus.

The Hepatitis C Real Options (HERO) study is an ongoing, randomized study aimed at investigating the effectiveness of different models of curative HCV treatment among PWID. The HERO study is the largest prospective study to date (754 PWID) and will have follow-up over a 3-year period to determine reinfection [72]. The HERO study has the potential to help identify specific risk factors for reinfection among active PWID which can be used for harm reduction efforts.

Treatment as prevention

Treatment as prevention is proven strategy to reduce transmission in HIV-infected persons [73] and is an emerging concept in HCV. Mathematical models suggest that HCV could be significantly decreased to near elimination levels of <5% in communities with HCV prevalence <50% by providing DAA therapy among populations with the highest transmission risks, namely PWID and men who have sex with men [74]. An example of treatment as prevention is the TraP HepC project in Iceland, which was initiated in 2016. All HCV RNA positive persons were offered DAA therapy, and among the 722 persons who initiated treatment SVR was achieved in 89%. Early reports indicate that universal access has now led to a marked reduction of HCV prevalence among PWIDs and the incarcerated in Iceland [75]. A similar pattern of reduced HCV infection was also found to be true in a population of HIV/HCV coinfected MSM in the Netherlands. Unrestricted DAA availability after 2016 was followed by a 51% decrease in acute HCV infections among HIV-positive MSM, while other infections related to sexual activity increased during the same time period [76]. Proactive treatment of populations most at risk of transmission, such as PWID, will be needed to reach HCV elimination targets.

Another innovative way to reduce the risk of HCV transmission as well as reduce deaths from opioid use involves HCV/HIV testing in combination with overdose prevention and response training at outreach facilities, and in a study done in Bronx, New York, there was high participant acceptability of such an intervention [77]. SSPs and MOUD programs are extremely valuable tools in preventing HCV transmission in PWID. In a Cochrane review of such programs, the combination of SSPs and MOUD was associated with the greatest reduction in HCV transmission [78].

Policy issues and restrictions

The implementation of new and innovative drug policies in the United States could facilitate a reduction of HCV among PWID in the United States. A clear example is Portugal where decriminalization of the purchase, possession, and consumption of drugs in 2001 coincided with a significant decrease in the number of people infected with HCV, as well as other infectious diseases related to drug use (i.e., HIV) [79].

Overall, a wide adoption of evidence-based strategies could help mitigate HCV risk and improve treatment among PWID, yet their implementation in the United States is scarce and partially obstructed by the current policies. There remain restrictions by payers on who can be treated; and restrictive criteria in Medicaid programs currently exclude persons with lower stages of liver fibrosis, persons actively using drugs, and restrictive prescriber eligibility, and these policies were largely driven by the profoundly expensive HCV medications [80]. The National Viral Hepatitis Roundtable and the Center for Health Law and Policy Innovation of Harvard Law School launched in October 2019 an update to "Hepatitis C: Sate of Medicaid Access," an interactive project grading all 50 state Medicaid programs, as well as the

District of Columbia and Puerto Rico, according to access to curative HCV treatments for HCV, the nation's deadliest infectious disease. Although Medicaid access to HCV antiviral medications has improved over the last few years, more than half of all state Medicaid programs still impose some restrictions on provider type, fibrosis level, and illicit drug use.

Another example of policy that supports treatment scale-up to achieve elimination is Australia's National Drug Strategy. In 2016, the Australian Government offered unrestricted access to DAA therapy with no restriction based on liver disease stage, drug and alcohol use, and incarcerated status. Additionally, any medical practitioner regardless of specialty could prescribe DAAs. This treatment-for-all, in combination with harm reduction strategies including government-funded syringe service programs and MOUD, could result in HCV elimination in Australia. As a consequence, recent mathematical modeling studies have proposed that Australia will meet the WHO targets of HCV elimination by 2028 [81].There is evidence that scaling-up HCV treatment to 80% of the PWID infected could reduce prevalence HCV among PWID by at least 45% [82]. Unfortunately, neither HCV testing nor care are routine practices implemented in North America [83].

Cost-effectiveness studies

Treating HCV among PWID is highly cost-effective independent of the type of regimen provided. For example, studies conducted with older generation therapies (e.g., pegylated-interferon and ribavirin) were shown to be cost-effective among PWID [84], despite the considerable side effects and low cure rates of interferon-based regimes. New DAA-containing regimens are cost-effective in various adult populations [85]. A recent meta-analysis reviewing 92 results from 10 studies evidenced that DAA treatment is cost-effective at a $100 000/QALY threshold, independent of the presence of cirrhosis and prior treatment history [86]. In the PREVAIL study, investigators analyzed the cost-effectiveness of SIT, GT, and DOT for HCV in OAT programs using trial results. GT and DOT models were found to be cost-effective alternatives to SIT, and these interventions could be adopted widely at OAT programs nationwide.

Conclusions

PWID have a high prevalence of chronic HCV and are a major source of new infections within the community. Highly effective and well tolerated, interferon free, all oral and pan-genotypic regimens have revolutionized the HCV treatment paradigm. These regimens are equally effective in PWID as they are in the general population. However, the majority of PWID in the United States have not initiated treatment and therefore have not achieved SVR. SVR is tantamount to HCV cure and leads to a significant improvement in hepatic and all-cause morbidity and mortality. HCV reinfection after SVR in PWID is low, and can be decreased even further with "wrap around" services including SSPs, MOUD, and co-located models of care. If DAA scale-up in PWID is supported by policy makers and payers, HCV eradication may become a reality.

References

[1]   Ly KN, Hughes EM, Jiles RB, Holmberg SD. Rising mortality associated with hepatitis C virus in the United States, 2003-2016. Clin Infect Dis 2016;62(10):1287−8.

[2]   Dowell D, Haegerich TM, Chou R. CDC guideline for prescribing opioids for chronic pain—United States, 2016. MMWR (Morb Mortal Wkly Rep) 2016;65(1):1−49.

[3]   Prescription Drug Monitoring Program. PDMP Maps and Tables. https://www.pdmpassist.org/content/pdmp-maps-and-tables.

[4]   Cicero TJ, Ellis MS, Harney J. Shifting patterns of prescription opioid and heroin abuse in the United States. N Engl J Med 2015;373(18):1789−90.

[5]   CDC. Hepatitis C questions and answers for health professionals. 2019. https://www.cdc.gov/hepatitis/hcv/hcvfaq.htm. Accessed February 6, 2020.

[6]   Peters PJ, Pontones P, Hoover KW, et al. HIV infection linked to injection use of oxymorphone in Indiana, 2014−2015. N Engl J Med 2016;375(3):229−39.

[7]   Zibbell JE, Iqbal K, Patel RC, et al. Increases in hepatitis C virus infection related to injection drug use among persons aged ≤30 Years — Kentucky, Tennessee, Virginia, and West Virginia, 2006−2012. MMWR (Morb Mortal Wkly Rep) 2015;64(17):453−8.

[8]   Larney S, Grebely J, Hickman M, De Angelis D, Dore GJ, Degenhardt L. Defining populations and injecting parameters among people who inject drugs: implications for the assessment of hepatitis C treatment programs. Int J Drug Pol 2015;26(10):950−7.

[9]   Edlin BR, Eckhardt BJ, Shu MA, Holmberg SD, T. S. Toward a more accurate estimate of the prevalence of hepatitis C in the United States. Hepatology 2015;62(5):1353−63.

[10] Smith BD, Morgan RL, Beckett GA, et al. Recommendations for the identification of chronic hepatitis C virus infection among persons born during 1945−1965. MMWR Recomm Rep (Morb Mortal Wkly Rep) 2012;61(14):1−32.

[11] Suryaprasad AG, White JZ, Xu F, et al. Emerging epidemic of hepatitis C virus infections among young nonurban persons who inject drugs in the United States, 2006−2012. Clin Infect Dis 2014;59(10):1411−9.

[12] Morse A, Barritt ASIV, Jhaveri R. Individual state hepatitis C data supports expanding screening beyond baby boomers to all adults. Gastroenterology 2018;154(6):1850−1. e1852.

[13] Nelson PK, Mathers BM, Cowie B, et al. Global epidemiology of hepatitis B and hepatitis C in people who inject drugs: results of systematic reviews. Lancet 2011; 378(9791):571−83.

[14] Grebely J, Larney S, Peacock A, et al. Global, regional, and country-level estimates of hepatitis C infection among people who have recently injected drugs. Addiction 2019; 114(1):150−66.

[15] Kapadia S, Aponte-Melendez Y, Fong C, et al. Hepatitis C treatment wanted yet not received: barriers to receiving HCV treatment among people who inject drugs. Open Forum Infect Dis 2018;5(Suppl. 1):S654−5.

[16] Hoofnagle JH. Course and outcome of hepatitis C. Hepatology 2002;36(S21-S29).

[17] Smith DJ, Combellick J, Jordan AE, Hagan H. Hepatitis C virus (HCV) disease progression in people who inject drugs (PWID): a systematic review and meta-analysis. Int J Drug Pol 2015;26(10):911−21.

[18] Lingala S, Ghany MG. Natural history of hepatitis C. Gastroenterol Clin N Am 2015; 44(4):717−34.

[19] Di Bisceglie AM, Shiffman ML, Everson GT, et al. Prolonged therapy of advanced chronic hepatitis C with low-dose peginterferon. N Engl J Med 2008;359(23):2429−41.

[20] Degenhardt L, Larney S, Randall D, Burns L, Hall W. Causes of death in a cohort treated for opioid dependence between 1985 and 2005. Addiction 2014;109(1):90−9.

[21] Kimber J, Stoové M, Maher L. Mortality among people who inject drugs: ten-year follow-up of the hepatitis C virus cohort. Drug Alcoh Rev 2019;38(3):270−3.

[22] Mathers BM, Degenhardt L, Bucello C, Lemon J, Wiessing L, Hickman M. Mortality among people who inject drugs: a systematic review and meta-analysis. Bull World Health Organ 2013;91:102−23.

[23] Degenhardt L, Charlson F, Stanaway J, et al. Estimating the burden of disease attributable to injecting drug use as a risk factor for HIV, hepatitis C, and hepatitis B: findings from the Global Burden of Disease Study 2013. Lancet Infect Dis 2016;16(12):1385−98.

[24] Viral hepatitis: statistics and surveillance. Centers for Disease Control 2018. https://www.cdc.gov/hepatitis/statistics/index.htm. Accessed September 29, 2018.

[25] Verna EC, Brown Jr RS. Hepatitis C virus and liver transplantation. Clin Liver Dis 2006; 10(4):919−40.

[26] Hernandez MD, Sherman KE. HIV/hepatitis C coinfection natural history and disease progression. Curr Opin HIV AIDS 2011;6(6):478−82.

[27] Rein DB, Wittenborn JS, Weinbaum CM, Sabin M, Smith BD, Lesesne SB. Forecasting the morbidity and mortality associated with prevalent cases of pre-cirrhotic chronic hepatitis C in the United States. Dig Liver Dis 2011;43(1):66−72.

[28] Davis GL, Alter MJ, El-Serag H, Poynard T, Jennings LW. Aging of hepatitis C virus (HCV)-infected persons in the United States: a multiple cohort model of HCV prevalence and disease progression. Gastroenterology 2010;138(2):513−21.

[29] Ly KN, Xing J, Klevens RM, Jiles RB, Ward JW, Holmberg SD. The increasing burden of mortality from viral hepatitis in the United States between 1999 and 2007. Ann Intern Med 2012;156(4):271−8.

[30] Ly KN, Hughcs EM, Jilcs RB, Holmbcrg SD. Rising mortality associated with hepatitis C virus in the United States, 2003-2013. Clin Infect Dis 2016;62(10):1287−8.

[31] AASLD-ISDA. HCV guidance: recommendations for testing, managing, and treating hepatitis C. 2018. https://www.hcvguidelines.org/. Accessed September 18, 2019.

[32] Akiyama MJ, Lipsey D, Heo M, et al. Low hepatitis C reinfection following direct-acting antiviral therapy among people who inject drugs on opioid agonist therapy. Clin Infect Dis 2020;70(12):2695−702.

[33] CDC. Testing for HCV infection: an update of guidance for clinicians and laboratorians. MMWR (Morb Mortal Wkly Rep) 2013;62(18):362−5.

[34] Martinello M, Grebely J, Petoumenos K, et al. HCV reinfection incidence among individuals treated for recent infection. J Viral Hepat 2017;24(5):359−70.

[35] Centers for Medicare and Medicaid Services. Tests waived granted status under CLIA. Baltimore, MD: Centers for Medicare and Medicaid Services. https://www.cms.gov/Regulations-and-Guidance/Legislation/CLIA/Downloads/waivetbl.pdf. Accessed September 29, 2018

[36] Afdhal NH, Bacon BR, Patel K, et al. Accuracy of fibroscan, compared with histology, in analysis of liver fibrosis in patients with hepatitis B or C: a United States multicenter study. Clin Gastroenterol Hepatol 2015;13(4):772−9. e773.

[37] Castéra L, Vergniol J, Foucher J, et al. Prospective comparison of transient elastography, Fibrotest, APRI, and liver biopsy for the assessment of fibrosis in chronic hepatitis C. Gastroenterol Clin 2005;128(2):343–50.

[38] Chou R, Wasson N. Blood tests to diagnose fibrosis or cirrhosis in patients with chronic hepatitis C virus infection: a systematic review. Ann Intern Med 2013; 159(4):807–20.

[39] Heimbach JK, Kulik LM, Finn RS, et al. AASLD guidelines for the treatment of hepatocellular carcinoma. Hepatology 2018;67(1):358–80.

[40] Younossi ZM, Kanwal F, Saab S, et al. The impact of hepatitis C burden: an evidence-based approach. Aliment Pharmacol Therapeut 2014;39(5):518–31.

[41] Ioannou GN, Green PK, Berry K. HCV eradication induced by direct-acting antiviral agents reduces the risk of hepatocellular carcinoma. J Hepatol 2018;68(1):25–32.

[42] Carey KJ, Huang W, Linas BP, Tsui JI. Hepatitis C virus testing and treatment among persons receiving buprenorphine in an office-based program for opioid use disorders. J Subst Abuse Treat 2016;66:54–9.

[43] Foster GR, Dore GJ, Wang S, et al. Glecaprevir/pibrentasvir in patients with chronic HCV and recent drug use: an integrated analysis of 7 phase III studies. Drug Alcohol Depend 2019;194:487–94.

[44] Dore GJ, Altice F, Litwin AH, et al. Elbasvir–grazoprevir to treat hepatitis C virus infection in persons receiving opioid agonist therapy: a randomized trial. Ann Intern Med 2016;165(9):625–34.

[45] Grebely J, Dalgard O, Conway B, et al. Sofosbuvir and velpatasvir for hepatitis C virus infection in people with recent injection drug use (SIMPLIFY): an open-label, single-arm, phase 4, multicentre trial. Lancet Gastroenterol Hepatol 2018;3(3):153–61.

[46] Graf C, Mucke MM, Dultz G, et al. Efficacy of direct-acting antivirals for chronic hepatitis C virus infection in people who inject drugs or receive opioid substitution therapy: a systematic review and meta-analysis. Clin Infect Dis 2020;70(11):2355–65.

[47] Iversen J, Grebely J, Catlett B, Cunningham P, Dore GJ, Maher L. Estimating the cascade of hepatitis C testing, care and treatment among people who inject drugs in Australia. Int J Drug Pol 2017;47:77–85.

[48] Mehta SH, Genberg BL, Astemborski J, et al. Limited uptake of hepatitis C treatment among injection drug users. J Community Health 2008;33(3):126–33.

[49] Asher AK, Portillo CJ, Cooper BA, Dawson-Rose C, Vlahov D, Page KA. Clinicians' views of hepatitis C virus treatment candidacy with direct-acting antiviral regimens for people who inject drugs. Subst Use Misuse 2016;51(9):1218–23.

[50] Grebely J, Oser M, Taylor LE, Dore GJ. Breaking down the barriers to hepatitis C virus (HCV) treatment among individuals with HCV/HIV coinfection: action required at the system, provider, and patient levels. J Infect Dis 2013;207(Suppl. 1):S19–25.

[51] Swan D, Long J, Carr O, et al. Barriers to and facilitators of hepatitis C testing, management, and treatment among current and former injecting drug users: a qualitative exploration. AIDS Patient Care STDS 2010;24(12):753–62.

[52] Yehia BR, Schranz AJ, Umscheid CA, Lo Re III V. The treatment cascade for chronic hepatitis C virus infection in the United States: a systematic review and meta-analysis. PLoS One 2014;9(7):e101554.

[53] Yehia BR, Schranz A, Craig Umscheild C, Vincent LR. The treatment cascade for people with chronic hepatitis C virus infection in the United States. In: Paper presented at: conference on retroviruses and opportunistic infections; 2014 [Boston, MA].

[54] Morris MD, Mirzazadeh A, Evans JL, et al. Treatment cascade for hepatitis C virus in young adult people who inject drugs in San Francisco: low number treated. Drug Alcohol Depend 2019;198:133–5.

[55] Doyle JS, Aspinall EJ, Hutchinson SJ, et al. Global policy and access to new hepatitis C therapies for people who inject drugs. Int J Drug Pol 2015;26(11):1064–71.

[56] Schillie S, Wester C, Osborne M, Wesolowski L, Ryerson AB. CDC recommendations for hepatitis C screening among adults - United States, 2020. MMWR Recomm Rep (Morb Mortal Wkly Rep) 2020;69(2):1–17.

[57] Ramers CB, Lewis R, Reyes L, Kuo A, Wyles DL. Initial results of a community-based rapid hepatitis C testing and linkage to care program. In: Conference on retroviruses and opportunistic infections; March 3-6, 2014; 2015 [Boston, MA].

[58] Ward KM, Falade-Nwulia O, Moon J, et al. A randomized controlled trial of cash incentives or peer support to increase HCV treatment for persons with HIV who use drugs: the CHAMPS study. Open Forum Infect Dis 2019;6(4):ofz166.

[59] Norton BLSR, Agyemang DJ, Litwin AH. Contingency management improves HCV linkage to care in persons who inject drugs: a pilot study. Oslo, Norway: International Network on Hepatitis in Substance Users (INHSU); 2016.

[60] Hochstatter KR, Hull SJ, Stockman LJ, et al. Using database linkages to monitor the continuum of care for hepatitis C virus among syringe exchange clients: experience from a pilot intervention. Int J Drug Pol 2017;42:22–5.

[61] Akiyama MJ, Columbus D, MacDonald R, et al. Linkage to hepatitis C care after incarceration in jail: a prospective, single arm clinical trial. BMC Infect Dis 2019;19(1):703.

[62] Butner JL, Gupta N, Fabian C, Henry S, Shi JM, Tetrault JM. Onsite treatment of HCV infection with direct acting antivirals within an opioid treatment program. J Subst Abuse Treat 2017;75:49–53.

[63] Schutz A, Moser S, Schwanke C, et al. Directly observed therapy of chronic hepatitis C with ledipasvir/sofosbuvir in people who inject drugs at risk of nonadherence to direct-acting antivirals. J Viral Hepat 2018;25(7):870–3.

[64] Scherz N, Bruggmann P, Brunner N. Direct-acting antiviral therapy for hepatitis C infection among people receiving opioid agonist treatment or heroin assisted treatment. Int J Drug Pol 2018;62:74–7.

[65] Akiyama MJ, Norton BL, Arnsten JH, Agyemang L, Heo M, Litwin AH. Intensive models of hepatitis C care for people who inject drugs receiving opioid agonist therapy: a randomized controlled trial. Ann Intern Med 2019;170(9):594–603.

[66] Arora S, Thornton K, Murata G, et al. Outcomes of treatment for hepatitis C virus infection by primary care providers. N Engl J Med 2011;364(23):2199–207.

[67] Federally Qualified Health Centers, Centers for Medicare and Medicaid. http://www.raconline.org/racmaps/mapfiles/federally-qualified-health-centers.jpg. Accessed 6 January 2014.

[68] Norton BL, Steinman M, Yu K, Deluca J, Cunningham CO, Litwin AH. High HCV cure rates for drug users treated with DAAs at an urban primary care clinic. Boston, MA: Conference on Retroviruses and Opportunistic Infections; 2016.

[69] Islam N, Krajden M, Shoveller J, et al. Incidence, risk factors, and prevention of hepatitis C reinfection: a population-based cohort study. Lancet Gastroenterol Hepatol 2017;2(3):200–10.

[70] Falade-Nwulia O, Sulkowski MS, Merkow A, Latkin C, Mehta SH. Understanding and addressing hepatitis C reinfection in the oral direct-acting antiviral era. J Viral Hepat 2018;25(3):220–7.

[71] Hajarizadeh B, Cunningham EB, Valerio H, et al. SAT-233-Hepatitis C virus reinfection following antiviral treatment among people who inject drugs: a systematic review, meta-analysis, and meta-regression. J Hepatol 2019;70(1):e733.

[72] Litwin AH, Jost J, Wagner K, et al. Rationale and design of a randomized pragmatic trial of patient-centered models of hepatitis C treatment for people who inject drugs: the HERO study. Contemp Clin Trials 2019;87(1).

[73] Cohen MS, Chen YQ, McCauley M, et al. Prevention of HIV-1 infection with early antiretroviral therapy. N Engl J Med 2011;365(6):493−505.

[74] Martin NK, Vickerman P, Grebely J, et al. Hepatitis C virus treatment for prevention among people who inject drugs: modeling treatment scale-up in the age of direct-acting antivirals. Hepatology 2013;58(5):1598−609.

[75] Runarsdottir V, Tyrfingsson T, Fridriksdottir RH, et al. Universal access to direct acting antiviral treatment and high engagement in care results in a major drop in hepatitis C viremia in people who inject drugs: results from TraPHepC in Iceland. Miami, FL: AASLD/EASL HCV; 2019.

[76] Boerekamps A, van den Berk GE, Lauw FN, et al. Declining hepatitis C virus (HCV) incidence in Dutch human immunodeficiency virus-positive men who have sex with men after unrestricted access to HCV therapy. Clin Infect Dis 2018;66(9):1360−5.

[77] Aronson ID, Bennett A, Marsch LA, Bania TC. Mobile technology to increase HIV/HCV testing and overdose prevention/response among people who inject drugs. Front Public Health 2017;5(217).

[78] Platt L, Minozzi S, Reed J, et al. Needle syringe programmes and opioid substitution therapy for preventing hepatitis C transmission in people who inject drugs. Cochrane Database Syst Rev 2017;9(9).

[79] European Monitoring Centre for Drugs and Drug Addiction. Portugal, Country Drug Report 2017. https://www.emcdda.europa.eu/system/files/publications/4508/TD0116918 ENN.pdf. Accessed February 6, 2020

[80] National Viral Hepatitis Roundtable, Hepatitis C: The State of Medicaid Access, 2017 National Summary Report. https://nvhr.org/sites/default/files/.users/u33/State%20of%20HepC_2017.pdf. Accessed February 6, 2020

[81] Kwon JA, Dore GJ, Grebely J, et al. Australia on track to achieve WHO HCV elimination targets following rapid initial DAA treatment uptake: a modelling study. J Viral Hepat 2019;26(1):83−92.

[82] Stone J, Martin NK, Hickman M, et al. Modelling the impact of incarceration and prison-based hepatitis C virus (HCV) treatment on HCV transmission among people who inject drugs in Scotland. Addiction 2017;112(7):1302−14.

[83] Morris MD, Brown B, Allen SA. Universal opt-out screening for hepatitis C virus (HCV) within correctional facilities is an effective intervention to improve public health. Int J Prison Health 2017;13(3/4):192−9.

[84] Martin NK, Vickerman P, Miners A, et al. Cost-effectiveness of hepatitis C virus antiviral treatment for injection drug user populations. Hepatology 2012;55(1):49−57.

[85] Chhatwal J, He T, Lopez-Olivo MA. Systematic review of modelling approaches for the cost effectiveness of hepatitis C treatment with direct-acting antivirals. Pharmacoeconomics 2016;34(6):551−67.

[86] He T, Lopez-Olivo MA, Hur C, Chhatwal J. Systematic review: cost-effectiveness of direct-acting antivirals for treatment of hepatitis C genotypes 2-6. Aliment Pharmacol Therapeut 2017;46(8):711−21.

Opioid use disorder and Chronic Hepatitis B

Kali Zhou, MD, MAS [1], **Norah Terrault, MD, MPH** [2]

[1]*Assistant Professor, Division of Gastrointestinal and Liver Diseases, Keck School of Medicine of University of Southern California, Los Angeles, CA, United States;* [2]*Professor, Division of Gastrointestinal and Liver Diseases, Keck School of Medicine, University of Southern California, Los Angeles, CA, United States*

Introduction

Chronic hepatitis B virus (HBV) infection affects over 240 million individuals worldwide [1]. Detection of the disease is dependent on active surveillance and testing by healthcare providers. Due to the high risk of transmission, the Center for Disease Control (CDC) recommends HBV screening in all individuals with opioid use disorders [2]. Prompt identification of chronic infection and vaccination of susceptible persons at initial point of contact with the healthcare system is a priority. HBV diagnosis and prevention strategies should be coupled with effective harm reduction programs [3]. Safe and well-tolerated oral antiviral therapy is available and is highly efficacious at suppressing viral replication and ameliorating long-term complications; however, there is at present no cure [4]. Successful navigation of chronically infected individuals through the HBV care cascade (Fig. 7.1) is critical to reduce HBV-related morbidity and mortality.

Natural history of hepatitis B virus infection

A heterogeneous disease, chronic HBV infection can manifest in many ways, from long-term inactive disease with little impact on life expectancy to severe acute hepatitis that leads to liver failure and death in the absence of liver transplantation. Risk of chronic HBV infection following exposure differs by age. Spontaneous resolution of hepatitis B after exposure is high among healthy adults but lower in adults who are immunocompromised.

The course of chronic hepatitis B is characterized by variable periods of high viral replication and active hepatitis (liver inflammation and injury) and more quiescent periods with low viral replication and inactive liver disease (Fig. 7.2). The initial immune-tolerant phase (high viral replication, low activity) is typically absent or very short when infected in adulthood versus lasting decades in those infected as neonates or youngsters. Progression through the different phases of infection is not linear

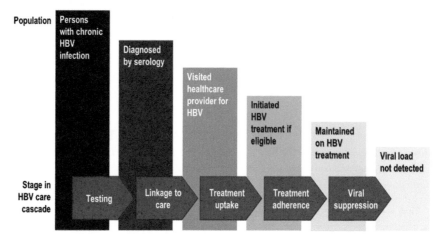

FIGURE 7.1 Care Cascade for Chronic Hepatitis B Infection.

The first step in optimizing outcomes of persons infected with chronic hepatitis B is identifying those who are infected. Once diagnosed, hepatitis B surface antigen (HBsAg)-positive persons need to be linked with a hepatitis B virus (HBV)-knowledgeable provider who can then determine if and when treatment is indicated. If treatment is not indicated at initial assessment, ongoing monitoring is necessary, as the need for treatment can change over time.

and all adults do not experience all phases during their lifetime. Roughly 30% of individuals with chronic HBV infection have an active disease phenotype marked by fluctuating periods of viral activity and subsequent hepatic inflammation (elevated alanine aminotransferase [ALT]) and intervening periods of viral quiescence [5]. Over time, usually on the order of decades, the repetitive injury to the liver leads to the formation of liver fibrosis and ultimately cirrhosis in about 15%−25%. On the other hand, about 20%−30% of chronically infected individuals are inactive carriers, with low HBV DNA and normal hepatic enzyme levels, and possess a much more benign course of disease with minimal risk of cirrhosis over their lifetime unless coexisting liver diseases are present. Risk of HBV-related complications of cirrhosis and hepatocellular carcinoma (HCC) positively correlates with the level of HBV viremia.

Once chronic infection is established, spontaneous resolution is highly infrequent at all ages, with hepatitis B surface antigen (HBsAg) loss occurring at a rate of ∼1% per year [6]. Furthermore, unlike other hepatotropic viruses, HBV integrates its DNA into hepatocytes and can be directly carcinogenic, leading to the development of liver cancer in the absence of fibrosis. Screening for liver cancer, therefore, is a critical aspect of clinical management in specific subpopulations of chronically infected individuals. Thus the vast majority of persons with chronic hepatitis B will require management of their infection over their lifetime, with the need for regular monitoring to determine indications for and duration of therapy. These considerations present unique challenges in the care of HBV-infected individuals with opioid use disorders.

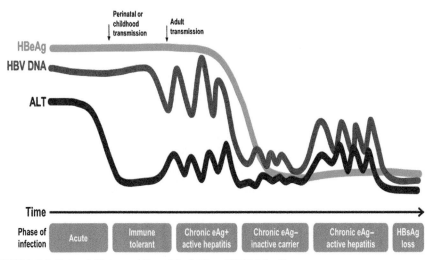

FIGURE 7.2 Natural History of Hepatitis B Virus (HBV) Infection.

There are several different phases of chronic HBV infection. Acute infection leads to chronic infection in only ~5% of healthy adults but the rates of chronicity are higher in those exposed as infants and young children or in immunocompromised adults. Once chronic infection is established, there will be periods of high viral replication and active hepatitis (liver inflammation and injury) and more quiescent periods of low viral replication and inactive liver disease. Hepatitis B e-antigen (HBeAg) is associated with higher levels of HBV replication. Periods of active hepatitis, if prolonged or untreated, can lead to progressive liver fibrosis, cirrhosis, and higher risk for liver cancer. For this reason, those patients with active hepatitis are the target group for treatment.

Hepatitis B virus infection epidemiology, with focus on persons who inject drugs

Globally there are an estimated 15.6 million persons who inject drugs (PWID) in the adult population, [7]. Substantial regional variation exists with respect to global HBV prevalence among PWID, reflecting the HBV endemicity of the region (Fig. 7.3). While overall approximately 9.1% of PWID are HBsAg positive, the proportion is highest (20%) in East and Southeast Asia and lowest in Latin America and Western Europe (2.8% and 3.2%, respectively). The estimated HBV prevalence among PWID in North America is intermediate at about 5% [7].

Injection drug use (IDU) accounts for the majority of HBV infections among those born in the United States. Unlike hepatitis C virus (HCV), prevention of HBV infection is achievable through widespread availability of a highly effective HBV vaccine. However, those born or infected before the introduction of universal birth-dose vaccination in the United States in 1991 remain at risk for acquisition of HBV and subsequent complications [8]. In fact, the rise of opioid use disorders has been an important vector for the ongoing spread of HBV. In the past decade, acute

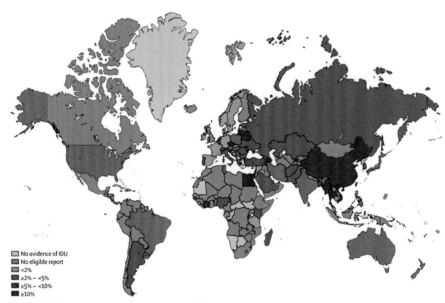

No evidence of IDU
No eligible report
<2%
≥2% – <5%
≥5% – <10%
≥10%

FIGURE 7.3 Global Prevalence of Hepatitis B Surface Antigen (HBsAg) Among Persons Who Inject Drugs (PWID).

A systematic review estimated that 4.8% of all PWID in North America were chronically infected. *IDU*, injection drug use.

Source: Degenhardt L, Peacock A, Colledge S, et al. Global prevalence of injecting drug use and sociodemographic characteristics and prevalence of HIV, HBV, and HCV in people who inject drugs: a multistage systematic review. Lancet Glob Health 2017;5:e1192—e1207.

HBV outbreaks among the IDU population have been reported in the Appalachian states and have signified a shift in the incident disease burden from urban to nonurban communities [9]. Among those with opioid use disorders, transmission most commonly occurs through sharing needles, with sexual transmission being a secondary risk factor, which can be related to unsafe behaviors such as the exchange of sex for drugs [10,11]. In addition, incarceration occurs at higher rates among opioid users and is an established risk factor for HBV acquisition [12]. Coinfection with human immunodeficiency virus (HIV), HCV, and hepatitis delta virus (HDV) is also more frequent among opioid users because of the shared routes of transmission, and these coinfections increase the risk of progression to end-stage liver disease [13,14].

Acute hepatitis B

Acute HBV infection may be accompanied by nonspecific symptoms such as fatigue, myalgias, nausea, and uncommonly jaundice, while symptoms are typically absent in those with chronic infection. Although usually self-limited, acute HBV infection can have severe consequences. Acute or fulminant liver *failure* due to

HBV, defined as coagulopathy and encephalopathy within 8 weeks of symptom onset, occurs in 0.1%–0.5% of acute cases and spontaneous recovery without liver transplantation is infrequent even with prompt administration of antiviral therapy [15]. Factors associated with a higher likelihood of acute liver failure among acutely infected PWID include concomitant alcohol use, methamphetamine use, HBV genotype D, and certain HBV mutations [16].

Epidemiologic data on acute HBV incidence in opioid use disorders are sparse and lacks disaggregation by drug type. Outbreaks are commonly related to sharing of injection equipment including filters and water used to prepare/rinse syringes [17]. An enhanced population-based surveillance strategy employed by six states (Colorado, Connecticut, Minnesota, Oregon, Tennessee, and New York) identified 2220 acute HBV cases between 2006 and 2011 with an average annual incidence rate of 0.86 per 100,000 persons [18]. There was a decline in cases over time in all sites except Tennessee where the incidence peaked at 2.26 per 100,000 persons in 2011. The majority of cases were US-born, white, male, and aged 30–49 years (mean, 44 years). IDU, particularly of heroin, is the main driver for acute HBV infection in US regions with increasing incidence [9]. Between 2006 and 2013, over 3000 cases of acute HBV infection were reported to CDC from the Appalachian states of Kentucky, Tennessee, and West Virginia alone, representing an increase of 113% in these three states. Over this period, the proportion of cases increased among those of white race, aged 30–39 years, and in nonurban counties (defined as population under 50,000). Report of IDU as a risk factor for HBV transmission increased as well (53% between 2006 and 2009 vs. 75% between 2010 and 2013), mirroring a rise in admissions for prescription opioid and heroin use disorders among young adults in these three states [9]. The escalating incidence of acute HBV in the 30- to 49-year age group may reflect susceptibility due to a lack of inclusion in routine or catch-up HBV vaccination and a growing engagement in risky behaviors. Outbreaks are reported in other states, with Massachusetts reporting a 78% increase in acute HBV cases in 2017 and North Carolina seeing a 56% increase between 2014 and 2016 [19], highlighting the need for broader vaccination efforts.

Natural history studies reveal that ∼90% of adults with acute HBV infection will clear HBsAg within 3–6 months, but delayed clearance of up to 2 years has also been described [20–22]. In a prospective study of acute hepatitis from Europe (most reported sex as a risk factor), the median time to HBsAg clearance was 67 days (interquartile range [IQR], 32–132 days) and median time to hepatitis B surface antibody (anti-HBs) >10 IU/L was 109 days (IQR, 49–169.5 days) [21]. In another study from Japan, HBV genotype A was found to be associated with delayed clearance of HBsAg (mean, 6.7 vs. 3.4 months), with 23% clearing HBsAg 6 months after the onset of acute hepatitis [22]. By definition, chronic HBV infection means the presence of HBsAg for 6 months or more, but in the case of documented acute HBV infection, a longer period of follow-up may be needed to establish chronicity with certainty.

Resolved and occult hepatitis B

In the United States, approximately 3.9% of the population, an estimated 10.8 million individuals, has evidence of resolved HBV infection [23]. Resolved HBV infection is very common in PWID exposed in adulthood. This reflects the high rate (>95%) of spontaneous clearance of HBV infection after acute infection among healthy adults. Risk of HBV exposure increases with the length of IDU. Therefore resolved HBV infection can be found in as high as 95% of those with greater than 30 years of use [24]. Although resolved infection is generally regarded as benign, the presence of positive hepatitis B core antibody (anti-HBc) has been associated with 1.3-fold increased all-cause mortality in the United States, which may be attributable to coexisting high-risk behaviors rather than liver-related complications [25]. However, reactivation of HBV infection (reversion to HBsAg positivity or reappearance of HBV DNA) in the setting of immunosuppression is an important risk in those with resolved hepatitis B. The risk not only is highest (>10%) with the use of anti-CD20 therapy (i.e., rituximab, ocrelizumab) and hematopoietic stem cell transplantation but also exists with exposure to cytotoxic chemotherapy, biologics, and high-dose corticosteroid therapy (1%–10%) [26].

Occult HBV infection is defined as absent serum HBsAg, but presence of serum anti-HBc and detectable HBV DNA, albeit in very low concentrations. Theories for lack of circulating HBsAg include gene mutations that lead to HBsAg nondetectability and, more likely, robust immune control of virus leading to low HBV replication. High prevalence of this form of HBV infection has been reported among PWID, although prevalence measures are dependent on the sensitivity (lower limit of detection [LLD]) of the assay used. Among 188 HCV-positive PWID in Baltimore, Maryland, HBV DNA was detected in 45% using an enhanced PCR assay (LLD 15 copies/mL) compared with 0% when using an older COBAS PCR assay (LLD 200 copies/mL) [27]. In another study from Taiwan, 41% of 301 HBsAg-negative PWID had positive results for serum HBV DNA (mean, 4.0 log copies/mL) [28]. No mutations were found in 20 randomly selected samples. In both studies, occult infection was associated with older age, likely a reflection of duration of IDU and cumulative HBV exposure. While treatment is not indicated, occult infection has been linked to infrequent events of HBV transmission, fibrosis progression (particularly with HCV coinfection), HCC, and reactivation [29].

Chronic hepatitis B

Current US estimates of HBV-infected individuals range from 0.8 to 2.2 million, many of whom are immigrants from endemic regions of Asia and sub-Saharan Africa [30]. The seroprevalence of chronic HBV infection (positive HBsAg) has been relatively stable over the past two decades among US adults at 0.3%, based on the National Health and Nutrition Examination Survey (NHANES), although likely an underestimate because of the exclusion of military, incarcerated, and homeless population from sampling [23]. Population-based estimates of HBV prevalence among self-reported PWID in NHANES are not available and other estimates of

HBsAg seroprevalence among PWID have ranged from 3.5% to 20%, attributable to the study design (i.e., convenience sampling, recruitment site) and cohort differences [31]. The higher prevalence of resolved versus chronic infection reflects the considerable burden of HBV exposure coupled with a high likelihood of clearance.

Data suggest that the trend in HBV exposure over time among PWID has largely declined. The proportion of anti-HBc-positive cases in cross-sectional sampling of IDU individuals in the Urban Health Study in San Francisco decreased from 68% in 1987 to 45% between 1998 and 2000 [24]. Increased uptake of HBV vaccination is one explanation, as only 1% had serologic evidence of vaccination in the early period compared with 12% in the later period. Similarly, in a cross-sectional sampling of PWID residing in Seattle, anti-HBc prevalence declined from 43% to 15% between 1994 and 2004, with coexisting increases seen in self-reported needle-exchange use, condom use, and vaccination uptake [32].

HBV-related mortality

About 1800 individuals die from the sequelae of chronic HBV infection yearly in the United States, including HCC and complications of cirrhosis [33]. Mortality rates are much higher among those with opioid use disorders and IDU than the general population; most commonly early deaths are from drug overdose, suicide, traumatic injuries, and complications of HIV [34]. The risk of liver-related mortality is estimated to be 17-fold higher among PWID as compared with the general population. Viral hepatitis accounts for three-quarters of those who die from liver disease, with chronic alcohol use contributing in up to 40% [35]. Historically, the impact of HBV infection on life expectancy among IDU individuals was much less than that of chronic HCV infection [35]. But the long latency of viral hepatitis means liver disease has emerged as a major contributor to mortality only as opiate-dependent populations have aged, particularly as life expectancy with HIV infection has lengthened with improved therapies. In a large Australian cohort of PWID, liver disease was the underlying cause of or contributed to 17% of deaths over 30 years; there was a clear uptrend over time, with 0 deaths per 1000 person-years between 1980 and 1984 to 5 deaths per 1000 person-years between 2005 and 2006, overtaking death rates from overdose [36] (Fig. 7.4).

Hepatitis B and other coinfections in persons who inject drugs

Coinfection with HIV, HCV, and/or HDV is frequently encountered among those with opioid use disorders because of the shared means of transmission. Age at first injection, incarceration, men who have sex with men (MSM), and greater number of lifetime partners have all been identified as risk factors for coinfection [13,37]. The interplay of viral dynamics in those with coinfection can have significant bearing on clinical outcomes, most notably the risk of cirrhosis, HCC, and liver-related mortality.

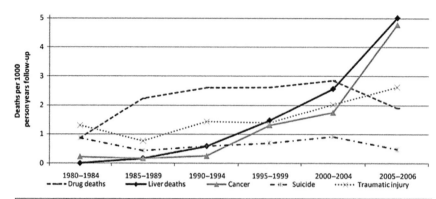

	1980–1984 deaths per 1000 PY (95% CI)	1985–1989 deaths per 1000 PY (95% CI)	1990–1994 deaths per 1000 PY (95% CI)	1995–1999 deaths per 1000 PY (95% CI)	2000–2004 deaths per 1000 PY (95% CI)	2005–2006 deaths per 1000 PY (95% CI)
Drug induced	0.87(0.24–2.22)	2.23(1.46–3.27)	2.61(1.77–3.71)	2.62(1.77–3.74)	2.85(1.93–4.00)	1.91(0.83–3.77)
Liver related	0.0(0.00–0.02)	0.17(0.02–0.62)	0.59(0.24–1.21)	1.48(0.86–2.38)	2.57(1.71–3.72)	5.02(3.11–7.68)
Cancer	0.22(0.01–1.21)	0.17(0.02–0.62)	0.25(0.05	1.31(0.73–2.16)	1.75(1.05–2.73)	4.78(2.92–7.39)
Suicide	0.87(0.24–2.22)	0.43(0.14–1.00)	0.59(0.24–1.21)	0.7(0.30–1.38)	0.92(0.44–1.69)	0.48(0.06–1.73)
Traumatic injury	1.3(0.48–2.83)	0.77(0.35–1.47)	1.43(0.83–2.29)	1.4(0.80–2.27)	2.02(1.27–3.06)	2.63(1.31–4.71)

FIGURE 7.4 Trends in Mortality Among Persons Who Inject Drugs (PWID).

In a large Australian cohort of PWID, liver disease was the underlying cause of or contributed to 17% of deaths over 30 years with an upward trend evident over time. This encompasses liver disease from all causes, including chronic viral hepatitis (hepatitis C virus and hepatitis B virus). *CI*, confidence interval; *PY*, person-years.

Source: Mathers BM, Degenhardt L, Bucello C, et al. Mortality among people who inject drugs: a systematic review and meta-analysis. Bull World Health Organ 2013;91:102–123.

Human immunodeficiency virus

HBV screening is recommended in all HIV-infected persons, and all PWID and MSM who are HBsAg-positive should be tested for HIV [4]. Among HIV-infected cohorts, rates of coinfection with HBV can be as high as 20% in endemic regions compared with 5%–8% in nonendemic regions, related to the age of exposure and likelihood of chronicity [14,38]. In nonendemic regions, HBV infection may precede HIV infection because of the more efficient transmission of HBV. MSM are a much stronger determinant of HBV infection risk than IDU among HIV-infected adults in nonendemic regions [39]. In comparison, IDU accounts for most cases of HCV/HIV coinfection. Concurrent HIV infection influences the natural history of HBV infection: those with lower CD4 counts are more likely to develop chronic infection after exposure, experience HBV reactivation, and develop cirrhosis and HCC [14]. Conversely, HBV infection appears to have little impact on HIV natural history, with no differences seen in progression to AIDS and response to antiretroviral therapy between HIV monoinfected and HIV/HBV coinfected persons [40]. Among HIV-infected PWID, HIV care models provide an ideal opportunity to integrate HBV testing, vaccination, and treatment.

Hepatitis C virus

Over 60% of HCV-infected adults in the United States have evidence of prior HBV infection while dual infection with chronic HBV is present in 6% [41]. In one study performed in New York City, the strongest predictors of coinfection were Asian race, IDU, and the number of lifetime sexual partners. PWID were eight times more likely to have HBV/HCV coinfection than those who did not report IDU [41] and simultaneous acute infection is more common [42]. Dual infection with HBV and HCV substantially increases the rates of liver disease progression compared with monoinfection with either virus [43,44]. Coexisting HCV infection appears to induce suppression of HBV replication, but the specific mechanism underlying this phenomenon is still unknown. The complex interaction between the two viruses is evident in the context of HCV therapy where HBV reactivation has been reported during and after HCV treatment, leading to guideline recommendations to screen for HBsAg before the initiation of HCV direct-acting antivirals (DAAs) [4,45].

Hepatitis D virus

Unlike HIV and HCV, HDV is unique in that it requires HBV proteins for viral assembly and proliferation within a human host. HDV can be acquired either at the same time as HBV (acute coinfection) or in a host with established chronic HBV infection (superinfection). Acute superinfection carries an increased risk of acute liver failure and can be mistaken for an HBV flare. In about half of patients, HBV DNA levels are low when HDV RNA levels are high; thus the index of suspicion for HDV should be high when ALT levels are elevated despite a low level of HBV DNA [46]. The estimate of HDV-infected persons in the United States ranges from 3% to 12%, with the accuracy of estimates limited by the relatively low uptake of testing in clinical settings [47,48]. However, much higher rates of HBV/HDV coinfection in the United States have been detected among PWID, ranging from 36% to 50% [49,50], which is comparable to rates in HDV-endemic regions such as Central Africa and Mongolia [51]. The combination of HBV and HDV results in the most rapidly progressive form of hepatitis, with progression to cirrhosis within 2 years in 10%−15% of affected individuals and a threefold higher risk of HCC [51]. The high prevalence of HDV among PWID and worse prognosis reinforce the need to screen for HDV infection among all HBsAg-positive persons.

Hepatitis B virus screening and diagnosis
Awareness and knowledge

Awareness of hepatitis B infection among PWID is glaringly low. Less than 40% of the adult US population are aware of their HBV infection and this percentage drops to 15% among PWID [52,53]. Concordance between self-reported and serologic evidence of HBV status, including immunization status, is very poor and self-report should not be relied on for estimates of disease burden or clinical decision-making. Between 46% and 95% of PWID without self-report of HBV infection had serologic evidence of exposure [54]. Furthermore, knowledge regarding HBV transmission and risk factors is lacking. Among 493 inner-city PWID, only one-third were aware that there was no cure for HBV infection and 55% were aware that a vaccine was available [55]. In comparison, over 85% knew there was no cure and no vaccine for HIV infection—a marker of the success of numerous HIV prevention programs that have been implemented in high-risk populations. In another survey of participants in a syringe exchange program, only 49% were aware HBV was transmitted through sharing needles despite 33% reporting testing positive for HBV [56]. Increased knowledge on hepatitis was associated with known infection, substance abuse treatment, and less risky injection behaviors, suggesting good retention of knowledge after engagement with hepatitis-related healthcare systems and providers. With the rising burden of IDU in nonurban settings, a study found that PWID in urban (vs. nonurban) areas were not more knowledgeable despite increased access to harm reduction services [57]. While most implementation studies in PWID have focused on the integration of HCV-specific patient education and testing into opiate substitution and drug treatment programs, these measures would likely produce similar success in boosting HBV awareness, testing, and vaccination (when appropriate) among PWID.

Screening

The initial test to screen for infection is a qualitative HBsAg test. In PWID, total anti-HBc and anti-HBs should also be tested at initial screening to determine past exposure and immune status, respectively. The gold standard test for HBsAg is a laboratory-based enzyme-linked immunoassay, which may not be ideal for those with opioid use disorders, who for many reasons may be unable or unwilling to follow-up on testing results.

Point-of-care (POC) tests are valuable alternatives in these populations, whereby results can be divulged at the time of testing and where convenient for the patient [58]. For HBV in particular, POC testing for immunity is of equal significance to diagnosis, as subsequent delivery of vaccine has benefits. Currently, POC immunologic rapid diagnostic tests (high sensitivity and specificity in research studies) for HBV have yet to be approved by the US Food and Drug Administration (FDA) and are not clinically available. Capillary whole-blood dried blood spot (DBS) testing is an alternate test increasingly utilized in resource-limited settings because it allows for multiple tests to be performed on a single sample, enables easy collection (important for persons with difficult venous access) and transportation of samples, and has good test characteristics. The disadvantage of DBS testing is that it is not a POC test; that is, results are not immediate and a second consultation is still required for decision-making.

Diagnosis

Diagnosis is made on the basis of serologic markers of infection (Table 7.1). If concern for acute infection exists (marked serum aminotransferase level elevation), the serologic test for diagnosis is a positive IgM-specific anti-HBc. Chronic infection is characterized by the persistence of HBsAg for at least 6 months. Those with a positive anti-HBc and anti-HBs with negative HBsAg have spontaneously cleared the infection and are immune. An isolated positive anti-HBc can represent occult infection (positive HBV DNA), resolved infection (either spontaneously or with treatment) with waned anti-HBs titers (negative HBV DNA), or a false-positive result, although the latter is very unlikely in PWID. Those with negative HBsAg and anti-HBc but positive anti-HBs are vaccinated, with anti-HBs titers ≥10 IU/L, signifying adequate immunity.

Testing for hepatitis B e-antigen (HBeAg) and hepatitis B e-antibody (anti-HBe) helps determine the phase of infection and the level of HBV DNA at which treatment should be initiated (see the section Treatment of hepatitis B). Serial measurements of HBV DNA and ALT levels (performed typically every 3—6 months for the first year)

Table 7.1 Serologic markers of HBV infection.

HBsAg	Anti-HBc IgM	Anti-HBc total	Anti-HBs	Interpretation	Comment
−	−	−	−	Never infected	
−	−	−	+	Vaccinated	Immune if anti-HBs titers ≥10 IU/L
+/−	+	−	−	Acute infection	Can be anti-HBc positive only during window period
+	−	+	−	Chronic infection	HBsAg positive for at least 6 months
−	−	+	+/−	Resolved infection	Anti-HBs can be negative with waned titers Also seen with spontaneous or treatment-induced HBsAg loss in chronically infected people
−	−	+	−	Occult infection	Occult if low-level HBV DNA is detected May also be a false-positive result, particularly among individuals without risk factors Also seen with spontaneous or treatment-induced HBsAg loss without anti-HBs seroconversion

Anti-HBc, *hepatitis B core antibody;* anti-HBs, *hepatitis B surface antibody;* HBsAg, *hepatitis B surface antigen;* HBV, *hepatitis B virus.*

are frequently necessary to establish the baseline phase of infection because of the fluctuating nature of HBV infection. Additional HBV studies such as HBV genotype and testing for the presence of HBV mutations are not recommended in routine clinical practice. Testing for coexisting HIV, HCV, and HDV infection should be performed. Although there is growing interest in the utility of quantitative HBsAg levels in classifying phase of infection, use of this serologic marker has not yet been standardized or incorporated into guidelines [58].

Prevention: Hepatitis B virus vaccination

Safe and highly effective vaccines are available for HBV. The HBV vaccine, consisting of highly purified HBsAg protein, induces endogenous production of anti-HBs and stimulates memory T cells. There are three commercially available FDA-approved vaccines in the United States: Engerix-B (three doses; GlaxoSmithKline Biologicals), Recombivax HB (three doses; Merck & co), and Heplisav-B (two doses; Dynavax Technologies); the last vaccine was approved in 2017. Additionally, a three-dose combined hepatitis A virus/HBV vaccine, Twinrix (GlaxoSmithKline Biologicals), which includes the Engerix-B vaccine, is available (Table 7.2).

Among PWID, a substantial proportion remain susceptible to HBV infection. In a surveillance study of 2077 PWID in German cities, 43% were found to lack antibodies to HBV [52]. A seroprevalence study in San Diego yielded similar results, with 47% of the 517 PWID found to be HBV susceptible (anti-HBs <10 IU/mL) [59]. These results highlight the need for a broad application of HBV vaccination in this at-risk group and the perils of relying on self-report to determine the need for vaccination. Thus all PWID should undergo serologic testing for HBV immunity (unless a written record of vaccination or positive titers are available) and offered vaccination if not immune. The standard timing of the three-dose regimen is at 0, 1, and 6 months and the two-dose regimen is at 0 and 1 month. Clinicians should err toward vaccination if uncertainty regarding immunity exists. While not routine, confirmation of immunity with testing of anti-HBs titers can be considered 1−2 months after vaccination in all PWID, and is recommended if HIV-positive, due to the high risk of infection and the potential for lower vaccine efficacy. Modeling studies have shown that both HBV screening and vaccination are cost-effective in PWID in the United States [60].

Efficacy and safety of hepatitis B virus vaccines

Completion of HBV vaccination produces adequate lifelong antibody response (anti-HBs titers of ≥ 10 IU/L) in over 90% of healthy adults. Similar efficacy has been reported among the different three-dose formulations. The newer two-dose vaccine demonstrated comparable efficacy to traditional vaccines [61]. However, PWID are one distinct population in whom HBV vaccine response may be attenuated. Reported seroprotection rates among PWID have ranged between 55% and 97% [62].

Table 7.2 Comparison of FDA-approved hepatitis B virus vaccines.

Vaccine	Dose	Schedule	Efficacy[c]	Adverse effects
Hepatitis B				
Engerix-B (GSK)	Birth to 19 yrs: 0.5 mL IM ≥20 yrs: 1 mL IM[a,b]	3 doses (0, 1, and 6 mos)	88%—96%	Injection-site soreness (22%) and fatigue (14%)
Recombivax HB (Merck)	Birth to 19 yrs: 0.5 mL IM ≥20 yrs: 1 mL IM[a,b]	3 doses (0, 1, and 6 mos)	96%	Injection-site reactions (18%) and systemic adverse reactions (15%)
Heplisav-B (Dynavax)	≥18 yrs: 0.5 mL IM	2 doses (0 and 1 mo)	96%	Injection-site pain (23%—39%), fatigue (11%—17%), and headache (8%—17%)
Hepatitis A/B				
Twinrix (GSK)	≥18 yrs: 0.5 mL IM	3 doses (0, 1, and 6 mos)	98.5%	Injection-site soreness (35%—41%), redness (8%—11%), headache (13%—22%), and fatigue (11%—14%)

IM, *intramuscular.*
[a] *Can be administered subcutaneously in those at risk of hemorrhage with lower efficacy.*
[b] *Alternate (higher) dosing available for patients on hemodialysis and can also be considered in immunocompromised patients.*
[c] *In adult populations (aged 18 years or more).*

Nonstandardized timing of anti-HBs measurement may impact estimates, with highest rates seen when testing for anti-HBs is performed 2 months following the third dose (peak of immune response) [62]. Older age, active drug use, and coinfection, including HIV infection, have been linked with lower responses in individual studies. Safety concerns regarding the HBV vaccine are minimal. Anaphylaxis is extremely rare, estimated at 1 per 1.1 million doses [63]. Although various conditions have been reported (i.e., Guillain-Barré syndrome, alopecia, multiple sclerosis, and other neurologic disorders), no causal link between these conditions and the vaccine has been established.

Vaccine uptake and adherence

While willingness to receive HBV vaccination is high among those with opioid use disorders [64], barriers such as inconvenience, lack of perceived benefits, and the number of injections contribute to persistently inadequate rates of vaccination coverage. A population-based study demonstrated that while unvaccinated status decreased overall among US adults at high risk for HBV infection between 2003−04 and 2013−14 (83.2%−69.4%), no significant change was seen over time among those who reported IDU (80% unvaccinated) [65]. Consistent with this finding, across heterogeneous PWID communities that have been sampled over time, evidence of immunity is seen in less than 30% [11,66,67]. Higher rates are found in women, younger individuals, higher levels of education, and those with greater contact with healthcare personnel, such as HIV-infected and opiate substitution therapy users [65−68]. Adherence to a multidose regimen is an additional obstacle. Studies have shown an approximate 20% drop-off with each additional dose of the vaccine, with completion rates as high as 60% and as low as 9% [69−71].

Strategies to improve hepatitis B virus vaccination rates among persons who inject drugs

Various strategies exist and should be employed to combat challenges in vaccine efficacy, the uptake of HBV vaccine, and adherence to vaccination schedule among PWID. Consensus recommendations from the WHO on enhancing vaccine uptake and efficacy among PWID have been published [72]. Opportunities to vaccinate PWID are few: prioritizing delivery of the first dose without assurance of completion and vaccinating without the knowledge of immune status are suboptimal but sometimes necessary tactics.

There are two potential methods to counteract lower vaccine efficacy. One is administration of additional doses if titers are insufficient after the standard regimen, which leads to immunity in 25%−50% after one extra dose and in 44%−100% after three extra doses [63]. The other is administration of a higher- or double-dose vaccine, a strategy that has been well studied and efficacious in those with HIV infection. A trial in PWID that randomized participants in methadone maintenance therapy to either high- or low-dose vaccine with standard timing of administration demonstrated higher titers in the high-dose group but similar rates of seroconversion (∼70% at 1 year) with no increase in adverse events [73].

Convenience and accessibility are key to vaccine uptake. In a study of young adult PWID, vaccine uptake was highest when given immediately on-site and lowest when offered after receiving results [64]. Co-location of vaccine with services for PWID such as syringe exchange sites and drug treatment programs can also increase uptake [64,74,75]. Prisons can be expedient and practical locations for vaccine administration. In addition, financial incentives in the form of modest sums of money or vouchers increase vaccine uptake as well as completion [71,76]. Both co-delivery of vaccine with syringe exchange programs and contingency management through monetary incentives have been demonstrated to be cost-effective and even cost-saving strategies in PWID [77,78].

Lastly, adherence to multiple injections can be boosted through a rapid or accelerated vaccination schedule. Accelerated schedules (at 0, 1, and 2 months) result in noninferior seroprotection rates in active drug users compared to standard regimens

[79,80]. Long-term effectiveness characterized by a decline in anti-HBs titers is also similar [81]. Furthermore, studies have shown that accelerated regimens directly lead to higher rates of vaccine completion [82]. The recently approved two-dose vaccine, Heplisav-B (Dynavax Technologies), given at 0 and 1 month is well suited for PWID in whom rapid achievement of protective anti-HBs titers is desired.

Treatment of hepatitis B
Acute hepatitis B

Approximately one in three patients with acute hepatitis B will be symptomatic, with the proportion higher in older than younger adults [83]. Symptoms are primarily fatigue, anorexia, nausea, and mild right upper quadrant discomfort. Aminotransferase levels are typically greater than five times the upper limits of normal (>200 U/L) but can be above 1000 U/L. The severity of hepatitis is influenced by the size of the infectious inoculum, viral genotype and mutations, and the robustness of the immune response [84]. Serial monitoring of aspartate transaminase and ALT levels as well as markers of liver function (prothrombin time and total bilirubin) is essential to guide management (Table 7.3). HBV DNA levels can be used to gauge

Table 7.3 Elements of management of acute hepatitis B.

Management strategy	Specifics
Establish diagnosis	HBsAg positive, anti-HBc IgM positive, HBV DNA positive Assess for concurrent viral infections: anti-HIV, anti-HCV, and anti-HDV
Serial monitoring of AST/ALT levels and liver function tests (bilirubin and INR)	Frequency is determined by severity: From weekly to daily If bilirubin or INR increased above normal, frequency of monitoring should be increased
Clinical management of symptoms	Fluids/hydration Bed rest as needed
Avoidance of other hepatotoxic substances	Minimize the use of acetaminophen Avoid alcohol
Assessment for extrahepatic manifestations	Renal panel, complete blood count, physical examination
If severe or protracted course	Start antiviral therapy with entecavir or tenofovir
If severe hepatitis with evidence of acute liver failure with hepatic encephalopathy, ascites, or rising INR or bilirubin	Hospitalize and determine if liver transplant is an option Consider the use of N-acetylcysteine

ALT, *alanine aminotransferase;* Anti-HBc, *hepatitis B core antibody;* AST, *aspartate aminotransferase;* HBsAg, *hepatitis B surface antigen;* HBV, *hepatitis B virus;* HCV, *hepatitis C virus;* HDV, *hepatitis delta virus;* HIV, *human immunodeficiency virus;* INR, *international normalized ratio.*

evolution of the acute infection but are of limited prognostic value. The severity of hepatitis is correlated with the likelihood of spontaneous resolution of the acute infection; those who are symptomatic and with more marked elevation of bilirubin and/or prothrombin time are most likely to achieve spontaneous clearance and HBV immunity (HBsAg loss, anti-HBs acquisition). On the other hand, patients with more severe hepatitis are also at the highest risk of acute liver failure.

For most patients with acute hepatitis B without signs of acute liver failure, hospitalization is not necessary and treatment is not indicated. Severe hepatitis, manifested by marked elevation of bilirubin or any elevation of prothrombin time, should prompt initiation of antiviral therapy and close monitoring, typically in a hospital setting. Treatment with antiviral therapy is recommended in this setting [4]; however, data to support benefit are lacking [85]. For persons who are eligible for liver transplantation, antiviral therapy prior to transplant reduces the risk of recurrent HBV infection after transplant. Although liver transplantation is an effective treatment with over 80% 5-year survival, for those with opioid use disorder, access to liver transplantation is likely to be limited because substance abuse disorders are a common exclusion criteria for liver transplantation at US centers. Thus for many opioid drug users, management of acute liver failure with supportive care and adjuvant therapies, such as *N*-acetylcysteine, is recommended [86].

Elimination of other causes of liver injury during an acute infection is crucial. In a case-control study of an outbreak of acute hepatitis B among IDU individuals in the United States, higher mortality was associated with the use of alcohol, methamphetamines, and acetaminophen during their illness [16]. Extrahepatic manifestations are rare but reported, involving the kidney, joints, skin, and bone marrow. The presence of extrahepatic complications should prompt immediate initiation of antiviral therapy. For most patients with acute hepatitis B, antiviral therapy is not indicated.

If treatment is necessary, the preferred oral drugs are entecavir (ETV) or tenofovir disoproxil fumarate (TDF) or tenofovir alafenamide (TAF). Peginterferon should not be used. Once antiviral treatment is started, it should be continued until HBsAg is lost and anti-HBs >10 IU/L present. For those who do not clear HBsAg, the duration of antiviral therapy should be guided by the same rules as persons with chronic hepatitis B (see later discussion).

Given the safety and efficacy of current oral antivirals, ETV, TDF, and TAF, one must wonder why treatment of all persons with acute HBV infection is not recommended. There are two primary reasons. First, there are no data that show that antiviral therapy improves the outcomes of acute infection. Most will resolve spontaneously without treatment, so unnecessary treatment exposure is avoided. A systematic review with attempted network analysis found no evidence that antiviral therapy was a benefit, but acknowledged that study quality was poor [87]. Second, there is a mild concern that antiviral therapy may do harm by modifying the immune response to the virus and reducing the likelihood of spontaneous resolution. In a prospective randomized, placebo-controlled trial of patients with severe acute hepatitis B treated with lamivudine versus placebo, 67.7% treated with lamivudine versus

85% of placebo-treated patients had protective anti-HBs titers after 1 year ($P = .096$) [88]. In a systematic review and network analysis, the proportion of patients who evolved to chronic HBV infection was higher in lamivudine-treated than in untreated patients (odds ratio [OR] 1.99; 95% confidence interval [CI], 1.05−3.77) but not between ETV-administered and untreated patients (OR 0.58; 95% CI, 0.23−1.49) [87]. However, limitations of the network analysis include a modest number of treated patients, heterogeneity in acute hepatitis severity, and other factors such as timing of treatment that may have influenced outcomes. Regardless, this lingering concern that antiviral therapy might reduce the likelihood of clearance of HBV contributes to the reluctance to recommend antiviral therapy for all acutely infected persons.

Chronic hepatitis B

General approach

As there are no curative therapies for patients with chronic hepatitis B, management requires serial monitoring to determine if and when antiviral therapy is required. The goals of therapy are to prevent progression of liver disease and the complications of cirrhosis and liver cancer.

There are four preferred therapies, peginterferon and three oral drugs: ETV, TDF, and TAF [4]. The side effects associated with peginterferon make this a less appealing drug for providers and patients alike, although it does have the advantage of being of finite duration. The three nucleos(t)ide analogues (NAs) offer excellent safety and tolerability and a high genetic barrier to resistance; selecting one drug over another is dependent on HBV treatment history, the presence of coinfection with HIV, pregnancy status, and the presence of renal and bone diseases (Table 7.4). NAs are safe to use in patients with cirrhosis, including those with decompensation.

Staging of liver disease is important − both to determine the need for antiviral therapy and the need for HCC surveillance. All persons with cirrhosis are recommended to be on lifelong antiviral therapy and to undergo surveillance for HCC [4]. Screening for liver cancer extends to other groups at high risk for HCC in the absence of cirrhosis. Asian-American men aged >40 years, Asian-American women aged >50 years, and African-Americans aged >40 years, as well as those with HDV coinfection (any age), should undergo screening [4]. Recommended HCC surveillance is with ultrasonography and α-fetoprotein testing every 6 months.

Liver biopsy is rarely used to evaluate the stage of the disease; typically, it is reserved for scenarios where a coexisting liver condition is suspected (e.g., nonalcoholic fatty liver). Routine laboratory tests can serve to rule out cirrhosis; additionally, transient elastography is increasingly available and useful in measuring liver stiffness, which correlates with hepatic fibrosis severity (Table 7.5). Most adults who acquired HBV infection via IDU or sex will not have cirrhosis until after several decades of chronic infection, unless other cofactors for liver injury, such as alcohol or HCV, are present. Nonetheless, as PWID may have several concurrent risks for liver disease, periodic assessment of liver fibrosis stage using noninvasive methods is prudent.

Table 7.4 Treatment options for patients with chronic hepatitis B.

	Peginterferon	Entecavir	TDF	TAF
Route	Subcutaneous	Oral	Oral	Oral
Dose	α2a: 180 µg/wk α2b: 1.5 mg/ kg/wk	0.5 mg daily (adjust if CrCl <50)	300 mg daily (adjust if CrCl <50)	25 mg daily (adjust if CrCl <15)
Coexisting conditions				
Pregnancy	−	−	+	−
HIV infection	+	−[a]	+	+
Renal disease	+	+	−	+
Osteoporosis	+	+	−	+
HBV-related factors				
Prior lamivudine exposure	+	−	+	+
Cirrhosis	−	+	+	+
Decompensation	−	+	+	+

HBV, *hepatitis B virus;* HIV, *human immunodeficiency virus;* TAF, *tenofovir alafenamide;* TDF, *tenofovir disoproxil fumarate.*
[a] *Unless on fully suppressive antiretroviral therapy.*

Table 7.5 Recommended initial and follow-up assessments of patients with chronic hepatitis B and not on treatment.

	Initial	Follow-up
Laboratory tests	CBC, liver and renal panel, HBsAg, HBeAg/Ab, HBV DNA Anti-HCV, anti-HDV, anti-HIV	AST/ALT, every 3–6 months HBV DNA, every 3–6 months ■ reduce frequency to every 6–12 months if normal ALT and HBV DNA <2000 IU/mL Repeat HCV, HDV, and HIV if there is concern for new exposure
Staging of liver fibrosis	APRI[a] or FIB-4[a] Transient elastography	
Others	HBV genotype HAV total/IgG Ultrasonography of the abdomen AFP	Ultrasonography and AFP every 6 months in case of the following: ■ Cirrhosis ■ Asian American, aged >40 years if men and aged >50 years if women ■ African-American men aged >40 years ■ HDV coinfection

AFP, *α-fetoprotein;* ALT, *alanine aminotransferase;* Anti-HBc, *hepatitis B core antibody;* APRI, *AST-to-platelet ratio index;* AST, *aspartate aminotransferase;* CBC, *complete blood count;* FIB-4, *fibrosis-4;* HAV, *hepatitis A virus;* HBeAg/Ab, *hepatitis B e-antigen/antibody;* HBsAg, *hepatitis B surface antigen;* HBV, *hepatitis B virus;* HCV, *hepatitis C virus;* HDV, *hepatitis delta virus;* HIV, *human immunodeficiency virus.*
[a] *https://www.mdcalc.com.*

When to start and when to stop treatment

The patients targeted for chronic hepatitis B treatment are those with "active" inflammation and injury of the liver, as these individuals are at risk for progression to cirrhosis and liver failure [4]. Active disease is defined by ALT level elevation (typically twice the upper limits of normal) in conjunction with HBV DNA above 2000 IU/mL if HBeAg negative and above 20,000 IU/mL if HBeAg positive. Thus by measuring HBeAg, HBV DNA, and ALT levels, decisions regarding the need for treatment can be made. If a patient's ALT or HBV DNA levels do not meet the thresholds for treatment, serial follow-up of ALT and HBV DNA levels at 3- to 6-month intervals is recommended to detect elevations that might lead to future treatment. Once treatment starts, monitoring of HBV DNA every 6 months is necessary to monitor for adherence and in the case of nonadherence, to monitor the emergence of HBV resistance. Of note, repeat testing for HCV, HDV, and HIV may be warranted annually in those engaged in at-risk behaviors (sex or IDU).

Nonspecialists caring for patients with chronic HBV may consider using a more simplified algorithm (Fig. 7.5). Baseline testing to exclude other viral coinfections is

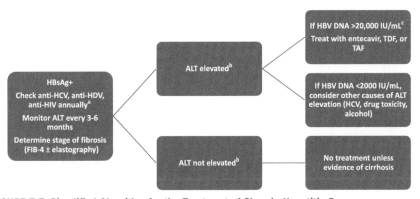

FIGURE 7.5 Simplified Algorithm for the Treatment of Chronic Hepatitis B.

At initial evaluation, all hepatitis B surface antigen (HBsAg)-positive patients with opioid use disorder should undergo hepatitis B e-antigen (HBeAg), anti-HCV, anti-HDV, anti-HIV, and HBV DNA testing to guide subsequent management. Additionally, the stage of liver disease needs to be determined, as all patients with cirrhosis are recommended to be on long-term antiviral therapy. For those without cirrhosis, monitoring of alanine aminotransferase (ALT) levels at initial presentation and every 3–6 months is a simple means to determine when antiviral therapy is needed. For those with elevated ALT levels (typically >60 U/mL for women and >70 U/L for men), the HBV DNA level should be checked to confirm >2000 IU/mL. If both ALT and HBV DNA levels are elevated above these thresholds, antiviral therapy is indicated. It is also useful to perform repeat HBeAg testing at the time of starting antiviral therapy. *FIB-4*, fibrosis 4; *HBV*, hepatitis B virus; *HCV*, hepatitis C virus; *HDV*, hepatitis delta virus; *TAF*, tenofovir alafenamide; *TDF*, tenofovir disoproxil fumarate. [a]If ongoing risk behaviors present. [b]Normal ALT ranges from 19 to 25 U/L for men and 25 to 35 UL for men. [c]If HBV DNA <20,000 but >2000 IU/mL, then consider treatment if HBeAg negative.

performed in addition to ALT and HBV DNA measurement. Thereafter monitoring can rely on ALT alone, as this will trigger the need to evaluate HBV DNA and HBeAg to see if treatment criteria are met.

As highlighted previously, all patients with cirrhosis should be treated with antiviral therapy regardless of ALT or HBV DNA levels and treated indefinitely [4]. For patients without cirrhosis on treatment, the duration of therapy is dependent on HBeAg status. For those who are HBeAg negative at treatment start, treatment should be continued until HBsAg loss occurs. In contrast, for patients who are HBeAg positive at the start of therapy, treatment is continued until HBeAg is lost and anti-HBe gained (seroconversion) and then for at least an additional year (consolidation phase) before stopping. Although virologic relapse may occur after discontinuation of antiviral therapy, the likelihood of relapse in patients who seroconvert from HBeAg to anti-HBe on antiviral therapy is low if they are under the age of 40 years and have completed at least a year of consolidation therapy. Monitoring for relapse after treatment discontinuation is necessary; retreatment may be needed.

Resistance to HBV therapy is infrequent when current preferred therapies are used: ETV, TDF, and TAF. For patients with a history of HBV treatment, whether known or unknown, TDF or TAF should be used rather than ETV because of the concern that prior lamivudine exposure increases the risk of resistance to ETV. Resistance to ETV in treatment-naïve patients is only 1% after 5 years, but in case of prior lamivudine exposure, resistance to ETV at 5 years reaches 50% [89]. Resistance to TDF and TAF is extremely rare [90].

Treatment of hepatitis B virus infection in pregnancy

There are unique management issues that arise for HBsAg-positive women during pregnancy. Preventing mother-to-child transmission of HBV is critically important and the provision of hepatitis B immunoglobulin and HBV vaccination within hours of birth is highly effective in preventing transmission [91]. However, even with prophylaxis of the newborn, HBV transmission can occur if the mother's level of HBV DNA is high during the last trimester of pregnancy [4]. For this reason, all women are recommended to be tested for HBsAg in pregnancy and if positive, HBV DNA should be measured in the second trimester. Those mothers with HBV DNA levels >200,000 IU/mL should be treated with TDF, starting at week 28 of gestation and continued until delivery. The combination of antiviral therapy of mothers with high viremia coupled with hepatitis B immunoglobulin administration and vaccine prophylaxis of the infants provides the highest level of protection against perinatal transmission of HBV, with studies showing a reduction in transmission rate from 7% to 0% [92].

Pregnancy can be the first time when women are diagnosed with hepatitis B, so this represents a unique opportunity to engage women in longitudinal care for their chronic viral infection. Studies have highlighted the gaps in care following a pregnancy diagnosis of hepatitis. Using claims data from 2011 to 2014, 1190 pregnancies were associated with a new HBV diagnosis, but only 42% received HBV-directed care either before or after delivery [93]. Insuring that women diagnosed with HBV during pregnancy receive ongoing management post partum is an essential step in improving the HBV cascade of care.

Treatment of hepatitis B infection in patients with other viral infections (HIV, HCV, and HDV)

The presence of viral coinfections increases the complexity of managing chronic hepatitis B.

For HBV patients with HIV, treatment of HIV should be initiated as soon as the diagnosis is made and an antiretroviral regimen should be used that includes tenofovir plus lamivudine or emtricitabine, as these drugs have activity against HIV and HBV [94]. HBV DNA levels should be checked at baseline, although the levels of HBV DNA or ALT are not used to determine if treatment is given. All HIV patients with HBV should be on long-term suppressive therapy. In the rare patient who cannot be on a TDF or TAF plus lamivudine or emtricitabine backbone, the other option is to use ETV for treatment of HBV infection, but because ETV does have HIV activity, it should only be used in patients who are on a fully suppressive antiretroviral therapy regimen.

All HBsAg-positive patients with confirmed HCV viremia should undergo treatment with HCV DAAs [95]. The approach to HCV management in coinfected patients is similar to patients with HCV monoinfection in terms of the need for pretreatment staging of fibrosis and genotype to guide the specific drugs chosen and the duration of treatment. Availability of pangenotypic DAA regimens eliminates the need for genotype testing, but staging to assess for the presence versus absence of advanced fibrosis/cirrhosis is required. Additionally, as clearance of HCV with therapy can lead to reactivation of HBV infection, assessment of HBV DNA levels prior to and at the end of treatment is needed. If HBV DNA is quantifiable before treatment, it is prudent to start HBV therapy concurrent with HCV DAA therapy to minimize the risk of HBV reactivation. If HBV DNA level is undetectable at baseline, monitoring is recommended at the end of treatment and at SVR 12 (sustained virologic response at week 12 post-treatment) to assess for HBV reactivation (reappearance and progressive rise in HBV DNA levels) and the need for HBV therapy.

HDV infection occurs only in HBsAg-positive patients and is a challenging coinfection to manage because of the lack of effective therapies. Peginterferon has a modest effect in normalizing ALT levels and reducing HDV RNA levels, but relapse after treatment discontinuation is high. Additionally, tolerability of peginterferon is difficult, especially because treatment is typically given in 12 months' duration. Newer drugs that specifically target HDV entry and replication are under development. Patients with HDV infection are at higher risk of cirrhosis and liver cancer, and it is recommended that all patients with HDV infection undergo surveillance of liver cancer with ultrasonography with or without α-fetoprotein levels every 6 months [4].

Additional considerations for treating hepatitis B virus infection in persons with opioid use disorders

First and foremost, PWID should be appropriately vaccinated in order to prevent HBV acquisition, particularly those within age groups born before recommendations for universal perinatal HBV vaccination were made. Awareness and knowledge regarding chronic hepatitis B is low among PWID, including persons with opioid use disorders. As knowledge is linked with readiness for treatment, there is need for consideration of how best to engage PWID for monitoring of disease and treatment, if needed. Unlike HCV infection, management is lifelong and not restricted to a finite treatment course. As the risk for resistance to anti-HBV therapy may be increased with poor adherence, assessment of willingness for treatment is important. Colocation of hepatitis and substance use treatment would be an important means of improving adherence and efficacy of HBV infection treatment.

References

[1] Ott JJ, Stevens GA, Groeger J, et al. Global epidemiology of hepatitis B virus infection: new estimates of age-specific HBsAg seroprevalence and endemicity. Vaccine 2012;30: 2212—9.

[2] Weinbaum CM, Mast EE, Ward JW. Recommendations for identification and public health management of persons with chronic hepatitis B virus infection. Hepatology 2009;49:S35—44.

[3] Hagan H, Des Jarlais D, Friedman S, et al. Reduced risk of hepatitis B and hepatitis C among injection drug users in the Tacoma syringe exchange program. Am J Public Health 1995;85.

[4] Terrault NA, Lok AS, McMahon BJ, et al. Update on prevention, diagnosis, and treatment and of chronic hepatitis B: AASLD 2018 hepatitis B guidance. Hepatology 2018; 67:1560—99.

[5] Di Bisceglie AM, Lombardero M, Teckman J, et al. Determination of hepatitis B phenotype using biochemical and serological markers. J Viral Hepat 2017;24:320—9.

[6] Zhou K, Contag C, Whitaker E, et al. Spontaneous loss of surface antigen among adults living with chronic hepatitis B virus infection: a systematic review and pooled meta-analyses. Lancet Gastroenterol Hepatol 2019;4:227—38.

[7] Degenhardt L, Peacock A, Colledge S, et al. Global prevalence of injecting drug use and sociodemographic characteristics and prevalence of HIV, HBV, and HCV in people who inject drugs: a multistage systematic review. Lancet Glob Health 2017;5:e1192—207.

[8] Edlich RF, Diallo AO, Buchanan L, et al. Hepatitis B virus: a comprehensive strategy for eliminating transmission in the United States. J Long Term Eff Med Implants 2003;13:117—25.

[9] Harris AM, Iqbal K, Schillie S, et al. Increases in acute hepatitis B virus infections - Kentucky, Tennessee, and West Virginia, 2006-2013. MMWR Morb Mortal Wkly Rep 2016;65:47—50.

[10] Seal KH, Ochoa KC, Hahn JA, et al. Risk of hepatitis B infection among young injection drug users in San Francisco: opportunities for intervention. West J Med 2000;172: 16—20.

[11] Kuo I, Sherman SG, Thomas DL, et al. Hepatitis B virus infection and vaccination among young injection and non-injection drug users: missed opportunities to prevent infection. Drug Alcohol Depend 2004;73:69—78.

[12] Smith JM, Uvin AZ, Macmadu A, et al. Epidemiology and treatment of hepatitis B in prisoners. Curr Hepatol Rep 2017;16:178—83.

[13] Reimer J, Lorenzen J, Baetz B, et al. Multiple viral hepatitis in injection drug users and associated risk factors. J Gastroenterol Hepatol 2007;22:80—5.

[14] Thio CL. Hepatitis B and human immunodeficiency virus coinfection. Hepatology 2009;49:S138—45.

[15] Schiodt FV, Davern TJ, Shakil AO, et al. Viral hepatitis-related acute liver failure. Am J Gastroenterol 2003;98:448—53.

[16] Garfein RS, Bower WA, Loney CM, et al. Factors associated with fulminant liver failure during an outbreak among injection drug users with acute hepatitis B. Hepatology 2004; 40:865—73.

[17] Vogt TM, Perz JF, Van Houten Jr CK, et al. An outbreak of hepatitis B virus infection among methamphetamine injectors: the role of sharing injection drug equipment. Addiction 2006;101:726—30.

[18] Iqbal K, Klevens RM, Kainer MA, et al. Epidemiology of acute hepatitis B in the United States from population-based surveillance, 2006-2011. Clin Infect Dis 2015;61: 584—92.

[19] https://www.hhs.gov/hepatitis/blog/2018/02/21/the-rise-in-acute-hepatitis-b-infection-in-the-us.html.

[20] Menzo S, Minosse C, Vincenti D, et al. Long-term follow-up of acute hepatitis B: new insights in its natural history and implications for antiviral treatment. Genes (Basel) 2018;9.

[21] Wiegand J, Wedemeyer H, Franke A, et al. Treatment of severe, nonfulminant acute hepatitis B with lamivudine vs placebo: a prospective randomized double-blinded multicentre trial. J Viral Hepat 2014;21:744—50.

[22] Ito K, Yotsuyanagi H, Yatsuhashi H, et al. Risk factors for long-term persistence of serum hepatitis B surface antigen following acute hepatitis B virus infection in Japanese adults. Hepatology 2014;59:89—97.

[23] Roberts H, Kruszon-Moran D, Ly KN, et al. Prevalence of chronic hepatitis B virus (HBV) infection in U.S. Households: National health and Nutrition Examination survey (NHANES), 1988-2012. Hepatology 2016;63:388—97.

[24] Tseng FC, O'Brien TR, Zhang M, et al. Seroprevalence of hepatitis C virus and hepatitis B virus among San Francisco injection drug users, 1998 to 2000. Hepatology 2007;46: 666—71.

[25] Jinjuvadia R, Liangpunsakul S, Antaki F. Past exposure to hepatitis B: a risk factor for increase in mortality? J Clin Gastroenterol 2014;48:267—71.

[26] Perrillo RP, Gish R, Falck-Ytter YT. American Gastroenterological Association Institute technical review on prevention and treatment of hepatitis B virus reactivation during immunosuppressive drug therapy. Gastroenterology 2015;148:221—244 e3.

[27] Torbenson M, Kannangai R, Astemborski J, et al. High prevalence of occult hepatitis B in Baltimore injection drug users. Hepatology 2004;39:51—7.

[28] Lin CL, Liu CJ, Chen PJ, et al. High prevalence of occult hepatitis B virus infection in Taiwanese intravenous drug users. J Med Virol 2007;79:1674—8.

[29] Raimondo G, Pollicino T, Cacciola I, et al. Occult hepatitis B virus infection. J Hepatol 2007;46:160—70.

[30] Kowdley KV, Wang CC, Welch S, et al. Prevalence of chronic hepatitis B among foreign-born persons living in the United States by country of origin. Hepatology 2012;56:422−33.

[31] Nelson PK, Mathers BM, Cowie B, et al. Global epidemiology of hepatitis B and hepatitis C in people who inject drugs: results of systematic reviews. Lancet 2011;378: 571−83.

[32] Burt RD, Hagan H, Garfein RS, et al. Trends in hepatitis B virus, hepatitis C virus, and human immunodeficiency virus prevalence, risk behaviors, and preventive measures among Seattle injection drug users aged 18-30 years, 1994-2004. J Urban Health 2007;84:436−54.

[33] Ly KN, Xing J, Klevens RM, et al. The increasing burden of mortality from viral hepatitis in the United States between 1999 and 2007. Ann Intern Med 2012;156:271−8.

[34] Mathers BM, Degenhardt L, Bucello C, et al. Mortality among people who inject drugs: a systematic review and meta-analysis. Bull World Health Organ 2013;91:102−23.

[35] Degenhardt L, Whiteford HA, Ferrari AJ, et al. Global burden of disease attributable to illicit drug use and dependence: findings from the Global Burden of Disease Study 2010. Lancet 2013;382:1564−74.

[36] Gibson A, Randall D, Degenhardt L. The increasing mortality burden of liver disease among opioid-dependent people: cohort study. Addiction 2011;106:2186−92.

[37] Fisher DG, Reynolds GL, Jaffe A, et al. Hepatitis and human immunodeficiency virus co-infection among injection drug users in Los Angeles County, California. J Addict Dis 2006;25:25−32.

[38] Spradling PR, Richardson JT, Buchacz K, et al. Prevalence of chronic hepatitis B virus infection among patients in the HIV Outpatient Study, 1996-2007. J Viral Hepat 2010; 17:879−86.

[39] Sanchez MA, Scheer S, Shallow S, et al. Epidemiology of the viral hepatitis-HIV syndemic in San Francisco: a collaborative surveillance approach. Public Health Rep 2014; 129(Suppl. 1):95−101.

[40] Konopnicki D, Mocroft A, de Wit S, et al. Hepatitis B and HIV: prevalence, AIDS progression, response to highly active antiretroviral therapy and increased mortality in the EuroSIDA cohort. AIDS 2005;19:593−601.

[41] Bini EJ, Perumalswami PV. Hepatitis B virus infection among American patients with chronic hepatitis C virus infection: prevalence, racial/ethnic differences, and viral interactions. Hepatology 2010;51:759−66.

[42] Yan BM, Lee SS. Acute coinfection with hepatitis B and hepatitis C viruses. Can J Gastroenterol 2005;19:729−30.

[43] Crespo J, Lozano J, de la Cruz F, et al. Prevalence and significance of hepatitis C viremia in chronic active hepatitis B. Am J Gastroenterol 1994;89:1147−51.

[44] Fong T-L, Shindo M, Feinstone S, et al. Detection of replicative intermediates of hepatitis C viral RNA in liver and serum of patients with chronic hepatitis C. J Clin Invest 1991;88:1058−60.

[45] Bersoff-Matcha SJ, Cao K, Jason M, et al. Hepatitis B virus reactivation associated with direct-acting antiviral therapy for chronic hepatitis C virus: a review of cases reported to the U.S. Food and Drug Administration adverse event reporting system. Ann Intern Med 2017;166:792−8.

[46] Schaper M, Rodriguez-Frias F, Jardi R, et al. Quantitative longitudinal evaluations of hepatitis delta virus RNA and hepatitis B virus DNA shows a dynamic, complex replicative profile in chronic hepatitis B and D. J Hepatol 2010;52:658−64.

[47] Kushner T, Serper M, Kaplan DE. Delta hepatitis within the Veterans Affairs medical system in the United States: prevalence, risk factors, and outcomes. J Hepatol 2015; 63:586−92.

[48] Gish RG, Yi DH, Kane S, et al. Coinfection with hepatitis B and D: epidemiology, prevalence and disease in patients in Northern California. J Gastroenterol Hepatol 2013;28: 1521−5.

[49] Kucirka LM, Farzadegan H, Feld JJ, et al. Prevalence, correlates, and viral dynamics of hepatitis delta among injection drug users. J Infect Dis 2010;202:845−52.

[50] Mahale P, Aka PV, Chen X, et al. Hepatitis D viremia among injection drug users in San Francisco. J Infect Dis 2018;217:1902−6.

[51] Koh C, Heller T, Glenn JS. Pathogenesis of and new therapies for hepatitis D. Gastroenterology 2019;156:461−476 e1.

[52] Haussig JM, Nielsen S, Gassowski M, et al. A large proportion of people who inject drugs are susceptible to hepatitis B: results from a bio-behavioural study in eight German cities. Int J Infect Dis 2018;66:5−13.

[53] Kim HS, Yang JD, El-Serag HB, et al. Awareness of chronic viral hepatitis in the United States: an update from National Health and Nutrition Examination Survey. J Viral Hepat 2019;26(5):596−602.

[54] Topp L, Day C, Dore GJ, et al. Poor criterion validity of self-reported hepatitis B infection and vaccination status among injecting drug users: a review. Drug Alcohol Rev 2009;28:669−75.

[55] Heimer R, Clair S, Grau LE, et al. Hepatitis-associated knowledge is low and risks are high among HIV-aware injection drug users in three US cities. Addiction 2002;97:1277−87.

[56] Carey J, Perlman DC, Friedmann P, et al. Knowledge of hepatitis among active drug injectors at a syringe exchange program. J Subst Abuse Treat 2005;29:47−53.

[57] Grau LE, Zhan W, Heimer R. Prevention knowledge, risk behaviours and seroprevalence among nonurban injectors of southwest Connecticut. Drug Alcohol Rev 2016; 35:628−36.

[58] Coffin CS, Zhou K, Terrault NA. New and old biomarkers for diagnosis and management of chronic hepatitis B virus infection. Gastroenterology 2019;156:355−368 e3.

[59] Collier MG, Drobeniuc J, Cuevas-Mota J, et al. Hepatitis A and B among young persons who inject drugs-vaccination, past, and present infection. Vaccine 2015;33:2808−12.

[60] Chahal HSP, M.G, Harris AM, McCabe D, Volberding P, Kahn JG. Cost-effectiveness of hepatitis B virus infection screening and treatment or vaccination in 6 high-risk populations in the United States. Open Forum Infect Dis 2019;6.

[61] Jackson S, Lentino J, Kopp J, et al. Immunogenicity of a two-dose investigational hepatitis B vaccine, HBsAg-1018, using a toll-like receptor 9 agonist adjuvant compared with a licensed hepatitis B vaccine in adults. Vaccine 2018;36:668−74.

[62] Kamath GR, Shah DP, Hwang LY. Immune response to hepatitis B vaccination in drug using populations: a systematic review and meta-regression analysis. Vaccine 2014;32: 2265−74.

[63] Mast EE, Margolis HS, Fiore AE, et al. A comprehensive immunization strategy to eliminate transmission of hepatitis B virus infection in the United States: recommendations of the Advisory Committee on Immunization Practices (ACIP) part 1: immunization of infants, children, and adolescents. MMWR Recomm Rep 2005;54:1−31.

[64] Campbell JV, Garfein RS, Thiede H, et al. Convenience is the key to hepatitis A and B vaccination uptake among young adult injection drug users. Drug Alcohol Depend 2007;91(Suppl. 1):S64−72.

[65] Yeo YH, Le MH, Chang ET, et al. The prevalence of undetectable vaccine-induced immunity against hepatitis B virus in US adults at high risk for infection. Hepatology 2018;69(4):1385−97.

[66] Lum PJ, Hahn JA, Shafer KP, et al. Hepatitis B virus infection and immunization status in a new generation of injection drug users in San Francisco. J Viral Hepat 2008;15:229−36.

[67] Deacon RM, Topp L, Wand H, et al. Correlates of susceptibility to hepatitis B among people who inject drugs in Sydney, Australia. J Urban Health 2012;89:769−78.

[68] Lu PJ, Byrd KK, Murphy TV, et al. Hepatitis B vaccination coverage among high-risk adults 18-49 years, U.S., 2009. Vaccine 2011;29:7049−57.

[69] Stitzer ML, Polk T, Bowles S, et al. Drug users' adherence to a 6-month vaccination protocol: effects of motivational incentives. Drug Alcohol Depend 2010;107:76−9.

[70] Altice FL, Bruce RD, Walton MR, et al. Adherence to hepatitis B virus vaccination at syringe exchange sites. J Urban Health 2005;82:151−61.

[71] Weaver T, Metrebian N, Hellier J, et al. Use of contingency management incentives to improve completion of hepatitis B vaccination in people undergoing treatment for heroin dependence: a cluster randomised trial. Lancet 2014;384:153−63.

[72] Walsh N, Verster A, Rodolph M, et al. WHO guidance on the prevention of viral hepatitis B and C among people who inject drugs. Int J Drug Policy 2014;25:363−71.

[73] Shi J, Feng Y, Gao L, et al. Immunogenicity and safety of a high-dose hepatitis B vaccine among patients receiving methadone maintenance treatment: a randomized, double-blinded, parallel-controlled trial. Vaccine 2017;35:2443−8.

[74] Ramasamy P, Lintzeris N, Sutton Y, et al. The outcome of a rapid hepatitis B vaccination programme in a methadone treatment clinic. Addiction 2010;105:329−34.

[75] Charuvastra A, Stein J, Schwartzapfel B, et al. Hepatitis B vaccination practices in state and federal prisons. Public Health Rep 2001;116:203−9.

[76] Seal KH, Kral AH, Lorvick J, et al. A randomized controlled trial of monetary incentives vs. outreach to enhance adherence to the hepatitis B vaccine series among injection drug users. Drug Alcohol Depend 2003;71:127−31.

[77] Hu Y, Grau LE, Scott G, et al. Economic evaluation of delivering hepatitis B vaccine to injection drug users. Am J Prev Med 2008;35:25−32.

[78] Rafia R, Dodd PJ, Brennan A, et al. An economic evaluation of contingency management for completion of hepatitis B vaccination in those on treatment for opiate dependence. Addiction 2016;111:1616−27.

[79] Hwang LY, Grimes CZ, Tran TQ, et al. Accelerated hepatitis B vaccination schedule among drug users: a randomized controlled trial. J Infect Dis 2010;202:1500−9.

[80] Tran TQ, Grimes CZ, Lai D, et al. Effect of age and frequency of injections on immune response to hepatitis B vaccination in drug users. Vaccine 2012;30:342−9.

[81] Shah DP, Grimes CZ, Nguyen AT, et al. Long-term effectiveness of accelerated hepatitis B vaccination schedule in drug users. Am J Public Health 2015;105:e36−43.

[82] Bowman S, Grau LE, Singer M, et al. Factors associated with hepatitis B vaccine series completion in a randomized trial for injection drug users reached through syringe exchange programs in three US cities. BMC Public Health 2014;14:820.

[83] John TJ, Ninan GT, Rajagopalan MS, et al. Epidemic hepatitis B caused by commercial human immunoglobulin. Lancet 1979;1:1074.

[84] Tillmann HL, Patel K. Therapy of acute and fulminant hepatitis B. Intervirology 2014;57:181−8.

[85] Dao DY, Seremba E, Ajmera V, et al. Use of nucleoside (tide) analogues in patients with hepatitis B-related acute liver failure. Dig Dis Sci 2012;57:1349−57.

[86] Lee WM, Hynan LS, Rossaro L, et al. Intravenous N-acetylcysteine improves transplant-free survival in early stage non-acetaminophen acute liver failure. Gastroenterology 2009;137:856−64. e1.

[87] Mantzoukis K, Rodriguez-Peralvarez M, Buzzetti E, et al. Pharmacological interventions for acute hepatitis B infection: an attempted network meta-analysis. Cochrane Database Syst Rev 2017;3:CD011645.

[88] Kumar M, Satapathy S, Monga R, et al. A randomized controlled trial of lamivudine to treat acute hepatitis B. Hepatology 2007;45:97−101.

[89] Tenney DJ, Rose RE, Baldick CJ, et al. Long-term monitoring shows hepatitis B virus resistance to entecavir in nucleoside-naive patients is rare through 5 years of therapy. Hepatology 2009;49:1503−14.

[90] Park ES, Lee AR, Kim DH, et al. Identification of a quadruple mutation that confers tenofovir resistance in chronic hepatitis B patients. J Hepatol 2019;70(6):1093−102.

[91] Jourdain G, Ngo-Giang-Huong N, Harrison L, et al. Tenofovir versus placebo to prevent perinatal transmission of hepatitis B. N Engl J Med 2018;378:911−23.

[92] Pan CQ, Duan Z, Dai E, et al. Tenofovir to prevent hepatitis B transmission in mothers with high viral load. N Engl J Med 2016;374:2324−34.

[93] Harris AM, Isenhour C, Schillie S, et al. Hepatitis B virus testing and care among pregnant women using commercial claims data, United States, 2011-2014. Infect Dis Obstet Gynecol 2018;2018:4107329.

[94] AIDS Info. Guidelines for the use of antiretroviral agents in adults and adolescents living with HIV. 2019.

[95] AASLD-IDSA. Recommendations for testing, managing, and treating hepatitis C. 2018. http://www.hcvguidelines.org.

Opioid use disorder and endocarditis

8

Christopher F. Rowley, MD, MPH [1], Audrey Li, MD [2]

[1]*Assistant Professor Medicine, Beth Israel Deaconess Medical Center, Boston, MA, United States;*
[2]*Clinical Fellow in Medicine, Beth Israel Deaconess Medical Center, Boston, MA, United States*

Opioid use disorder and endocarditis

The increasing use of opioids over the past decade has resulted in a crisis of over-dose and death in the United States that has also been accompanied by an increase in infectious complications related to injection drug use (IDU). It has been well described in the medical literature that there is an increased risk of hepatitis C and HIV infections in people who inject drugs (PWID) [1], even if knowledge gaps related to these infections exist among PWID [2], but the dramatic increase in endocarditis secondary to IDU has been striking to those who practice in regions of the country affected by the opioid epidemic. Providers are seeing this entity with great frequency [3], and treating endocarditis in this population has unique challenges that if not addressed, it may impact the ability to be successful with treatment. This chapter will attempt to identify the specific issues related to the populations of patients with endocarditis secondary to injecting opioids and aims to provide strategies to address the unique issues inherent in this group of patients to ensure the best possible clinical outcome.

From an epidemiologic perspective, it remains difficult to estimate the number of cases of infective endocarditis (IE) related to IDU. It has been estimated there are 3–10 cases of endocarditis per 100,000 people and that the number of cases of IE overall is up to 50,000 cases per year in the United States [4], with an increasing proportion of those cases secondary to IDU [5]. Given the ongoing national health crisis secondary to opioid use disorder (OUD), it is likely that the total number of cases is on the rise. And while overdose deaths from drug use, and opioids in particular, are rightfully identified as a national public health emergency, our inability to characterize the true impact of serious infections related to IDU on these patients mitigates our ability to grasp the vast extent of this healthcare crisis. These infections, seemingly rising to rates unforeseen previously, represent a highly morbid and potentially lethal health condition that requires prolonged antibiotic therapy and often results in cardiac surgery for valvular repair. Failure to address the underlying substance use disorder in these patients, specifically OUD, is a common occurrence leading to possible reinfection from continued IDU or death after hospital discharge from drug overdose. We will review the epidemiology of endocarditis in persons who inject drugs, the treatment strategies to cure these infections, and the opportunities to engage with these patients while hospitalized to potentially initiate a plan to engage them in OUD treatment.

How does endocarditis occur in PWID?

Endocarditis has long been known to be a consequence of IDU with many studies dating back at least to the 1950s describing the increasing rates of infections due to IDU, with a focus typically on right-sided endocarditis given the frequency of these cardiac valves being involved [6–8]. The risk of infection in these individuals is multifactorial and relates to the drug product, the practice of injection itself, and the susceptibility of the host (Table 8.1).

Table 8.1 Mechanisms of infection in endocarditis, by stage of injection drug use process.

Contaminated drug product	Spore-producing organisms including *Clostridium* spp. Fungi including *Candida* spp. *Bacillus* spp. *Pseudomonas aeruginosa*
Adulterated drug product Products are commonly "cut" with substances that lead to local tissue injury, thus impacting local immune function and predisposing to infection	Talc Baking soda Acid
Unsterile water If acquired as solid product, substances require dissolution prior to use; this is often performed with unsterile water	*Pseudomonas aeruginosa* *Burkholderia* spp. Other gram-negative organisms, including anaerobes
Oral flora Needles or syringes sometimes are licked prior to use for a variety of reasons, including drug sampling, needle sharpening, or habit.	*Streptococci* *Candida* spp. HACEK organisms[a] Anaerobic organisms
Skin flora	*S. aureus* *Streptococci* Coagulase-negative *Staphylococci* Polymicrobial
Host impaired immunity	Hepatitis C HIV Potential opioid-induced immune response reduction

[a] *Haemophilus* spp., *Aggregatibacter actinomycetemcomitans*, *Cardiobacterium hominis*, *Eikenella corrodens*, *Kingella kingaote*

The pathology of endocarditis results in the establishment of bacteria on the cardiac valves but the initial structural abnormality of the cardiac valve is typically a sterile vegetation composed of fibrin and platelets to which bacteria adhere [9]. The proposed mechanism of disease begins with impurities in the heroin or drug product that may damage the cardiac valves (or the valves already have preexisting abnormalities) through repetitive injury to the tricuspid valve causing endothelial damage as this is the first valve to encounter the foreign material when injecting into the venous system [10]. Aside from causing direct mechanical damage, injected diluents can cause vasospasm and damage to the intima layer of the endothelium, leading to thrombus formation and platelet aggregation [11]. Different organisms have been reported to affect valves with differing frequency [12] due to the propensity of the individual bacteria to adhere to damaged valves and subsequently colonize this inflamed endothelium producing cytokines and tissue factor which serves to recruit monocytes and platelets [9,13].

The process itself of injecting heroin, for example, is complex and comes with attendant risks at different stages of the injecting process. There are many different factors that are at play both with respect to the effects of heroin and other impurities on the ability of the individual to clear bacteria as well as the actual process of injecting opioids can result in the introduction of bacterial or fungal pathogens leading to disease.

Opioids are often "cut" with impurities which refers to substances added to increase the weight of the drug product being sold but often does not necessarily contain an active drug (although, the addition of synthetic fentanyl to heroin is likely responsible for many overdose deaths in this current epidemic [14]). These impurities such as talc or baking soda, when injected, may cause local vascular injury which, in conjunction with poor skin antisepsis, can lead to localized or systemic infection. Heroin that is adulterated in this fashion may be limited in its potency requiring the person to inject with greater frequency, enhancing the potential of infectious complications. In addition, the opioid may not have been produced in a sterile fashion and there have been reports of heroin contaminated with spore-producing bacteria [15,16], leading to well-described outbreaks of severe infectious complications of IDU [16].

The typically solid preparation of the heroin product is subsequently dissolved often with the use of a spoon or an aluminum can in the presence of water and/or heat. The source of the water may range from sterile water to water from a toilet and with it the organisms that may become intermixed with the opioid preparation will then be injected [17]. Infections that result from gram-negative bacteria that live in water sources have been well described [18–20], and the possibility that these organisms are present needs to be considered when treating individuals empirically for life-threatening bacterial infections.

Candida species and other fungi are a relatively rare cause of IE but well known to occur in PWID [21,22] due to environmental contamination. Recent reports from both Denver, CO, and Massachusetts [23,24] point to *Candida* species increasing in frequency in this population as a cause of both fungemia and endocarditis. Also, syringe tips often will be put into the mouth of the individual prior to injecting for multiple reasons such as habit, to test the drug prior to injecting, or to ensure that the bevel of the needle remains sharp [25]. This has the potential to introduce mouth pathogens into the bloodstream once the syringe is introduced [26] into the vein or skin. In addition, a sterile site is often not prepared on the skin with the use of an alcohol pad, and with any penetration of the skin by use of an injectable device can lead to infection typically with skin pathogens, mostly prominently *Staphylococcus aureus* and *Streptococcal* species of bacteria.

In addition to infectious agents being introduced through injecting drugs, opioids have been demonstrated to affect the immune system broadly as organs and tissue throughout the body contain opioid receptors, not solely limited to the central nervous system, suggesting a greater overall role in human health. In vitro data suggest opioids have broad effects on all aspects of the immune system including both adaptive and innate immunity [27], but the research is far from conclusive to suggest either a clear detrimental or beneficial effect on overall immune health [28,29]. While case series and cohort studies have suggested an increased risk for certain infections [30−33], more rigorous studies will need to be undertaken to determine the interplay between opioids and the immune system, the impact of length of opioid treatment on these immune effects, and whether all opioid analgesics have the same properties with respect to immune activity.

The host may be uniquely susceptible to bacterial infections as hepatitis C virus (HCV) antibody positivity is seen in roughly 70% of PWID, and the majority of these individuals likely have active disease without having cleared the infection [34]. While it is unclear to what degree these individuals with HCV are at increased risk for serious bloodstream infections or endocarditis, HCV does appear to represent an additional risk for *S. aureus* infection [35]. In those select individuals with HCV and resulting cirrhosis, their immune function will be compromised in various regards, but characteristically they will have more complications from infection than healthy individuals given defects in innate immunity, phagocytosis, and impaired humoral immunity [36]. Increasing numbers of HIV infections have been seen in different areas of the country [37,38] with the outbreak of HIV infections in Scott County, IN [39,40], being the most dramatic demonstration of an HIV infection cluster related to IDU. Obviously, HIV infection has long been seen in individuals with a history of IDU, and serious bacterial infections which occur in individuals with HIV which can result in endocarditis [41]; however, the risk of serious bacterial infections can be mitigated with early antiretroviral treatment [42,43].

Increasing rates and epidemiology of infective endocarditis secondary to injection drug use

Several recent studies [5,44−47] have clearly demonstrated that the rates of endocarditis secondary to IDU have increased over the past 15 years, all of them showing dramatic increases that coincide with the national opioid epidemic [48,49]. In fact, the sharp increase in cases of endocarditis could serve as a method to mark this new epidemic of IDU as an increase in endocarditis seen in the early 2000s was associated was associated increase in positive opioid toxicology and new HCV infections [50]. There remains, however, a limited ability to capture exact number of cases of endocarditis related to IDU given the dependence on discharge data or the use of surrogate markers for IDU such as hepatitis C status [5,47,51] given the lack of an International Classification of Disease (ICD)-9 or ICD-10 code for IDU and no reporting requirements at either the state or national level which could provide actual numbers of patients with this condition. In addition, gaps in recording data fail to account for long-term morbidity, for example, when a patient suffers a devastating embolic stroke from IDU. Regardless of the failure to systematically capture the number of cases of endocarditis, the number of cases certainly is increasing anecdotally and in the available medical literature, and the total numbers of cases that are being discussed likely represent an underestimation of the real number of infections.

An increase in hospitalizations for IE in PWID was seen by Wurcel et al. with 12% of admissions for endocarditis at community hospitals were secondary to IDU in 2013 compared with 7% in 2000 [44]. Similarly, in North Carolina, annual hospitalizations for IE associated with IDU increased from 0.92 to 10.95 per 100,000 persons between 2007 and 2017 using data gathered from hospital discharges [5] and in a national survey based on hospital discharge data, endocarditis secondary to IDU increased from 15.3% to 29.1% of IE cases between 2010 and 2015 [46].

The incidence of *S. aureus* infections has increased over the last half-century worldwide and this pathogen is the most common cause of IE in developed countries, with the incidence of *S. aureus* infection being even greater in those with IE from IDU, with well over half of the cases in PWID being due to *S. aureus* [52,53], far greater than in those who do not inject drugs. Infection with *S. aureus* puts patients with IDU-IE at increased risk of severe sepsis, multiorgan dysfunction, major neurological events, and death [54−56] given the higher rates of vegetations > 1 cm and extracardiac emboli compared with non-IDU patients. Other gram-positive organisms besides *S. aureus*, gram-negative bacteria, fungal organisms, and polymicrobial infections all have been shown to cause endocarditis in this population[20,24,57,58].

The International Collaboration on Endocarditis-Prospective Cohort Study (ICE-PCS) investigators found most cases of IE in a pooled international population involve vegetations on either the aortic (38%) or mitral valves (41%) compared with the tricuspid valve (12%) [52]. However, in those individuals with IDU-related endocarditis, a far higher percentage of them have right-sided disease [59,60]. The mechanism behind this phenomenon remains elusive [11,60]. But, more recently, right-sided endocarditis is by no means the exclusive presentation for those with IDU-associated endocarditis as several studies have demonstrated a relatively high rate of left-sided involvement as well in individuals who inject drugs [53,54,56,61,62]. Historically, there were more men than women with IE secondary to IDU [63,64], and while this seems to continue to be the case, the gap is narrowing as there is an increase in the number of women with this condition [44,53], a fact that is likely trending with the increase in women who use opioids [65].

IDU-associated endocarditis: diagnosis and treatment

Persons who inject drugs are at high risk for bloodstream infections, and early recognition and diagnosis of endocarditis is paramount to potentially mitigate sequelae of the infection. Individuals presenting with fever and with a history of IDU should be strongly considered as possibly having a bloodstream infection with the need to rule out endocarditis. The early treatment of this condition may prevent complications such as the development of a paravalvular abscess, embolic phenomena, or possibly valve destruction that may require a surgical intervention in order to treat.

The diagnosis relies on the use of the universally accepted, modified Duke criteria (Table 8.2) [66,67] that include major and minor criteria to categorize cases as definite, probable, or unlikely IE, and this well-accepted method has been shown to retain its accuracy in diagnosing endocarditis in PWID [68,69]. Two to three sets of blood cultures, ideally drawn prior to the administration of antibiotics, with each

Table 8.2 Modified Duke criteria for diagnosis of infective endocarditis (IE)[66,67,70,71].

Major criteria	Blood culture positivity • Typical organisms consistent with IE from 2 separate blood cultures OR • Persistently positive blood cultures taken >12 h apart OR • Three or more positive cultures taken over a period >1 h
	Evidence of endocardial involvement • Echocardiogram positive for IE (*vegetation, abscess, new partial dehiscence of prosthetic valve*, or *new valvular regurgitation*)
Minor criteria	Predisposition to IE • Predisposing heart condition • Preexisting valvular abnormality • injection drug use
	Fever >38°C/100.4°F
	Vascular phenomena • Janeway lesions • Mycotic aneurysm • Arterial emboli • Conjunctival hemorrhages • Septic pulmonary infarcts • Intracranial hemorrhage Immunologic phenomena • Osler's nodes • Rheumatoid factor • Roth's sports • Glomerulonephritis
	Microbiologic evidence • Blood culture positivity not meeting major criteria OR • Serologic evidence of active infection with organisms consistent with IE
Definite IE	2 major criteria OR 1 major + 3 minor criteria OR 5 minor criteria
Possible IE	1 major + 1 minor criteria OR 3 minor criteria

blood culture drawn from a different anatomical site, provide the greatest yield with respect to determining the organism responsible for the condition. Obtaining blood cultures can be very difficult at times in PWID due to sclerosis of veins secondary to the frequent injection of intravenous (IV) drugs, and this difficulty in obtaining blood cultures risks contamination. An echocardiogram to look for valvular vegetations is included in the modified Duke criteria with additional criteria including fever, elevated inflammatory markers, and recovery of an organism that is a typical cause of endocarditis. The diagnosis of endocarditis can be challenging but given that PWID are at significant risk for this condition, ongoing evaluation needs to continue. Transthoracic echocardiogram is often applied as the first modality to evaluate for valvular lesions and if negative, a transesophageal echocardiogram (TEE) is often required to detect infection involving a cardiac valve.

In individuals who have continued bacteremia, but no clear evidence of endocarditis on initial TEE, a repeat TEE 5—7 days after the initial study is recommended [70]. Once the diagnosis of IE is made, treatment decisions can follow largely well-accepted treatment guidelines from the American Heart Association (AHA), the European Society of Cardiology (ESC), and the British Society for Antimicrobial Chemotherapy (BSAC) [67,70,71].

Treatment of IDU infective endocarditis

Empiric treatment of IE in patients who have endocarditis, or bacteremia with a concern for endocarditis, needs to account for the likely pathogens. Therefore, it is important that broad antibiotic therapy to cover gram-positive pathogens (particularly methicillin-resistant and methicillin-sensitive *S. aureus* given the highest likelihood that *S. aureus* is the causative agent), but also empiric treatment for gram-negative bacteria, including *Pseudomonas* [20,72], is initiated in the population of patients who inject drugs. This would be a necessary expansion of typical empiric coverage for those who do not inject drugs which may not be as broad with respect to the gram-negative coverage. While empiric treatment is determined on a case-by-case basis, regimens such as vancomycin and either meropenem, a third or fourth generation cephalosporin (ceftazidime or cefepime), or an extended spectrum beta-lactamase inhibitor with activity against *Pseudomonas* provide the requisite broad antimicrobial therapy in this setting.

Each of the IE guidelines has addressed the topic of empiric antimicrobial treatment slightly differently. The AHA approach to empiric treatment has a statement that simply recognizes that therapy initially is usually broad, will likely be narrowed, and infectious diseases consultation should take place at the time of the initiation of empiric antibiotic therapy. The BSAC guideline provides explicit recommendations for native valve, empiric treatment for endocarditis in an individual who injects drugs and is septic which includes vancomycin dosed as per local guidelines and meropenem 2 g intravenously q8h to cover staphylococci (including methicillin-resistant staphylococci), streptococci, enterococci, HACEK, *Enterobacteriaceae*, and *Pseudomonas aeruginosa*. The ESC recommends that consideration be given to the type of drug and solvent used as well as the infection location, while ensuring that *S. aureus* is covered. If the patient is injecting pentazocine, *Pseudomonas* is emphasized as a potential pathogen and must be included as a target of empiric treatment due to outbreaks of this pathogen [73,74], while if brown heroin was injected, *Candida* spp. should be covered [58].

Once the microbiologic diagnosis of IE has been established in PWID, the treatment is antibiotic therapy typically for 4 to 6 weeks with much of the historical data suggesting this should be parenteral therapy. The guidelines again provide similar detailed guidance that is organism specific with the most common causative agents in this population in both those with native and prosthetic valves.

Surgical interventions

Surgical indications for IE have been developed and assessment by the surgical team should occur early in the course of a hospitalization and with IE, surgery occurs in up to 50% of the patients affected [67]. The generally defined indications for which prompt evaluation and consideration for cardiac surgery are listed in Table 8.3. These include large valvular vegetations, valve rupture, paravalvular abscess, difficult to treat organisms, new embolic phenomena despite appropriate treatment, and heart failure that fails to respond to medical therapy.

The decision to intervene surgically in patients with endocarditis is often reached through a multidisciplinary approach involving the cardiothoracic surgical team, internal medicine providers, and cardiologists, taking into account the risk of the surgical procedure and weighing the benefit that the patient is likely to experience from the procedure.

Table 8.3 Indications for surgical evaluation and treatment in patients with IE[67,70,71].

Heart failure
    In IE of the aortic or
    mitral valve
	Severe regurgitation causing refractory cardiogenic shock or pulmonary edema
	Fistula into a cardiac chamber or pericardium causing refractory cardiogenic shock or pulmonary edema

Uncontrolled infection	Increase in vegetation size despite appropriate antimicrobial therapy Infection caused by fungi or drug resistant bacteria Persistent fever and positive blood cultures >7–10 days
Prevention of embolism	Persistent vegetation after systemic embolization Anterior mitral leaflet vegetation, particularly with size >10 mm ≥1 Embolic events during first 2 weeks of antimicrobial therapy
Perivalvular extension	Valvular dehiscence, rupture, or fistula New heart block Large abscess or extension of abscess despite appropriate antimicrobial therapy

The ESC IE guidelines specifically include recommendations regarding surgery in PWID as it relates to right-sided endocarditis [70]. They suggest that avoiding surgery for this condition is advised given the risk of relapse related to opioid use and the chances of recurrent infection. These guidelines are consistent with US practice as clinical data support the relative infrequency of the necessity of surgical intervention for right-sided endocarditis as it is successfully medically managed in the vast majority of cases.

Timing of cardiac surgery for endocarditis

There has been a great deal of discussion in the medical literature about the appropriate timing of surgery for endocarditis [75–77]. Several studies have demonstrated that early surgery is not associated with worse clinical outcomes and the US and European guidelines suggest there is no need to delay surgery in general once an indication for early surgery has been identified [67,70,78]. Even in patients with ischemic stroke, several studies have suggested that there is no apparent survival benefit in delaying surgery [79,80].

However, surgery will often be delayed when there is evidence of a large cerebral infarction or a hemorrhagic stroke given concerns for neurological compromise. Patients can bleed into the infarcted areas of the brain [81] or further bleed into the hemorrhage with the use of the cardiac bypass machine and the anticoagulation associated with that procedure. Much of the medical consensus currently suggests waiting at least 2 weeks and ideally up to four before considering surgery in patients with large cerebral infarction and for at least 4 weeks in those with intracerebral hemorrhage if possible [67,82].

In the patient with OUD, it would be expected that the timing of surgery would be consistent with those who do not inject drugs given that the recent thoracic surgery guidelines for the treatment of IE that suggest the same criteria are used for determining surgery whether the patient has a history of IDU or not [78]. While right-sided disease is successfully treated medically most of the time, stable patients with OUD with large emboli or stroke will occasionally be discharged from the hospital with the plan to complete much of their IV antibiotic therapy only to return at a future date for a planned cardiac surgery procedure. This may be a chance to engage the patient with treatment for their OUD prior to their surgery. Delays for other reasons, including not performing surgery until the patient engages in treatment for OUD, are sometimes considered without data supporting that this strategy motivates patients to engage in OUD treatment, and may not benefit either the patient's cardiovascular health or in overcoming their OUD.

Outcomes with surgery

Short-term clinical outcomes after surgery are supported by a recent metaanalysis of 13 studies that evaluated the 30-day mortality in patients who receive cardiac surgery for IDU-related endocarditis and demonstrated it is no different than surgical outcomes in those without drug-use associated endocarditis [85]. However, there are poor long-term health outcomes in patients with OUD who have surgery as part of their treatment for endocarditis with high 1 year mortality rates up to 22.5% in one study of 64 patients [54], while another had a 5-year mortality rate of 41% [83].

These high mortality rates are striking when considering the few medical comorbidities in these patients compared with the noninjecting endocarditis patients [84,85]. The reasons for this finding are possibly related to the severity of the disease, the aggressiveness of *S. aureus* (the organisms most likely to be responsible for endocarditis in OUD), late presentation to care, or possibly other unidentified factors. But, the far more likely driver of these poor outcomes is the recurrence of active drug use, subsequent reinfection and endocarditis, or even overdose death. Several studies have demonstrated that continued drug use after hospital discharge leads to frequent recurrence of infection, higher risk of valve complications, and overall higher mortality than expected for this cohort [83–86]. These data support both that necessary surgery should not be denied in PWID due to concerns about short-term clinical outcomes, but in addition, the postsurgical care addressing substance use should be considered to be one of the most important aspects of the comprehensive postoperative and long-term future care.

Data reporting on the impact of inpatient treatment of OUD while inpatient for the treatment of endocarditis on reducing morbidity and mortality are limited. One recent study however has demonstrated mortality benefit in patients who were able to be treated for their OUD while hospitalized [87]. While the numbers of patients who were treated for their OUD was small (only 40 out of 202), a statistically significant improvement in mortality was seen, and this represents one of the first clear examples of a hospital-based intervention for treatment of OUD in endocarditis.

Controversies regarding surgery

Surgical indications are fairly consistent for the treatment of endocarditis from both the US and European guidelines [67,70]. However, there can be barriers to surgery that relate to the underlying OUD with decisions made about surgery on occasion based on an individual provider's opinion about performing what they might consider to be futile care. The cardiovascular surgery guidelines state that "Although operative risk is not higher, drug-addicted patients have a greater probability of death in the year after operation than do nonaddicted patients. The injection drug use must be included and weighed in decision-making, and patient treatment must include drug rehabilitation [78]." This topic has been the subject of both the lay press and the medical literature as society struggles to grapple with ethical issues about providing care that is costly and often unsuccessful unless the underlying OUD is addressed, with questions being asked about how much care is too much given the cost and poor outcomes in many cases [88,89].

The care of a patient who has developed IE undoubtedly is best done with a team approach, particularly when surgery is necessary. An editorial accompanying the latest guidelines from cardiothoracic surgery (and a letter in response) regarding when to perform surgery commented specifically on the individual with IE from IDU [90,91]. The author rightly suggested that the use of addiction services within the hospital setting prior to the surgery with a plan to support the patient in their recovery both from the surgery and substance use disorder. However, the suggestion put forth that there is value in creating a contract between the surgeon and patient that outlines in advance that another operation may not be offered should the individual continue to engage in substance use is not based on data and represents bias some patients with OUD face even within the medical system. It is purported that a contract will provide "additional motivation to remain "clean" and can assist in decision making if reinfection occurs [90]." Similar contracts are not given to diabetics who are unable to manage their blood sugar or smokers who cannot stop smoking [91], other challenging health conditions where individual behaviors can have significant and poor consequences. More emphasis needs to be placed on trying to address the barriers that prevent the patient with OUD from achieving meaningful recovery.

A response providing the surgeon's perspective argued that just as antibiotics are required for treatment of endocarditis, addiction treatment is of equal importance [92]. While asking the patient to sign a contract may not be evidence-based, it can provide a tangible effort to show the importance of the dual nature of the care that is required. And, "the reassurance that surgeons need and are entitled to is that the patient with SUD has been evaluated by an addition medicine expert, addiction treatment is available and offered, and the patient has agreed to make a good faith effort [92]…" Efforts need to be universal to address addiction in this setting so that both the surgical issue and the underlying cause of that issue can be addressed.

The decision to considering limiting surgical interventions in patients with OUD has been likened to the approach that has been taken over the years with individuals who need a liver transplant. For example, a patient who has cirrhosis from underlying alcohol use disorder often will not be listed for a liver transplant unless they have been able to demonstrate a period of being alcohol-free. This selection process allows for the transplanted liver to be given in situations that are most likely to result in a successful transplantation, as livers to be transplanted represent a finite resource. In many situations, surgeons will operate on individuals during the first admission for endocarditis, but oftentimes a second surgery will not be undertaken [93].

Counter arguments to the approach of limiting surgical options in PWID recognize that, unlike procurement of livers for transplantation, cardiac valves do not represent a finite resource. And while it is a technically challenging procedure that is costly [94] and may expose healthcare personnel to risk including acquisition of viral infections such as HIV or hepatitis C, we as a society have not limited surgical care when it is obviously beneficial for other illnesses, such as cancer, which also has recurrence, and is many times related to substance use behaviors such as nicotine or alcohol. Our inability to provide a pathway toward meaningful OUD treatment often represents a failure of the healthcare system as it does not address the complex medical needs of patients with OUD. In addition, like many chronic medical conditions, OUD is characterized by periods of success/relapse, and while relapse in this situation can lead to serious infections such as endocarditis or prosthetic valve endocarditis, it does not represent a reason to no longer engage the person in care, which in many circumstances is life-saving care.

Some cardiac surgeons have taken the approach that waiting until the person has agreed to OUD treatment and has been successful in those efforts is the best strategy in patients who otherwise are clinically stable and whose surgery can be delayed. This approach may be an acceptable strategy in some individuals but in others, it may in fact be arbitrarily applied. Clearly, if this approach is to be taken, a robust program engaging the person in OUD treatment while in the hospital needs to be enacted, and many such programs do not exist at this time. An aggressive approach that allows for optimal treatment of both the infection and OUD is the ideal strategy to care for these patients [95] but developing such a system remains challenging, and while many hospitals are developing comprehensive teams to assist with these complex patients, this level of care is not yet universal, and therefore guidelines that force patients to start OUD treatment prior to receiving life-saving medical care cannot be universally or equally applied.

Location to receive parenteral antibiotics

Outpatient parenteral antimicrobial therapy (OPAT) allows patients the opportunities to be treated outside the hospital (at a skilled nursing facility or at home) for their extended course of antibiotics. There are opportunities for cost savings as patients do not need to remain in the acute care setting and a return to a more normal life in familiar surroundings while still being treated appropriately for a severe infection. It is not, however, without challenges as laboratory and clinical monitoring needs to be coordinated with service providers who may be outside of the hospital network. In one study, 33% of individuals discharged from two different academic medical centers experienced an adverse event during OPAT when being treated for complicated *S. aureus* bacteremia, with over 60% of those complications resulting in rehospitalization [96]. These data demonstrate that OPAT is a challenging endeavor for patients and there may be burdens unique to the OUD population requiring even greater resource utilization to be successful with OPAT, but there remains a significant bias at this time against even making OPAT available for these patients.

Many providers, healthcare systems, and visiting nurse companies do not allow for patients who inject drugs to safely return home with a peripherally inserted central venous catheter or a midline catheter for administration due to the risk of possible manipulation of the catheter for drug use. This results in the requirement in many circumstances that they entirety of IV antibiotics occur either in the hospital or in a facility that can monitor them. A survey of over 500 Infectious Diseases providers suggested that the majority of patients are treated for IE either in the hospital or an extended care facility for the entirety of their antibiotic course [3] which represents an incredible burden on both the inpatient and outpatient facilities and likely adds additional costs that must be absorbed by the medical system. A separate survey demonstrated that 95% of inpatient providers would consider using OPAT for patients without IDU, but if the patient is a PWID, that number dropped to 29% [97]. The most common barriers to discharging a patient with IDU on OPAT were socio-economic factors, willingness of infectious diseases physicians to follow as an outpatient, and concerns for misuse of peripherally inserted central catheters and adherence with antibiotic treatment. This results in many younger patients being asked to stay in a facility for many weeks, often after they are well enough to return home, simply for the administration of IV antibiotics. This additional burden of keeping patients away from their families or out of work increases stress and creates financial hardships on many occasions. It can add to the complex psychological issues that many patients with OUD are experiencing.

It is not clear that parenteral antibiotics need to be administered in a monitored setting for this patient population nor is it obvious that this significantly improves clinical outcomes compared to allowing patients to return home for the completion of their therapy. The concern that an indwelling catheter will be utilized by the PWID as a means of injecting drugs seems plausible, but data from several studies do not support that this happens in great numbers when OPAT is done with close supervision [98−100], nor is it clear that rates of access of IV lines is higher as an outpatient than in patients who are in a skilled nursing facility for the entirety of their antibiotic course [101]. The truth is likely that people will find ways to use drugs if they are so inclined whether an IV catheter is in place or not. No study has directly compared strategies for OPAT comparing those who use drugs and those who do not, nor does a study exists allowing patients to be randomized to different arms such as inpatient versus going home, with treatment provided for both their infection and OUD; data which are sorely lacking.

One recent study identified retrospectively hospitalized PWID, with IDU in the preceding 2 years, who were discharged with the need to complete at least 2 weeks of parenteral antibiotics which were being monitored by an OPAT program. Persons who inject drugs discharged home were not more likely to have complications than those discharged to an SNF/rehab [100]. Another study of 29 PWID who presented to an infusion center for daily antibiotic infusions reported success in that no patients were suspected of manipulating their PICC line. However, these patients were carefully selected and a seal was used over the PICC line that would be able to identify if the line was tampered with, but represents an alternative that needs to be considered in appropriate patients [98]. This decision in some cases is made by the treating provider as it is deemed to be in the patient's best interest; however, in other situations, there are no options as many home infusion companies may have developed policies that preclude them from giving antibiotics at home to a patient with a PICC line and a history of IDU. These decisions are not based on data and, there are significant gaps in the data about safe strategies that allow PWID to be discharged with a PICC line [102].

Other treatment issues

Short-course treatment options for right-sided endocarditis

Short-course treatment options for right-sided endocarditis were sought given the frequency of right-sided endocarditis in PWID and the above-mentioned challenges with parenteral antibiotics in this population. Several studies from the early 1990s demonstrated that 2 weeks of treatment for strictly right-sided endocarditis can be effective. Reports of three prospective, nonrandomized clinical trials support the use of a 2-week course of a penicillinase-resistant penicillin and an aminoglycoside antibiotic to treat uncomplicated, exclusively right-sided endocarditis caused by methicillin-susceptible *S. aureus* (MSSA) in PWID [103–106].

A subsequent study of 90 consecutive individuals with IDU and right-sided MSSA endocarditis randomized individuals to a regimen of cloxacillin alone or cloxacillin plus gentamicin. Treatment was successful in 34 of the 38 patients who received cloxacillin alone and 31 of the 36 patients who received cloxacillin plus gentamicin. Of the 37 patients who completed 2-week treatment with cloxacillin, 34 were cured and 3 needed prolonged treatment to cure the infection (1 patient died during treatment) which was equivalent to the group that received combination therapy. However, with the increasing data demonstrating that even low-dose gentamicin for a short period of time is associated with significant renal toxicity [107], the recommendation now for individuals who are candidates for short-course treatment for right-sided IE with MSSA is for the β-lactam antibiotic alone. It remains incumbent on the provider who is opting for a short-course regimen to continue to be vigilant that these patients remain uncomplicated with respect to their right-sided disease as there may be need for extension of therapy if complications ensue.

Long acting IV options

Dalbavancin and oritavancin have been approved for the treatment of complicated skin and soft tissue infections and represent two novel agents that are unique in that they have extremely long half-lives [108]. This allows infrequent administration of these medications while still achieve therapeutic drug levels. These novel lipoglycopeptides were approved by the Food and Drug Administration for the treatment of acute bacterial skin and skin structure infections (ABSSSIs) and have activity against several gram-positive pathogens, including methicillin-resistant and vancomycin-intermediate susceptible strains of staphylococci and viridans group and β-hemolytic *streptococci*, *Streptococcus pneumoniae*, *Enterococcus* species, and anaerobic gram-positive cocci and bacilli [108].

This has a great deal of appeal to providers caring for people with OUD given the concerns about long-term IV access. However, there have already been reports of treatment failures with this approach and caution is therefore advised [109–111]. It is likely that decisions will need to be made on a case-by-case basis, weighing the risk versus benefits. The largest study to date that suggests that this strategy may have promise required most patients to complete a standard treatment regimen through the period of bacteremia prior to changing to dalbavancin [112]. More clinicians in practice have resorted to using these medications for the treatment of endocarditis [3,113] particularly after the initial recommended IV therapy has been given while bacteremic. It is unclear if there will be randomized studies to support the use of long-acting glycopeptides for the treatment of endocarditis in individuals with or without IDU. A randomized trial had been planned to address this question in patients without OUD but was discontinued in 2017 by the sponsor after only enrolling one participant [114].

Dilemmas for treating providers—is oral therapy for endocarditis an option?

Not infrequently, the ID provider is asked to provide recommendations for oral therapy to the primary team caring for a patient who is otherwise clinically stable, and perhaps well into their IV antibiotic treatment for endocarditis. This often occurs because the patient is not being appropriately treated for their OUD while hospitalized, and does not want to stay hospitalized for an extended course of IV antibiotics while in withdrawal. It becomes very challenging to practice medicine where a provider must attempt to provide a treatment regimen that is effective but does not conform to current treatment guidelines; however, there are some minimal data to help guide potential decisions.

Recently, a trial was published that provides preliminary data to support switching to oral antibiotics in very stable individuals with left-sided IE. In the Partial Oral versus Intravenous Antibiotic Treatment of Endocarditis (POET) trial [115,116], individuals with left-sided IE were randomized to continuing IV therapy versus changing to highly effective oral antibiotics after they had been stabilized on at least 10 days of IV therapy. The trial found that oral therapy was noninferior to IV therapy with respect to incidence of clinically relevant embolic events, cardiac surgery, and bacteremia relapse, while the oral antibiotic group also had fewer deaths. The causes of the endocarditis were streptococcus species, *Enterococcus faecalis*, *S. aureus*, or coagulase negative staphylococci. Of note, there were no individuals with methicillin-resistant *S. aureus* (MRSA) and only 5 of the 400 participants in the study were PWID. Further considerations that may temper the enthusiasm for this strategy in PWID were the frequent visits required to the ID clinic over the course of the study and that several antibiotics used in the study are not available in the United States. However, once patients were randomized to the oral treatment group, they only remained in the hospital for 3 days compared with 19 days in the IV group, a definite appeal to many patients with OUD. While the results are certainly encouraging, further research will be required to evaluate this strategy. It will definitely provide some reassurance to providers who often are forced to consider alternative treatment strategies in patients with OUD [3]. These data can serve as one strategy when the clinical situation does not allow for guideline-based decision-making.

Two studies have evaluated the use of predominantly oral 4-week antibiotic regimens (featuring ciprofloxacin plus rifampin) for the therapy of uncomplicated right-sided MSSA IE in PWIDs. In each study, including one in which >70% of patients were HIV seropositive, cure rates were >90% [117,118]. While the relatively high rate of quinolone resistance in *S. aureus* isolates found today may make this strategy problematic, it does provide additional strategies to consider when providers are in situations where they must choose oral alternatives for treatment of this serious condition, which is preferably treated with IV therapy.

Retreatment of PWID with recurrent episodes of endocarditis

PWID who present with repeat infections is an unfortunate reality related to the relapsing-remitting nature of the underlying OUD. However, it also represents another opportunity to engage with patients whose overall poor health outcomes are most likely attributable to their ongoing OUD. Data from one hospital demonstrated that engagement with addiction services or psychiatry was less likely to occur with recurrent admissions perhaps reflecting perceptions of futility in trying to address addiction [119]. It is imperative that the retreatment of these individuals, even repeat surgical intervention, needs to be undertaken more systematically given the high-risk nature of this group. It should be expected that there will be relapses to drug use given the natural history of OUD, and health systems need to engage in longitudinal care of these patients with the chronic medical condition of OUD.

Addiction treatment for hospitalized patients: an opportunity to intervene

Failure to address OUD in hospitalized patients

IE cannot be disconnected from the disorder that led to the infection—IDU due to OUD. However, the failure to address OUD reliably, or connect patients to appropriate long-term follow-up, has been demonstrated in studies focused on endocarditis [119,120], as well as in PWID admitted to the hospital for any reason [121]. A major opportunity has been missed in the past, but engagement must ensue now in order to stem this current crisis.

Hospitalization as opportunity to intervene in OUD

There are increasing calls from a broad range of stakeholders to consider the hospital setting a time to engage patients to get started on OUD treatment [121–125]. While it is abundantly clear that treatment for OUD will require a longstanding relationship with a team of providers in an outpatient setting [126], opportunities abound to engage patients in all areas of the hospital to begin treatment. In emergency departments, research has suggested that brief interventions and initiation of buprenorphine treatment, either during the limited stay in the emergency department or a home-based buprenorphine induction, can lead to increase linkage to care over the following 30 days [127]. The success of this intervention has led to some states legislating that the referral or treatment of OUD be routine for all emergency departments [128]. As with all the interventions for OUD, the key is reliable linkage to care after patients are started on medication to treat OUD, and it will be key that the care continuum is established prior to discharge from emergency departments [129].

If there are demonstrable data showing that an intervention during the brief period of an ED visit can be beneficial, the typical lengthy hospital stay for an admission for treatment of IE represents possibly an even more opportune time to engage and work with the patient on their path to OUD treatment. Englander et al. demonstrated that over 50% of individuals who are hospitalized with substance use disorder are interested in being treated for their condition, with 54% (39 out of 72) of individuals with moderate or high-risk opioid use being interested in medication to treat OUD [130]. It has also been shown that during the course of a hospitalization, a patient will move forward through the stages of change, accepting their illness and becoming ready to begin treatment [131]. Though patients may not be ready or willing to engage during the initial phase of their hospitalization, evidence suggests that this is a fluid period and patients can change in their willingness to accept treatment. It becomes incumbent on the care team to continue to readdress OUD during the course of the hospitalization and offer treatment if the patient is receptive.

The development of a team approach, when feasible, appears to be associated with the most success. In these settings, it becomes important to engage the patient both from a provider level—a person who can write for the medication to treat OUD at the time of discharge—and wraparound services with either case management or social worker [132,133]. Some programs also enlist peer counselors to assist the patients as they begin OUD treatment, offering a voice from someone who has undergone a similar experience as the patient [134].

Medications for OUD treatment—all treatment options should be available to inpatients

There are limited options to medically treat OUD but all three medications (buprenorphine, naltrexone, and methadone) need to be available to all patients who have OUD (Table 8.4). Buprenorphine was approved in 2002 for the treatment of patients with OUD and it allows for an office-based approach for this condition [139,140]. The goal of starting buprenorphine while a patient remains in the inpatient setting is that it can allow the individual to be titrated to a dose that allows for the mitigation of symptoms of withdrawal, decrease cravings, and efficient commencement of OUD treatment. It provides the patient an opportunity for immediate engagement in OUD treatment, relieves withdrawal symptoms which often potentiate early hospital elopement, and allows for appropriate linkage to long-term follow-up.

Naltrexone is an opioid antagonist that has both an oral and intramuscular (IM) formulation. The IM medication is administered monthly and has been approved since 2006 for the treatment of alcohol dependence and approved in 2010 for opioid

Table 8.4 Medication options for opioid use disorder[133,135,139,141].

	Methadone	**Buprenorphine**	**Naltrexone**
Class	Full opioid receptor agonist	Partial opioid receptor agonist	Opioid receptor antagonist
Administration	Oral Once daily	Oral/sublingual Up to three times daily	Intramuscular Once monthly
Effect	Reduces opioid cravings and withdrawal symptoms	Reduces opioid cravings and withdrawal symptoms	Diminishes the reinforcing effects of opioids
Advantages	Ability to offer highly supervised care where additional services can be provided if needed	Available in office settings Comparatively safer profile	Available in office setting Long acting No addictive risk No risk of diversion
Disadvantages	Can only be utilized in specialized programs	8 h of training required to prescribe (or 24 h for advanced practice providers)	Requires prolonged period of abstinence (e.g., 7 days) prior to medication start, risking possible interim relapse

dependence. Treatment with naltrexone has recently been shown to be effective in treating patients with OUD over 24 weeks if they are able to be opioid free for a period of time [141]. In a patient with a protracted hospitalization, as is often the case with IE, this may be an option if it is deemed to be the best treatment for the patient. Long-term data on naltrexone are limited but the recent studies are encouraging that this may be an option that is equivalent to methadone and buprenorphine in the patient that prefers this option after medical detoxification that limit initial withdrawal symptoms.

Methadone clearly has the most data supporting its use for the treatment of OUD since the 1970s and has been a mainstay in providing patients with highly effective OUD treatment. There do remain challenges with how methadone is administered in the country—only at federally sanctioned methadone treatment centers—and there are calls for less restrictive settings given the extent of the current opioid epidemic [142—144]. However, there is no doubt of the efficacy of this medication as it has been studied extensively. In the hospital setting, methadone is often used to control withdrawal symptoms (30—40 mg); however, not all settings allow for the up titration of methadone to actual OUD treatment doses while in the inpatient setting (60—100 mg/day) [135]. The rationale for this strategy is to wean the individual off methadone over the course of the hospitalization (detoxification), and driving the patient to become opioid free. Alternatively, appropriate treatment dose methadone should be considered for inpatient OUD treatment in order to allow the patient to acquire medical care without opioid withdrawal symptoms, decrease their cravings for opioids, efficiently commence full OUD treatment, and hopefully mitigate the chances that these patients will want to leave the hospital before their inpatient treatment is complete or against medical advice.

Furthermore, detoxification rather than treatment creates a period of extreme vulnerability for the patient if they are discharged from the hospital without medications to treat their OUD and are discharged opioid free. Similar to prison settings [136] where individuals often become opioid free, at the time of release from prison (or release from a protracted hospital stay of up to six or more weeks in some cases of endocarditis), they have very low tolerance to opioids and resumption of IDU can lead to fatal overdose. Data from the prison system have shown that death rates in PWID in the early weeks from prison release are staggering with high mortality rates [136,137]. These data support improved OUD treatment and linkage prior to release from prison but should serve as a clear parallel for patients entrusted to our care for many weeks in the hospital setting and whose discharge must ensure a safe transition of care for OUD. The strategy to encourage an individual to become opioid free while hospitalized, though appropriate for some, is not a strategy that is supported by data—given that the chance of being opioid-free 6 months after ceasing all use is highly unlikely when only a strategy of detoxification is employed [138].

Transitions of care

Starting patients on OUD treatment while in the hospital is a key element to the multicomplex treatment of IE in PWID. The success of any medication initiated for OUD during the course of the hospitalization is only as good as the ability to transition the care to the outpatient setting. Methadone initiation in the hospital is a key element to OUD treatment; however, a seamless transition, often with a "warm handoff" to a methadone treatment program, is essential, as methadone cannot be written as a prescription for OUD. This link to an outpatient methadone clinic must be established as it is important from a time perspective that the patient is able to get their next daily dose of methadone to prevent withdrawal symptoms, cravings, and possibly relapse. This is challenging for many given the lack of proximity to methadone facilities throughout the Unites States, but this needs to be arranged prior to discharge from the hospital setting. In many settings, hospital initiation of buprenorphine may be more beneficial, given that a short-term prescription can be written upon hospital discharge that allows time to link the patient to an outpatient buprenorphine provider.

As the initial hospital course ends, the reality of returning to society can expose the patient to multiple challenges including financial, social, legal, and potentially returning to an environment that may trigger their drug use. This only adds to the complex dynamic that patients are experiencing as they recover from endocarditis, and attention to their vulnerability in this moment can be instrumental to their successful treatment of OUD.

Teaching harm reduction strategies prior to discharge

Harm reduction refers to strategies (Table 8.5) that attempt to decrease the negative consequences from drug use [145], and these interventions need to be included both as a set of guidelines to allow for safe drug use and also as means of engagement with the patient, such that they understand that the provider and health system are willing to meet the patient where they are. Whether a patient with IE has decided to enter OUD treatment during hospitalization (buprenorphine or treatment dose methadone), all patients should be taught strategies to both decrease the chance of new infections from their current IDU (or relapse) and prevent suffering from fatal overdose [146]. Providers need to actively engage patients in discussing safe injection practices and other harm reduction strategies.

While there remains controversy as to whether communities should adopt safe injection facilities, either within hospital settings or within a designated space in the community [147,148], there should be agreement that routine teaching about safe injection practices, availability of clean syringes and other paraphernalia, and education about community resources for all patients with a history of IDU at the time of discharge should be considered normal practice [149]. Many communities throughout the country have developed needle exchange programs that have been shown to decrease the risk of infection from HIV and hepatitis C infection [150,151]. There are currently no specific data supporting that needle exchange programs also reduce the incidence of IE, but there is a presumption that a clean syringe that is not overused can reduce risk of bacterial translocation and therefore IE. If harm reduction services are not available to patients in certain communities, teaching patients how to sterilize dirty needles is advised including the use of a diluted bleach solution to kill microorganisms. This requires expanding the typical role of an ID provider, but this advice can perhaps prevent the next infection.

In addition to safe injection practices, advice on avoiding injecting drugs alone as well as giving naloxone to the patient, friends, and family should become commonplace. A sharp increase in overdose deaths related to the introduction of fentanyl into the heroin supply in many parts of the country has resulted in patients unknowingly injecting fentanyl which leads to respiratory suppression and death [152]. Intranasal or intramuscular naloxone administration is a potentially life-saving intervention and access to this medication is one of the three areas of focus in the Department of Health and Human Services strategy to respond to the opioid crisis [153,154]. Naloxone is the only medication approved for the reversal of the effects of an opioid overdose and its administration represents a means to keep a patient from dying from an unintentional overdose until they have a chance to succeed in their OUD treatment. Increasing naloxone availability in the community has been shown to lower overdose deaths and it should be routine for all individuals with OUD who are being discharged from the hospital [155].

Table 8.5 Harm reduction strategies[145,146,159,160].

Engage without bias	Stigma decreases engagement Implicit and explicit bias Appropriate linkage to addiction care and medication

Safe injection practices	"Fix with a friend," or avoidance of solo injection drug use
	
	    While encouraging patients to work on recovery, be mindful that individuals may relapse with multiple starts/stops — hopefully with overall fewer days of drug use. In the interim, encourage patients to avoid injecting alone, in order to mitigate potential fatal overdose.
	
	Seek clean needles, or disinfect used needles if necessary
	
	    Discourage needle sharing or needle reuse; if access to new needles is unavailable, PWID should sterilize used needles with bleach or equivalent cleaning solution between uses
	
	Syringe services programs (SSP)
	
	    These community-based prevention programs provide services like linkage to substance use disorder treatment; access to/disposal of sterile syringes and injection equipment; vaccination, testing, and linkage to care for infectious diseases. SSPs protect the public by facilitating the safe disposal of used needles/syringes. Providing testing, counseling, and sterile injection supplies also prevents outbreaks of diseases like HIV, HCV, or STIs.
	
	Teaching sterile injection technique
	
	    In addition to syringe and needle targeted efforts as above, patients should be provided information surrounding cleaning the skin and other injection equipment ("cookers"), utilizing sterile water, caution with acidification of substance with citrus peels or juice (which can cause fungal infection), and counseling surrounding "cotton" or filter reuse.

Overdose education and naloxone distribution	Offer naloxone to patients at increased risk of overdose • Personal history of overdose • history of substance use disorder • Taking benzodiazepines with opioids • at risk for returning to high dose of opioids to which they are no longer tolerant (e.g., patients recently released from prison) • Taking high doses of opioids ($\geq$50 MME/day) Educate not only the patient, but also household members on overdose prevention and naloxone use Please note that distributing naloxone to third parties is regulated by state laws.

Outpatient based opioid treatment (OBOT) in ID clinic

Treatment of addiction within the Infectious Diseases clinic is a natural fit in many cases as buprenorphine prescribing can be seen as an opportunity to provide primary care for OUD and infectious diseases care in the same location [156,157]. This colocation of essential services treats both long-term disease processes and certainly makes it easier for patients to have both issues treated within the same physical clinic space. This model was successful in the past with clinics providing both HIV primary care and treatment for OUD with buprenorphine and ID clinics should again consider encouraging providers to become engaged in the treatment of OUD. In many ways, the current crisis reminds ID providers of the early days of the HIV epidemic where providers need to be enlisted to care for many stigmatized patients providing them the care they need, even when it occasionally is outside of the typical role the ID provider plays. The education of more ID providers in addiction treatment needs to occur and a recent manuscript served as a primer for providers in order to gain a level of familiarity with the concept, and offers instructions for a way forward [158]. The reality has been that "far too often … infections that we treat resolve while underlying substance use disorders are left to fester" [123].

Summary

The current opioid epidemic, and in particular, the increasing frequency of injection of these drugs, has led to a sharp increase in the number of cases of IE. Special care needs to be given to ensure that the concomitant treatment of OUD and treatment of IE occurs simultaneously. Emphasis should also be placed on harm reduction strategies both to prevent reinfection and to provide life-saving overdose reversal medication given the relapsing and remitting challenges in a patient's journey toward OUD treatment. As infectious diseases providers, it is incumbent on us to learn how to manage both infection and the OUD in order to give our patients the chance at the best possible outcomes from this serious infectious complication of IDU.

References

[1] Zibbell JE, Asher AK, Patel RC, Kupronis B, Iqbal K, Ward JW, et al. Increases in acute hepatitis C virus infection related to a growing opioid epidemic and associated injection drug use, United States, 2004 to 2014. Am J Public Health 2018;108(2): 175−81. https://doi.org/10.2105/AJPH.2017.304132. Epub 2017/12/22; PubMed PMID: 29267061; PubMed Central PMCID: PMCPMC5846578.

[2] Jost JJ, Tempalski B, Vera T, Akiyama MJ, Mangalonzo AP, Litwin AH. Gaps in HCV knowledge and risk behaviors among young suburban people who inject drugs. Int J Environ Res Public Health 2019;16(11). https://doi.org/10.3390/ijerph16111958. Epub 2019/06/05; PubMed PMID: 31159479.

[3] Rapoport AB, Fischer LS, Santibanez S, Beekmann SE, Polgreen PM, Rowley CF. Infectious diseases physicians' perspectives regarding injection drug use and related

infections, United States, 2017. Open Forum Infect Dis 2018;5(7):ofy132. https://doi.org/10.1093/ofid/ofy132. Epub 2018/07/19; PubMed PMID: 30018999; PubMed Central PMCID: PMCPMC6041812.

[4] Cahill TJ, Baddour LM, Habib G, Hoen B, Salaun E, Pettersson GB, et al. Challenges in infective endocarditis. J Am Coll Cardiol 2017;69(3):325—44. https://doi.org/10.1016/j.jacc.2016.10.066. Epub 2017/01/21; PubMed PMID: 28104075.

[5] Schranz AJ, Fleischauer A, Chu VH, Wu LT, Rosen DL. Trends in drug use-associated infective endocarditis and heart valve surgery, 2007 to 2017: astudy of statewide discharge data. Ann Intern Med 2018. https://doi.org/10.7326/M18-2124. Epub 2018/12/07; PubMed PMID: 30508432.

[6] Arbulu A, Kafi A, Thoms NW, Wilson RF. Right-sided bacterial endocarditis. New concepts in the treatment of the uncontrollable infection. Ann Thorac Surg 1973; 16(2):136—40. Epub 1973/08/01; PubMed PMID: 4200348.

[7] Stimmel B, Donoso E, Dack S. Comparison of infective endocarditis in drug addicts and nondrug users. Am J Cardiol 1973;32(7):924—9. Epub 1973/12/01; PubMed PMID: 4757232.

[8] Hussey HH, Katz S. Infections resulting from narcotic addiction; report of 102 cases. Am J Med 1950;9(2):186—93. Epub 1950/08/01; PubMed PMID: 15432465.

[9] Keynan Y, Rubinstein E. Pathophysiology of infective endocarditis. Curr Infect Dis Rep 2013;15(4):342—6. https://doi.org/10.1007/s11908-013-0346-0. Epub 2013/06/06; PubMed PMID: 23737237.

[10] Chambers HF, Morris DL, Tauber MG, Modin G. Cocaine use and the risk for endocarditis in intravenous drug users. Ann Intern Med 1987;106(6):833—6. Epub 1987/06/01; PubMed PMID: 3579070.

[11] Frontera JA, Gradon JD. Right-side endocarditis in injection drug users: review of proposed mechanisms of pathogenesis. Clin Infect Di 2000;30(2):374—9. https://doi.org/10.1086/313664. Epub 2000/02/15; PubMed PMID: 10671344.

[12] Barrau K, Boulamery A, Imbert G, Casalta JP, Habib G, Messana T, et al. Causative organisms of infective endocarditis according to host status. Clin Microbiol Infect 2004;10(4):302—8. https://doi.org/10.1111/j.1198-743X.2004.00776.x. Epub 2004/04/03; PubMed PMID: 15059118.

[13] Widmer E, Que YA, Entenza JM, Moreillon P. New concepts in the pathophysiology of infective endocarditis. Curr Infect Dis Rep 2006;8(4):271—9. Epub 2006/07/11; PubMed PMID: 16822370.

[14] Ciccarone D. Fentanyl in the US heroin supply: a rapidly changing risk environment. Int J Drug Policy 2017;46:107—11. https://doi.org/10.1016/j.drugpo.2017.06.010. Epub 2017/07/25; PubMed PMID: 28735776; PubMed Central PMCID: PMCPMC5742018.

[15] McGuigan CC, Penrice GM, Gruer L, Ahmed S, Goldberg D, Black M, et al. Lethal outbreak of infection with Clostridium novyi type A and other spore-forming organisms in Scottish injecting drug users. J Med Microbiol 2002;51(11):971—7. https://doi.org/10.1099/0022-1317-51-11-971. Epub 2002/11/27; PubMed PMID: 12448681.

[16] Dancer SJ, McNair D, Finn P, Kolsto AB. Bacillus cereus cellulitis from contaminated heroin. J Med Microbiol 2002;51(3):278—81. https://doi.org/10.1099/0022-1317-51-3-278. Epub 2002/03/02; PubMed PMID: 11871624.

[17] Phillips KT, Stein MD. Risk practices associated with bacterial infections among injection drug users in Denver, Colorado. Am J Drug Alcohol Abuse 2010;36(2):

92−7. https://doi.org/10.3109/00952991003592311. Epub 2010/03/27; PubMed PMID: 20337504; PubMed Central PMCID: PMCPMC4869685.

[18] Nnaoma C, Chika-Nwosuh O, Sossou C. A rare culprit of infective endocarditis in an IV drug user: *Burkholderia cepacia*. Case Rep Med 2019;2019:6403943. https://doi.org/10.1155/2019/6403943. Epub 2019/05/21; PubMed PMID: 31105761; PubMed Central PMCID: PMCPMC6481116.

[19] Williamson DA, McBride SJ. A case of tricuspid valve endocarditis due to *Burkholderia cepacia* complex. N Z Med J 2011;124(1340):84−6. Epub 2011/09/29; PubMed PMID: 21952388.

[20] Lorson WC, Heidel RE, Shorman MA. Microbial epidemiology of infectious endocarditis in the intravenous drug abuse population: aretrospective study. Infect Dis Ther 2019;8(1):113−8. https://doi.org/10.1007/s40121-019-0232-7. Epub 2019/01/24; PubMed PMID: 30673991; PubMed Central PMCID: PMCPMC6374230.

[21] Pierrotti LC, Baddour LM. Fungal endocarditis, 1995-2000. Chest 2002;122(1):302−10. https://doi.org/10.1378/chest.122.1.302. Epub 2002/07/13; PubMed PMID: 12114375.

[22] Leen CL, Brettle RP. Fungal infections in drug users. J Antimicrob Chemother 1991;28(Suppl. A):83−96. https://doi.org/10.1093/jac/28.suppl_a.83. Epub 1991/07/01; PubMed PMID: 1938709.

[23] Barter DM, Johnston HL, Williams SR, Tsay SV, Vallabhaneni S, Bamberg WM. Candida bloodstream infections among persons who inject drugs - Denver Metropolitan Area, Colorado, 2017-2018. MMWR Morb Mortal Wkly Rep 2019;68(12):285−8. https://doi.org/10.15585/mmwr.mm6812a3. Epub 2019/03/29; PubMed PMID: 30921302; PubMed Central PMCID: PMCPMC6448981 potential conflicts of interest. No potential conflicts of interest were disclosed.

[24] Poowanawittayakom N, Dutta A, Stock S, Touray S, Ellison 3rd RT, Levitz SM. Reemergence of intravenous drug use as risk factor for candidemia, Massachusetts, USA. Emerg Infect Dis 2018;24(4). https://doi.org/10.3201/eid2404.171807. Epub 2018/03/20; PubMed PMID: 29553923; PubMed Central PMCID: PMCPMC5875264.

[25] Deutscher M, Perlman DC. Why some injection drug users lick their needles: a preliminary survey. Int J Drug Policy 2008;19(4):342−5. https://doi.org/10.1016/j.drugpo.2007.06.006. Epub 2008/07/22; PubMed PMID: 18638706.

[26] Swisher LA, Roberts JR, Glynn MJ. Needle licker's osteomyelitis. Am J Emerg Med 1994;12(3):343−6. Epub 1994/05/01; PubMed PMID: 8179747.

[27] Liang X, Liu R, Chen C, Ji F, Li T. Opioid system modulates the immune function: a review. Transl Perioper Pain Med 2016;1(1):5−13. Epub 2016/03/18; PubMed PMID: 26985446; PubMed Central PMCID: PMCPMC4790459.

[28] Dublin S, Von Korff M. Prescription opioids and infection risk: research and caution needed. Ann Intern Med 2018;168(6):444−5. https://doi.org/10.7326/M18-0001. Epub 2018/02/13; PubMed PMID: 29435579.

[29] Plein LM, Rittner HL. Opioids and the immune system - friend or foe. Br J Pharmacol 2018;175(14):2717−25. https://doi.org/10.1111/bph.13750. Epub 2017/02/19; PubMed PMID: 28213891; PubMed Central PMCID: PMCPMC6016673.

[30] Wiese AD, Grijalva CG. The use of prescribed opioid analgesics & the risk of serious infections. Future Microbiol 2018;13:849−52. https://doi.org/10.2217/fmb-2018-0101. Epub 2018/06/14; PubMed PMID: 29896976; PubMed Central PMCID: PMCPMC6060396.

[31] Wiese AD, Griffin MR, Stein CM, Mitchel Jr EF, Grijalva CG. Opioid analgesics and the risk of serious infections among patients with rheumatoid arthritis: aself-controlled case series study. Arthritis Rheumatol 2016;68(2):323−31. https://doi.org/10.1002/art.39462. Epub 2015/10/17; PubMed PMID: 26473742; PubMed Central PMCID: PMCPMC4728045.

[32] Dublin S, Walker RL, Jackson ML, Nelson JC, Weiss NS, Von Korff M, et al. Use of opioids or benzodiazepines and risk of pneumonia in older adults: a population-based case-control study. J Am Geriatr Soc 2011;59(10):1899−907. https://doi.org/10.1111/j.1532-5415.2011.03586.x. Epub 2011/11/19; PubMed PMID: 22091503; PubMed Central PMCID: PMCPMC3223721.

[33] Wiese AD, Griffin MR, Schaffner W, Stein CM, Grijalva CG. Opioid analgesic use and risk for invasive pneumococcal diseases. Ann Intern Med 2018;169(5):355. https://doi.org/10.7326/L18-0295. Epub 2018/09/05; PubMed PMID: 30178014.

[34] Amini M, Poustchi H. Hepatitis C virus spontaneous clearance: immunology and genetic variance. Viral Immunol 2012;25(4):241−8. https://doi.org/10.1089/vim.2011.0052. Epub 2012/07/25; PubMed PMID: 22823386.

[35] Kaka AS, Filice GA, Kuskowski M, Musher DM. Does active hepatitis C virus infection increase the risk for infection due to *Staphylococcus aureus*? Eur J Clin Microbiol Infect Dis 2017;36(7):1217−23. https://doi.org/10.1007/s10096-017-2912-0. Epub 2017/02/06; PubMed PMID: 28160146.

[36] Albillos A, Lario M, Alvarez-Mon M. Cirrhosis-associated immune dysfunction: distinctive features and clinical relevance. J Hepatol 2014;61(6):1385−96. https://doi.org/10.1016/j.jhep.2014.08.010. Epub 2014/08/20; PubMed PMID: 25135860.

[37] Cranston K, Alpren C, John B, Dawson E, Roosevelt K, Burrage A, et al. Notes from the field: HIV diagnoses among persons who inject drugs - Northeastern Massachusetts, 2015-2018. MMWR Morb Mortal Wkly Rep 2019;68(10):253−4. https://doi.org/10.15585/mmwr.mm6810a6. Epub 2019/03/15; PubMed PMID: 30870405; PubMed Central PMCID: PMCPMC6421964 potential conflicts of interest. Nivedha Panneer reports stock ownership in Gilead. Shauna Onofrey reports that a family member works for and owns stock in Emergent Biosolutions. No other potential conflicts of interest were disclosed.

[38] Bradley H, Hogan V, Agnew-Brune C, Armstrong J, Broussard D, Buchacz K, et al. Increased HIV diagnoses in West Virginia counties highly vulnerable to rapid HIV dissemination through injection drug use: a cautionary tale. Ann Epidemiol 2019;34:12−7. https://doi.org/10.1016/j.annepidem.2019.02.012. Epub 2019/04/11; PubMed PMID: 30967302.

[39] Conrad C, Bradley HM, Broz D, Buddha S, Chapman EL, Galang RR, et al. Community outbreak of HIV infection linked to injection drug use of oxymorphone-Indiana, 2015. MMWR Morb Mortal Wkly Rep 2015;64(16):443−4. Epub 2015/05/01; PubMed PMID: 25928470; PubMed Central PMCID: PMCPMC4584812.

[40] Peters PJ, Pontones P, Hoover KW, Patel MR, Galang RR, Shields J, et al. HIV infection linked to injection use of oxymorphone in Indiana, 2014-2015. N Engl J Med 2016;375(3):229−39. https://doi.org/10.1056/NEJMoa1515195. Epub 2016/07/29; PubMed PMID: 27468059.

[41] Berger BJ, Hussain F, Roistacher K. Bacterial infections in HIV-infected patients. Infect Dis Clin North Am 1994;8(2):449−65. Epub 1994/06/01; PubMed PMID: 8089471.

[42] O'Connor J, Vjecha MJ, Phillips AN, Angus B, Cooper D, Grinsztejn B, et al. Effect of immediate initiation of antiretroviral therapy on risk of severe bacterial infections in HIV-positive people with CD4 cell counts of more than 500 cells per muL: secondary outcome results from a randomised controlled trial. Lancet HIV 2017;4(3):e105–12. https://doi.org/10.1016/S2352-3018(16)30216-8. Epub 2017/01/09; PubMed PMID: 28063815; PubMed Central PMCID: PMCPMC5337625.

[43] de Gaetano Donati K, Tumbarello M, Tacconelli E, Bertagnolio S, Rabagliati R, Scoppettuolo G, et al. Impact of highly active antiretroviral therapy (HAART) on the incidence of bacterial infections in HIV-infected subjects. J Chemother 2003; 15(1):60–5. https://doi.org/10.1179/joc.2003.15.1.60. Epub 2003/04/08; PubMed PMID: 12678416.

[44] Wurcel AG, Anderson JE, Chui KK, Skinner S, Knox TA, Snydman DR, et al. Increasing infectious endocarditis admissions among young people who inject drugs. Open Forum Infect Dis 2016;3(3):ofw157. https://doi.org/10.1093/ofid/ofw157. Epub 2016/11/02; PubMed PMID: 27800528; PubMed Central PMCID: PMCPMC5084714.

[45] Deo SV, Raza S, Kalra A, Deo VS, Altarabsheh SE, Zia A, et al. Admissions for infective endocarditis in intravenous drug users. J Am Coll Cardiol 2018;71(14):1596–7. https://doi.org/10.1016/j.jacc.2018.02.011. Epub 2018/04/07; PubMed PMID: 29622169.

[46] Rudasill SE, Sanaiha Y, Mardock AL, Khoury H, Xing H, Antonios JW, et al. Clinical outcomes of infective endocarditis in injection drug users. J Am Coll Cardiol 2019; 73(5):559–70. https://doi.org/10.1016/j.jacc.2018.10.082. Epub 2019/02/09; PubMed PMID: 30732709.

[47] Cooper HL, Brady JE, Ciccarone D, Tempalski B, Gostnell K, Friedman SR. Nationwide increase in the number of hospitalizations for illicit injection drug use-related infective endocarditis. Clin Infect Dis 2007;45(9):1200–3. https://doi.org/10.1086/522176. Epub 2007/10/06; PubMed PMID: 17918083; PubMed Central PMCID: PMCPMC2567828.

[48] Scholl L, Seth P, Kariisa M, Wilson N, Baldwin G. Drug and opioid-involved overdose deaths - United States, 2013-2017. MMWR Morb Mortal Wkly Rep 2018;67(5152): 1419–27. https://doi.org/10.15585/mmwr.mm675152e1. Epub 2019/01/04; PubMed PMID: 30605448; PubMed Central PMCID: PMCPMC6334822 potential conflicts of interest. No potential conflicts of interest were disclosed.

[49] Rudd RA, Seth P, David F, Scholl L. Increases in drug and opioid-involved overdose deaths - United States, 2010-2015. MMWR Morb Mortal Wkly Rep 2016;65(50–51): 1445–52. https://doi.org/10.15585/mmwr.mm655051e1. Epub 2016/12/30; PubMed PMID: 28033313.

[50] Keeshin SW, Feinberg J. Endocarditis as a marker for new epidemics of injection drug use. Am J Med Sci 2016;352(6):609–14. https://doi.org/10.1016/j.amjms.2016.10.002. Epub 2016/12/06; PubMed PMID: 27916216; PubMed Central PMCID: PMCPMC5482229.

[51] Bhat AG, Siddappa Malleshappa SK, Pasupula DK. Recognizing infective endocarditis and drug abuse through ICD codes in administrative databases. J Am Coll Cardiol 2019;73(22):2907–8. https://doi.org/10.1016/j.jacc.2019.02.077. Epub 2019/06/07; PubMed PMID: 31171101.

[52] Murdoch DR, Corey GR, Hoen B, Miro JM, Fowler Jr VG, Bayer AS, et al. Clinical presentation, etiology, and outcome of infective endocarditis in the 21st century: the

International Collaboration on Endocarditis-Prospective Cohort Study. Arch Intern Med 2009;169(5):463−73. https://doi.org/10.1001/archinternmed.2008.603. PubMed PMID: 19273776; PubMed Central PMCID: PMCPMC3625651.

[53] Leahey PA, LaSalvia MT, Rosenthal ES, Karchmer AW, Rowley CF. High morbidity and mortality among patients with sentinel admission for injection drug use-related infective endocarditis. Open Forum Infect Dis 2019;6(4):ofz089. https://doi.org/10.1093/ofid/ofz089. Epub 2019/04/06; PubMed PMID: 30949535; PubMed Central PMCID: PMCPMC6441563.

[54] Rabkin DG, Mokadam NA, Miller DW, Goetz RR, Verrier ED, Aldea GS. Long-term outcome for the surgical treatment of infective endocarditis with a focus on intravenous drug users. Ann Thorac Surg 2012;93(1):51−7. https://doi.org/10.1016/j.athoracsur.2011.08.016. PubMed PMID: 22054655.

[55] Nadji G, Remadi JP, Coviaux F, Mirode AA, Brahim A, Enriquez-Sarano M, et al. Comparison of clinical and morphological characteristics of *Staphylococcus aureus* endocarditis with endocarditis caused by other pathogens. Heart 2005;91(7):932−7. https://doi.org/10.1136/hrt.2004.042648. PubMed PMID: 15958364; PubMed Central PMCID: PMCPMC1768988.

[56] Thalme A, Westling K, Julander I. In-hospital and long-term mortality in infective endocarditis in injecting drug users compared to non-drug users: a retrospective study of 192 episodes. Scand J Infect Dis 2007;39(3):197−204. https://doi.org/10.1080/00365540600978856. PubMed PMID: 17366047.

[57] Lefort A, Chartier L, Sendid B, Wolff M, Mainardi JL, Podglajen I, et al. Diagnosis, management and outcome of Candida endocarditis. Clin Microbiol Infect 2012;18(4):E99−109. https://doi.org/10.1111/j.1469-0691.2012.03764.x. Epub 2012/02/15; PubMed PMID: 22329526.

[58] Bisbe J, Miro JM, Latorre X, Moreno A, Mallolas J, Gatell JM, et al. Disseminated candidiasis in addicts who use brown heroin: report of 83 cases and review. Clin Infect Dis 1992;15(6):910−23. https://doi.org/10.1093/clind/15.6.910. Epub 1992/12/01; PubMed PMID: 1457662.

[59] Sklaver AR, Hoffman TA, Greenman RL. Staphylococcal endocarditis in addicts. South Med J 1978;71(6):638−43. https://doi.org/10.1097/00007611-197806000-00009. Epub 1978/06/01; PubMed PMID: 663692.

[60] Moss R, Munt B. Injection drug use and right sided endocarditis. Heart 2003;89(5):577−81. Epub 2003/04/16; PubMed PMID: 12695478; PubMed Central PMCID: PMCPMC1767660.

[61] Carozza A, De Santo LS, Romano G, Della Corte A, Ursomando F, Scardone M, et al. Infective endocarditis in intravenous drug abusers: patterns of presentation and long-term outcomes of surgical treatment. J Heart Valve Dis 2006;15(1):125−31. PubMed PMID: 16480024.

[62] Faber M, Frimodt-Moller N, Espersen F, Skinhoj P, Rosdahl V. *Staphylococcus aureus* endocarditis in Danish intravenous drug users: high proportion of left-sided endocarditis. Scand J Infect Dis 1995;27(5):483−7. Epub 1995/01/01; PubMed PMID: 8588139.

[63] Mathew J, Addai T, Anand A, Morrobel A, Maheshwari P, Freels S. Clinical features, site of involvement, bacteriologic findings, and outcome of infective endocarditis in intravenous drug users. Arch Intern Med 1995;155(15):1641−8. Epub 1995/08/07; PubMed PMID: 7618988.

[64] Ruotsalainen E, Sammalkorpi K, Laine J, Huotari K, Sarna S, Valtonen V, et al. Clinical manifestations and outcome in *Staphylococcus aureus* endocarditis among injection drug users and nonaddicts: a prospective study of 74 patients. BMC Infect Dis 2006;6:137. https://doi.org/10.1186/1471-2334-6-137. PubMed PMID: 16965625; PubMed Central PMCID: PMCPMC1584240.

[65] Jones CM, Logan J, Gladden RM, Bohm MK. Vital signs: demographic and substance use trends among heroin users - United States, 2002-2013. MMWR Morb Mortal Wkly Rep 2015;64(26):719−25. PubMed PMID: 26158353.

[66] Li JS, Sexton DJ, Mick N, Nettles R, Fowler Jr VG, Ryan T, et al. Proposed modifications to the Duke criteria for the diagnosis of infective endocarditis. Clin Infect Dis 2000;30(4):633−8. https://doi.org/10.1086/313753. Epub 2000/04/19; PubMed PMID: 10770721.

[67] Baddour LM, Wilson WR, Bayer AS, Fowler Jr VG, Tleyjeh IM, Rybak MJ, et al. Infective endocarditis in adults: diagnosis, antimicrobial therapy, and management of complications: a scientific statement for healthcare professionals from the American heart association. Circulation 2015;132(15):1435−86. https://doi.org/10.1161/CIR.0000000000000296. PubMed PMID: 26373316.

[68] Cecchi E, Imazio M, Tidu M, Forno D, De Rosa FG, Dal Conte I, et al. Infective endocarditis in drug addicts: role of HIV infection and the diagnostic accuracy of Duke criteria. J Cardiovasc Med (Hagerstown) 2007;8(3):169−75. https://doi.org/10.2459/01.JCM.0000260824.14596.86. Epub 2007/02/22; PubMed PMID: 17312433.

[69] Palepu A, Cheung SS, Montessori V, Woods R, Thompson CR. Factors other than the Duke criteria associated with infective endocarditis among injection drug users. Clin Invest Med 2002;25(4):118−25. Epub 2002/09/11; PubMed PMID: 12220038.

[70] Habib G, Lancellotti P, Antunes MJ, Bongiorni MG, Casalta JP, Del Zotti F, et al. 2015 ESC guidelines for the management of infective endocarditis: the task force for the management of infective endocarditis of the European Society of Cardiology (ESC). Endorsed by: European Association for Cardio-Thoracic Surgery (EACTS), the European Association of Nuclear Medicine (EANM). Eur Heart J 2015;36(44):3075−128. https://doi.org/10.1093/eurheartj/ehv319. Epub 2015/09/01; PubMed PMID: 26320109.

[71] Gould FK, Denning DW, Elliott TS, Foweraker J, Perry JD, Prendergast BD, et al. Guidelines for the diagnosis and antibiotic treatment of endocarditis in adults: a report of the Working Party of the British Society for Antimicrobial Chemotherapy. J Antimicrob Chemother 2012;67(2):269−89. https://doi.org/10.1093/jac/dkr450. Epub 2011/11/17; PubMed PMID: 22086858.

[72] Reyes MP, Ali A, Mendes RE, Biedenbach DJ. Resurgence of Pseudomonas endocarditis in Detroit, 2006-2008. Medicine (Baltimore) 2009;88(5):294−301. https://doi.org/10.1097/MD.0b013e3181b8bedc. Epub 2009/09/12; PubMed PMID: 19745688.

[73] Shekar R, Rice TW, Zierdt CH, Kallick CA. Outbreak of endocarditis caused by *Pseudomonas aeruginosa* serotype O11 among pentazocine and tripelennamine abusers in Chicago. J Infect Dis 1985;151(2):203−8. https://doi.org/10.1093/infdis/151.2.203. Epub 1985/02/01; PubMed PMID: 3918121.

[74] Levin MH, Weinstein RA, Nathan C, Selander RK, Ochman H, Kabins SA. Association of infection caused by *Pseudomonas aeruginosa* serotype O11 with intravenous abuse of pentazocine mixed with tripelennamine. J Clin Microbiol 1984;20(4):

758−62. Epub 1984/10/01; PubMed PMID: 6436316; PubMed Central PMCID: PMCPMC271426.

[75] Lalani T, Cabell CH, Benjamin DK, Lasca O, Naber C, Fowler Jr VG, et al. Analysis of the impact of early surgery on in-hospital mortality of native valve endocarditis: use of propensity score and instrumental variable methods to adjust for treatment-selection bias. Circulation 2010;121(8):1005−13. https://doi.org/10.1161/CIRCULATIO-NAHA.109.864488. Epub 2010/02/18; PubMed PMID: 20159831; PubMed Central PMCID: PMCPMC3597944.

[76] Chatterjee S, Sardar P. Early surgery reduces mortality in patients with infective endo-carditis: insight from a meta-analysis. Int J Cardiol 2013;168(3):3094−7. https://doi.org/10.1016/j.ijcard.2013.04.078. Epub 2013/05/07; PubMed PMID: 23642830.

[77] Kim DH, Kang DH, Lee MZ, Yun SC, Kim YJ, Song JM, et al. Impact of early surgery on embolic events in patients with infective endocarditis. Circulation 2010;122(11 Suppl. l):S17−22. https://doi.org/10.1161/CIRCULATIONAHA.109.927665. Epub 2010/09/21; PubMed PMID: 20837909.

[78] Chairs ASToIECGWC, Pettersson GB, Coselli JS, Writing C, Pettersson GB, Coselli JS, et al. 2016 the American Association for Thoracic Surgery (AATS) consensus guidelines: surgical treatment of infective endocarditis: executive summary. J Thorac Cardiovasc Surg 2017;153(6):1241−58. https://doi.org/10.1016/j.jtcvs.2016.09.093. e29. Epub 2017/04/04; PubMed PMID: 28365016.

[79] Barsic B, Dickerman S, Krajinovic V, Pappas P, Altclas J, Carosi G, et al. Influence of the timing of cardiac surgery on the outcome of patients with infective endocarditis and stroke. Clin Infect Dis 2013;56(2):209−17. https://doi.org/10.1093/cid/cis878. Epub 2012/10/18; PubMed PMID: 23074311.

[80] Piper C, Wiemer M, Schulte HD, Horstkotte D. Stroke is not a contraindication for ur-gent valve replacement in acute infective endocarditis. J Heart Valve Dis 2001;10(6):703−11. Epub 2002/01/05; PubMed PMID: 11767174.

[81] Zhang J, Yang Y, Sun H, Xing Y. Hemorrhagic transformation after cerebral infarction: current concepts and challenges. Ann Transl Med 2014;2(8):81. https://doi.org/10.3978/j.issn.2305-5839.2014.08.08. Epub 2014/10/22; PubMed PMID: 25333056; PubMed Central PMCID: PMCPMC4200641.

[82] Kang DH. Timing of surgery in infective endocarditis. Heart 2015;101(22):1786−91. https://doi.org/10.1136/heartjnl-2015-307878. Epub 2015/08/20; PubMed PMID: 26285598.

[83] Osterdal OB, Salminen PR, Jordal S, Sjursen H, Wendelbo O, Haaverstad R. Cardiac surgery for infective endocarditis in patients with intravenous drug use. Interact Car-diovasc Thorac Surg 2016;22(5):633−40. https://doi.org/10.1093/icvts/ivv397. PubMed PMID: 26826713; PubMed Central PMCID: PMCPMC4892139.

[84] Nguemeni Tiako MJ, Mori M, Bin Mahmood SU, Shioda K, Mangi A, Yun J, et al. Recidivism is the leading cause of death among intravenous drug users who underwent cardiac surgery for infective endocarditis. Semin Thorac Cardiovasc Surg 2019;31(1):40−5. https://doi.org/10.1053/j.semtcvs.2018.07.016. Epub 2018/08/31; PubMed PMID: 30165237.

[85] Kim JB, Ejiofor JI, Yammine M, Ando M, Camuso JM, Youngster I, et al. Surgical out-comes of infective endocarditis among intravenous drug users. J Thorac Cardiovasc Surg 2016;152(3):832−41. https://doi.org/10.1016/j.jtcvs.2016.02.072. e1. Epub 2016/04/14; PubMed PMID: 27068439.

[86] Huang G, Barnes EW, Peacock Jr JE. Repeat infective endocarditis in persons who inject drugs: "take another little piece of my heart". Open Forum Infect Dis 2018; 5(12):ofy304. https://doi.org/10.1093/ofid/ofy304. Epub 2018/12/18; PubMed PMID: 30555849; PubMed Central PMCID: PMCPMC6288769.

[87] Rodger L, Glockler-Lauf SD, Shojaei E, Sherazi A, Hallam B, Koivu S, et al. Clinical characteristics and factors associated with mortality in first-episode infective endocarditis among persons who inject drugs. JAMA Netw Open 2018;1(7):e185220. https://doi.org/10.1001/jamanetworkopen.2018.5220. Epub 2019/01/16; PubMed PMID: 30646383; PubMed Central PMCID: PMCPMC6324402.

[88] Goodnaugh A. Injecting drugs can ruin a heart. How many second chances should a user get? The New York Times; 2018.

[89] Deas DS, Keeling B. Stop Draggin' My Heart Around: recidivism, intravenous drug use, and endocarditis. Semin Thorac Cardiovasc Surg 2018. https://doi.org/10.1053/j.semtcvs.2018.09.024. Epub 2018/10/03; PubMed PMID: 30278270.

[90] Vlahakes GJ. "Consensus guidelines for the surgical treatment of infective endocarditis": the surgeon must lead the team. J Thorac Cardiovasc Surg 2017;153(6):1259–60. https://doi.org/10.1016/j.jtcvs.2016.10.041. Epub 2016/12/28; PubMed PMID: 28024806.

[91] Wurcel AG, Yu S, Pacheco M, Warner K. Contracts with people who inject drugs following valve surgery: unrealistic and misguided expectations. J Thorac Cardiovasc Surg 2017;154(6):2002. https://doi.org/10.1016/j.jtcvs.2017.07.020. Epub 2017/11/15; PubMed PMID: 29132892.

[92] Hussain ST, Gordon SM, Streem DW, Blackstone EH, Pettersson GB. Contract with the patient with injection drug use and infective endocarditis: surgeons perspective. J Thorac Cardiovasc Surg 2017;154(6):2002–3. https://doi.org/10.1016/j.jtcvs.2017.08.004. Epub 2017/11/15; PubMed PMID: 29132891.

[93] Miljeteig I, Skrede S, Langorgen J, Haaverstad R, Josendal O, Sjursen H, et al. Should patients who use illicit drugs be offered a second heart-valve replacement? Tidsskr Nor Laegeforen 2013;133(9):977–80. https://doi.org/10.4045/tidsskr.12.0779. Epub 2013/05/09; PubMed PMID: 23652149.

[94] Libertin CR, Camsari UM, Hellinger WC, Schneekloth TD, Rummans TA. The cost of a recalcitrant intravenous drug user with serial cases of endocarditis: need for guidelines to improve the continuum of care. IDCases 2017;8:3–5. https://doi.org/10.1016/j.idcr.2017.02.001. Epub 2017/02/28; PubMed PMID: 28239556; PubMed Central PMCID: PMCPMC5320052.

[95] Ferraris VA, Sekela ME. Missing the forest for the trees: the world around us and surgical treatment of endocarditis. J Thorac Cardiovasc Surg 2016;152(3):677–80. https://doi.org/10.1016/j.jtcvs.2016.05.014. PubMed PMID: 27287673.

[96] Townsend J, Keller S, Tibuakuu M, Thakker S, Webster B, Siegel M, et al. Outpatient parenteral therapy for complicated *Staphylococcus aureus* infections: a snapshot of processes and outcomes in the real world. Open Forum Infect Dis 2018;5(11): ofy274. https://doi.org/10.1093/ofid/ofy274. Epub 2018/11/30; PubMed PMID: 30488039; PubMed Central PMCID: PMCPMC6251475.

[97] Fanucchi L, Leedy N, Li J, Thornton AC. Perceptions and practices of physicians regarding outpatient parenteral antibiotic therapy in persons who inject drugs. J Hosp Med 2016;11(8):581–2. https://doi.org/10.1002/jhm.2582. Epub 2016/04/05; PubMed PMID: 27043146.

[98] Ho J, Archuleta S, Sulaiman Z, Fisher D. Safe and successful treatment of intravenous drug users with a peripherally inserted central catheter in an outpatient parenteral antibiotic treatment service. J Antimicrob Chemother 2010;65(12):2641—4. https://doi.org/10.1093/jac/dkq355. Epub 2010/09/25; PubMed PMID: 20864497.

[99] Beieler AM, Dellit TH, Chan JD, Dhanireddy S, Enzian LK, Stone TJ, et al. Successful implementation of outpatient parenteral antimicrobial therapy at a medical respite facility for homeless patients. J Hosp Med 2016;11(8):531—5. https://doi.org/10.1002/jhm.2597. Epub 2016/04/28; PubMed PMID: 27120700.

[100] D'Couto HT, Robbins GK, Ard KL, Wakeman SE, Alves J, Nelson SB. Outcomes according to discharge location for persons who inject drugs receiving outpatient parenteral antimicrobial therapy. Open Forum Infect Dis 2018;5(5):ofy056. https://doi.org/10.1093/ofid/ofy056. Epub 2018/05/17; PubMed PMID: 29766017; PubMed Central PMCID: PMCPMC5941140.

[101] IDSA. 2018 IDSA clinical practice guideline for the management of outpatient parenteral antimicrobial therapy. Available from: https://www.idsociety.org/globalassets/idsa/practice-guidelines/2018-opat-ciy745.pdf.

[102] Suzuki J, Johnson J, Montgomery M, Hayden M, Price C. Outpatient parenteral antimicrobial therapy among people who inject drugs: a review of the literature. Open Forum Infect Dis 2018;5(9):ofy194. https://doi.org/10.1093/ofid/ofy194. Epub 2018/09/14; PubMed PMID: 30211247; PubMed Central PMCID: PMCPMC6127783.

[103] DiNubile MJ. Short-course antibiotic therapy for right-sided endocarditis caused by *Staphylococcus aureus* in injection drug users. Ann Intern Med 1994;121(11):873—6. Epub 1994/12/01; PubMed PMID: 7978701.

[104] Chambers HF, Miller RT, Newman MD. Right-sided *Staphylococcus aureus* endocarditis in intravenous drug abusers: two-week combination therapy. Ann Intern Med 1988;109(8):619—24. https://doi.org/10.7326/0003-4819-109-8-619. Epub 1988/10/15; PubMed PMID: 3421575.

[105] Torres-Tortosa M, de Cueto M, Vergara A, Sanchez-Porto A, Perez-Guzman E, Gonzalez-Serrano M, et al. Prospective evaluation of a two-week course of intravenous antibiotics in intravenous drug addicts with infective endocarditis. Grupo de Estudio de Enfermedades Infecciosas de la Provincia de Cadiz. Eur J Clin Microbiol Infect Dis 1994;13(7):559—64. Epub 1994/07/01; PubMed PMID: 7805683.

[106] Espinosa FJ, Valdes M, Martin-Luengo F, Arribas JP, Albaladejo J, Perez-Gracia A, et al. Right endocarditis caused by *Staphylococcus aureus* in parenteral drug addicts: evaluation of a combined therapeutic scheme for 2 weeks versus conventional treatment. Enferm Infecc Microbiol Clin 1993;11(5):235—40. Epub 1993/05/01; PubMed PMID: 8324018.

[107] Cosgrove SE, Vigliani GA, Fowler Jr VG, Abrutyn E, Corey GR, Levine DP, et al. Initial low-dose gentamicin for *Staphylococcus aureus* bacteremia and endocarditis is nephrotoxic. Clin Infect Dis 2009;48(6):713—21. https://doi.org/10.1086/597031. Epub 2009/02/12; PubMed PMID: 19207079.

[108] Roberts KD, Sulaiman RM, Rybak MJ. Dalbavancin and oritavancin: an innovative approach to the treatment of gram-positive infections. Pharmacotherapy 2015;35(10):935—48. https://doi.org/10.1002/phar.1641. Epub 2015/10/27; PubMed PMID: 26497480.

[109] Steele JM, Seabury RW, Hale CM, Mogle BT. Unsuccessful treatment of methicillin-resistant *Staphylococcus aureus* endocarditis with dalbavancin. J Clin Pharm Ther

2018;43(1):101–3. https://doi.org/10.1111/jcpt.12580. Epub 2017/06/20; PubMed PMID: 28628223.

[110] Kussmann M, Karer M, Obermueller M, Schmidt K, Barousch W, Moser D, et al. Emergence of a dalbavancin induced glycopeptide/lipoglycopeptide non-susceptible *Staphylococcus aureus* during treatment of a cardiac device-related endocarditis. Emerg Microb Infect 2018;7(1):202. https://doi.org/10.1038/s41426-018-0205-z. Epub 2018/12/06; PubMed PMID: 30514923; PubMed Central PMCID: PMCPMC6279813.

[111] Werth BJ, Jain R, Hahn A, Cummings L, Weaver T, Waalkes A, et al. Emergence of dalbavancin non-susceptible, vancomycin-intermediate *Staphylococcus aureus* (VISA) after treatment of MRSA central line-associated bloodstream infection with a dalbavancin- and vancomycin-containing regimen. Clin Microbiol Infect 2018; 24(4):429. https://doi.org/10.1016/j.cmi.2017.07.028. e1–e5. Epub 2017/08/08; PubMed PMID: 28782651.

[112] Tobudic S, Forstner C, Burgmann H, Lagler H, Ramharter M, Steininger C, et al. Dalbavancin as primary and sequential treatment for gram-positive infective endocarditis: 2-year experience at the general hospital of Vienna. Clin Infect Dis 2018;67(5):795–8. https://doi.org/10.1093/cid/ciy279. Epub 2018/04/17; PubMed PMID: 29659732.

[113] Bryson-Cahn C, Beieler AM, Chan JD, Harrington RD, Dhanireddy S. Dalbavancin as secondary therapy for serious *Staphylococcus aureus*infections in a vulnerable patient population. Open Forum Infect Dis 2019;6(2):ofz028. https://doi.org/10.1093/ofid/ofz028. Epub 2019/03/07; PubMed PMID: 30838225; PubMed Central PMCID: PMCPMC6388764.

[114] Efficacy and safety of dalbavancin compared to standard of care antibiotic therapy for the completion of treatment of patients with complicated bacteremia or infective endocarditis. ClinicalTrials.gov; 2019. Available from:https://clinicaltrials.gov/ct2/results?cond=endocarditis+&term=dalbavancin&cntry=&state=&city=&dist=.

[115] Iversen K, Ihlemann N, Gill SU, Madsen T, Elming H, Jensen KT, et al. Partial oral versus intravenous antibiotic treatment of endocarditis. N Engl J Med 2019;380(5): 415–24. https://doi.org/10.1056/NEJMoa1808312. Epub 2018/08/29; PubMed PMID: 30152252.

[116] Iversen K, Host N, Bruun NE, Elming H, Pump B, Christensen JJ, et al. Partial oral treatment of endocarditis. Am Heart J 2013;165(2):116–22. https://doi.org/10.1016/j.ahj.2012.11.006. Epub 2013/01/29; PubMed PMID: 23351813.

[117] Dworkin RJ, Lee BL, Sande MA, Chambers HF. Treatment of right-sided *Staphylococcus aureus* endocarditis in intravenous drug users with ciprofloxacin and rifampicin. Lancet 1989;2(8671):1071–3. Epub 1989/11/04; PubMed PMID: 2572799.

[118] Heldman AW, Hartert TV, Ray SC, Daoud EG, Kowalski TE, Pompili VJ, et al. Oral antibiotic treatment of right-sided staphylococcal endocarditis in injection drug users: prospective randomized comparison with parenteral therapy. Am J Med 1996;101(1): 68–76. Epub 1996/07/01; PubMed PMID: 8686718.

[119] Rosenthal ES, Karchmer AW, Theisen-Toupal J, Castillo RA, Rowley CF. Suboptimal addiction interventions for patients hospitalized with injection drug use-associated infective endocarditis. Am J Med 2016;129(5):481–5. https://doi.org/10.1016/j.amjmed.2015.09.024. PubMed PMID: 26597670.

[120] Gray ME, Rogawski McQuade ET, Scheld WM, Dillingham RA. Rising rates of injection drug use associated infective endocarditis in Virginia with missed opportunities

for addiction treatment referral: a retrospective cohort study. BMC Infect Dis 2018; 18(1):532. https://doi.org/10.1186/s12879-018-3408-y. Epub 2018/10/26; PubMed PMID: 30355291; PubMed Central PMCID: PMCPMC6201507.

[121] Blanchard J, Weiss AJ, Barrett ML, Stocks C, Owens PL, Coffey R, et al. Readmissions following inpatient treatment for opioid-related conditions. Subst Use Misuse 2019:1—9. https://doi.org/10.1080/10826084.2018.1517174. Epub 2019/01/09; PubMed PMID: 30618327.

[122] Suzuki J. Medication-assisted treatment for hospitalized patients with intravenous-drug-use related infective endocarditis. Am J Addict 2016;25(3):191—4. https://doi.org/10.1111/ajad.12349. PubMed PMID: 26991660.

[123] Rapoport AB, Rowley CF. Stretching the scope - becoming frontline addiction-medicine providers. N Engl J Med 2017;377(8):705—7. https://doi.org/10.1056/NEJMp1706492. Epub 2017/08/24; PubMed PMID: 28834479.

[124] Moreno JL, Wakeman SE, Duprey MS, Roberts RJ, Jacobson JS, Devlin JW. Predictors for 30-day and 90-day hospital readmission among patients with opioid use disorder. J Addict Med 2019. https://doi.org/10.1097/ADM.0000000000000499. Epub 2019/01/12; PubMed PMID: 30633044.

[125] Winetsky D, Weinrieb RM, Perrone J. Expanding treatment opportunities for hospitalized patients with opioid use disorders. J Hosp Med 2018;13(1):62—4. https://doi.org/10.12788/jhm.2861. Epub 2017/10/27; PubMed PMID: 29073311.

[126] Lagisetty P, Klasa K, Bush C, Heisler M, Chopra V, Bohnert A. Primary care models for treating opioid use disorders: what actually works? A systematic review. PLoS One 2017;12(10):e0186315. https://doi.org/10.1371/journal.pone.0186315. Epub 2017/10/19; PubMed PMID: 29040331; PubMed Central PMCID: PMCPMC5645096.

[127] D'Onofrio G, O'Connor PG, Pantalon MV, Chawarski MC, Busch SH, Owens PH, et al. Emergency department-initiated buprenorphine/naloxone treatment for opioid dependence: a randomized clinical trial. JAMA 2015;313(16):1636—44. https://doi.org/10.1001/jama.2015.3474. Epub 2015/04/29; PubMed PMID: 25919527; PubMed Central PMCID: PMCPMC4527523.

[128] Samuels EA, McDonald JV, McCormick M, Koziol J, Friedman C, Alexander-Scott N. Emergency department and hospital care for opioid use disorder: implementation of statewide standards in Rhode Island, 2017-2018. Am J Public Health 2019;109(2): 263—6. https://doi.org/10.2105/AJPH.2018.304847. Epub 2018/12/21; PubMed PMID: 30571304.

[129] Hawk K, D'Onofrio G. Emergency department screening and interventions for substance use disorders. Addict Sci Clin Pract 2018;13(1):18. https://doi.org/10.1186/s13722-018-0117-1. Epub 2018/08/07; PubMed PMID: 30078375; PubMed Central PMCID: PMCPMC6077851.

[130] Englander H, Weimer M, Solotaroff R, Nicolaidis C, Chan B, Velez C, et al. Planning and designing the improving addiction care team (IMPACT) for hospitalized adults with substance use disorder. J Hosp Med 2017;12(5):339—42. https://doi.org/10.12788/jhm.2736. Epub 2017/05/02; PubMed PMID: 28459904; PubMed Central PMCID: PMCPMC5542562.

[131] Pollini RA, O'Toole TP, Ford D, Bigelow G. Does this patient really want treatment? Factors associated with baseline and evolving readiness for change among hospitalized substance using adults interested in treatment. Addict Behav 2006;31(10):1904—18. https://doi.org/10.1016/j.addbeh.2006.01.003. Epub 2006/02/18; PubMed PMID: 16483724.

[132] Trowbridge P, Weinstein ZM, Kerensky T, Roy P, Regan D, Samet JH, et al. Addiction consultation services - linking hospitalized patients to outpatient addiction treatment. J Subst Abuse Treat 2017;79:1–5. https://doi.org/10.1016/j.jsat.2017.05.007. Epub 2017/07/05; PubMed PMID: 28673521; PubMed Central PMCID: PMCPMC6035788.

[133] Lee CS, Liebschutz JM, Anderson BJ, Stein MD. Hospitalized opioid-dependent patients: exploring predictors of buprenorphine treatment entry and retention after discharge. Am J Addict 2017;26(7):667–72. https://doi.org/10.1111/ajad.12533. Epub 2017/03/23; PubMed PMID: 28324627; PubMed Central PMCID: PMCPMC5608622.

[134] Waye KM, Goyer J, Dettor D, Mahoney L, Samuels EA, Yedinak JL, et al. Implementing peer recovery services for overdose prevention in Rhode Island: an examination of two outreach-based approaches. Addict Behav 2019;89:85–91. https://doi.org/10.1016/j.addbeh.2018.09.027. Epub 2018/10/03; PubMed PMID: 30278306; PubMed Central PMCID: PMCPMC6240389.

[135] Fareed A, Casarella J, Amar R, Vayalapalli S, Drexler K. Methadone maintenance dosing guideline for opioid dependence, a literature review. J Addict Dis 2010; 29(1):1–14. https://doi.org/10.1080/10550880903436010. Epub 2010/04/15; PubMed PMID: 20390694.

[136] Binswanger IA, Blatchford PJ, Mueller SR, Stern MF. Mortality after prison release: opioid overdose and other causes of death, risk factors, and time trends from 1999 to 2009. Ann Intern Med 2013;159(9):592–600. https://doi.org/10.7326/0003-4819-159-9-201311050-00005. Epub 2013/11/06; PubMed PMID: 24189594; PubMed Central PMCID: PMCPMC5242316.

[137] Marsden J, Stillwell G, Jones H, Cooper A, Eastwood B, Farrell M, et al. Does exposure to opioid substitution treatment in prison reduce the risk of death after release? A national prospective observational study in England. Addiction 2017;112(8): 1408–18. https://doi.org/10.1111/add.13779. Epub 2017/02/06; PubMed PMID: 28160345.

[138] Liebschutz JM, Crooks D, Herman D, Anderson B, Tsui J, Meshesha LZ, et al. Buprenorphine treatment for hospitalized, opioid-dependent patients: a randomized clinical trial. JAMA Intern Med 2014;174(8):1369–76. https://doi.org/10.1001/jamainternmed.2014.2556. Epub 2014/08/05; PubMed PMID: 25090173; PubMed Central PMCID: PMCPMC4811188.

[139] Raisch DW, Fye CL, Boardman KD, Sather MR. Opioid dependence treatment, including buprenorphine/naloxone. Ann Pharmacother 2002;36(2):312–21. https://doi.org/10.1345/aph.10421. Epub 2002/02/19; PubMed PMID: 11847954.

[140] Manlandro Jr JJ. Buprenorphine for office-based treatment of patients with opioid addiction. J Am Osteopath Assoc 2005;105(6 Suppl. 3):S8–13. Epub 2005/08/25; PubMed PMID: 16118361.

[141] Lee JD, Nunes Jr EV, Novo P, Bachrach K, Bailey GL, Bhatt S, et al. Comparative effectiveness of extended-release naltrexone versus buprenorphine-naloxone for opioid relapse prevention (X:BOT): a multicentre, open-label, randomised controlled trial. Lancet 2018;391(10118):309–18. https://doi.org/10.1016/S0140-6736(17)32812-X. Epub 2017/11/19; PubMed PMID: 29150198; PubMed Central PMCID: PMCPMC5806119.

[142] Samet JH, Botticelli M, Bharel M. Methadone in primary care - one small step for congress, one giant leap for addiction treatment. N Engl J Med 2018;379(1):7–8.

https://doi.org/10.1056/NEJMp1803982. Epub 2018/07/05; PubMed PMID: 29972744.

[143] Keen J, Oliver P, Mathers N. Methadone maintenance treatment can be provided in a primary care setting without increasing methadone-related mortality: the Sheffield experience 1997-2000. Br J Gen Pract 2002;52(478):387−9. Epub 2002/05/17; PubMed PMID: 12014536; PubMed Central PMCID: PMCPMC1314294.

[144] Fiellin DA, O'Connor PG, Chawarski M, Pakes JP, Pantalon MV, Schottenfeld RS. Methadone maintenance in primary care: a randomized controlled trial. JAMA 2001;286(14):1724−31. Epub 2001/10/12; PubMed PMID: 11594897.

[145] Hawk M, Coulter RWS, Egan JE, Fisk S, Reuel Friedman M, Tula M, et al. Harm reduction principles for healthcare settings. Harm Reduct J 2017;14(1):70. https://doi.org/10.1186/s12954-017-0196-4. Epub 2017/10/27; PubMed PMID: 29065896; PubMed Central PMCID: PMCPMC5655864.

[146] Stancliff S, Phillips BW, Maghsoudi N, Joseph H. Harm reduction: front line public health. J Addict Dis 2015;34(2−3):206−19. https://doi.org/10.1080/10550887.2015.1059651. Epub 2015/06/17; PubMed PMID: 26080038.

[147] Small D. Fools rush in where angels fear to tread Playing God with Vancouver's Supervised Injection Facility in the political borderland. Int J Drug Policy 2007;18(1):18−26. https://doi.org/10.1016/j.drugpo.2006.12.013. Epub 2007/08/11; PubMed PMID: 17689340.

[148] Hood JE, Behrends CN, Irwin A, Schackman BR, Chan D, Hartfield K, et al. The projected costs and benefits of a supervised injection facility in Seattle, WA, USA. Int J Drug Policy 2019;67:9−18. https://doi.org/10.1016/j.drugpo.2018.12.015. Epub 2019/02/26; PubMed PMID: 30802842.

[149] Sharma M, Lamba W, Cauderella A, Guimond TH, Bayoumi AM. Harm reduction in hospitals. Harm Reduct J 2017;14(1):32. https://doi.org/10.1186/s12954-017-0163-0. Epub 2017/06/07; PubMed PMID: 28583121; PubMed Central PMCID: PMCPMC5460456.

[150] Abdul-Quader AS, Feelemyer J, Modi S, Stein ES, Briceno A, Semaan S, et al. Effectiveness of structural-level needle/syringe programs to reduce HCV and HIV infection among people who inject drugs: a systematic review. AIDS Behav 2013;17(9):2878−92. https://doi.org/10.1007/s10461-013-0593-y. Epub 2013/08/27; PubMed PMID: 23975473.

[151] Jones CM. Syringe services programs: an examination of legal, policy, and funding barriers in the midst of the evolving opioid crisis in the U.S. Int J Drug Policy 2019;70:22−32. https://doi.org/10.1016/j.drugpo.2019.04.006. Epub 2019/05/07; PubMed PMID: 31059965.

[152] Colon-Berezin C, Nolan ML, Blachman-Forshay J, Paone D. Overdose deaths involving fentanyl and fentanyl analogs - New York City, 2000-2017. MMWR Morb Mortal Wkly Rep 2019;68(2):37−40. https://doi.org/10.15585/mmwr.mm6802a3. Epub 2019/01/18; PubMed PMID: 30653482; PubMed Central PMCID: PMCPMC6336189 potential conflicts of interest. No potential conflicts of interest were disclosed.

[153] Kerensky T, Walley AY. Opioid overdose prevention and naloxone rescue kits: what we know and what we don't know. Addiction Sci Clin Pract 2017;12(1):4. https://doi.org/10.1186/s13722-016-0068-3. Epub 2017/01/08; PubMed PMID: 28061909; PubMed Central PMCID: PMCPMC5219773.

[154] Mueller SR, Walley AY, Calcaterra SL, Glanz JM, Binswanger IA. A review of opioid overdose prevention and naloxone prescribing: implications for translating community programming into clinical practice. Subst Abus 2015;36(2):240−53. https://doi.org/10.1080/08897077.2015.1010032. Epub 2015/03/17; PubMed PMID: 25774771; PubMed Central PMCID: PMCPMC4470731.

[155] Walley AY, Xuan Z, Hackman HH, Quinn E, Doe-Simkins M, Sorensen-Alawad A, et al. Opioid overdose rates and implementation of overdose education and nasal naloxone distribution in Massachusetts: interrupted time series analysis. BMJ 2013; 346:f174. https://doi.org/10.1136/bmj.f174. Epub 2013/02/02; PubMed PMID: 23372174; PubMed Central PMCID: PMCPMC4688551.

[156] Weiss L, Netherland J, Egan JE, Flanigan TP, Fiellin DA, Finkelstein R, et al. Integration of buprenorphine/naloxone treatment into HIV clinical care: lessons from the BHIVES collaborative. J Acquir Immune Defic Syndr 2011;56(Suppl. 1):S68−75. https://doi.org/10.1097/QAI.0b013e31820a8226. Epub 2011/03/01; PubMed PMID: 21317597.

[157] Basu S, Smith-Rohrberg D, Bruce RD, Altice FL. Models for integrating buprenorphine therapy into the primary HIV care setting. Clin Infect Dis 2006;42(5): 716−21. https://doi.org/10.1086/500200. Epub 2006/02/01; PubMed PMID: 16447120.

[158] Westlake AA, Eisenberg MP. Infectious disease (ID) learning unit: what the ID clinician needs to know about buprenorphine treatment for opioid use disorder. Open Forum Infect Dis 2017;4(1):ofw251. https://doi.org/10.1093/ofid/ofw251. Epub 2017/05/10; PubMed PMID: 28480247; PubMed Central PMCID: PMCPMC5413994.

[159] Bell J, Belackova V, Lintzeris N. Supervised injectable opioid treatment for the management of opioid dependence. Epub 2018/08/23 Drugs 2018;78(13):1339−52. https://doi.org/10.1007/s40265-018-0962-y. PMID: 30132259.

[160] Wheeler E, Jones TS, Gilbert MK, Davidson PJ, Centers for disease C, prevention. opioid overdose prevention programs providing naloxone to laypersons - United States, 2014. MMWR Morb Mortal Wkly Rep 2015;64(23):631−5. Epub 2015/06/19. PMID: 26086633. PMCID: PMCPMC4584734.

Outpatient opioid use disorder treatment for the ID physician

9

Dharushana Muthulingam[1], Lynn M. Madden[1,2], Frederick L. Altice[3,4,5]

[1]*Department of Medicine, Section of Infectious Diseases, Yale School of Medicine, New Haven, CT, United States;* [2]*Department of Epidemiology of Microbial Diseases, Yale School of Public Health, New Haven, CT, United States;* [3]*Center for Interdisciplinary Research on AIDS (CIRA), Yale University, New Haven, CT, United States;* [4]*Academic Icon Professor of Medicine, University of Malaya, Kuala Lumpur, Malaysia;* [5]*Visiting Professor of Medicine, Sichuan University, Chengdu, China*

Infectious disease (ID) physicians have long treated the common complications of opioid use disorder (OUD) and injection drug use. Such complications encountered in patients with OUD include HIV, viral hepatitis (HBV, HCV), tuberculosis, skin and soft tissue infections (cellulitis, abscesses, necrotizing fasciitis), endovascular infections and complications (infective endocarditis, osteomyelitis, discitis), and internal abscesses (e.g., brain, epidural), among others. ID physicians, however, have not traditionally considered management of OUD as part of their clinical responsibilities. That said, in the context of the evolving opioid crisis and its relationship to managing IDs, it is crucial for ID physicians to better engage in OUD treatment. Treating OUD as ID physicians provides the opportunity to treat the primary medical condition driving these complications, similar to optimizing the immune system with antiretroviral therapy in HIV to prevent and treat opportunistic infections [1]. Untreated OUD in our patients undermines health outcomes, compromising mortality, ID management, and general physical and mental health [2]. Initiating evidence-based treatment can stabilize patients, improving their life functioning, health, and well-being. ID physicians who encounter patients during management of endocarditis or in their HIV and HCV clinical practice can use these key opportunities, or "teachable moments," [3] to diagnose OUD, initiate treatment (themselves or in strategic partnership with specialty care), maintain, and reevaluate their patients in the long term.

Benefits of opioid use disorder treatment

OUD is a chronic, relapsing condition that, when not managed, contributes to poor outcomes for OUD itself, and for the management of other medical and psychiatric conditions [4]. Long-term pharmacotherapy (also known as medication-assisted therapies) is the cornerstone of effective treatment for OUD and is superior to behavioral treatment alone [5]. These evidence-based medications act on *mu* and *kappa*

The Opioid Epidemic and Infectious Diseases. https://doi.org/10.1016/B978-0-323-68328-9.00009-6

opioid receptors to block the euphoric effects of other opioids, while reducing cravings and symptoms of opioid withdrawal [6]. Evidence-based medications include maintenance with methadone (pure opioid agonist), buprenorphine (partial opioid agonist/partial antagonist), and naltrexone (pure opioid antagonist). Opioid receptor agonists, like methadone and buprenorphine, consistently reduce overdose and related mortality [7], prevent relapse, improve social functioning, and improve mental and physical health. Initiation of pharmacotherapy by itself after nonfatal overdose is associated with a profound decrease in all-cause and opioid-related mortality [8]. This includes improved mortality from infective endocarditis [9], as well as improvements along the entire HIV treatment cascade and in Hepatitis C treatment [10]. Opioid agonist treatment increases HIV treatment engagement, including engagement in HIV care, initiation onto and adherence with ART retention, and viral suppression, as well as decreases ART drop-out relative to matched patients with HIV not on opioid agonist therapy [11]. Opioid antagonist treatment with extended-release naltrexone has been shown to reduce relapse [12,13] overdose [13] and improve HIV viral suppression [14]. OUD treatment is also a primary prevention of HIV [11,15] and HCV by reducing or eliminating the frequency of injection[16]. Thus, ID specialists can be more effective when they are able to engage their patients in treatment for OUD.

To treat opioid use disorder successfully, recognize that it is a chronic, relapsing and remitting disease of the brain

OUD is a chronic, relapsing condition that can be successfully managed over a lifetime. Despite effective treatments, however, relapse is common and expected, similar to patients with diabetes with poorly controlled glucose after eating a high caloric meal. Relapse rates for OUD are similar to those of other chronic diseases such as diabetes, hypertension, and asthma, which also require both pharmacologic and behavioral treatment modalities [17]. Practitioners may perceive that relapse during treatment is a failure, but this is not accurate. Successful treatment requires ongoing evaluation and treatment modification. Similar to diabetes and HIV, relapse indicates the need to adjust, restart, or change treatment. Treatment must keep patients engaged, as multiple episodes of treatment may be needed, and adequate treatment length is critical for good outcomes. A central predictor of retention in treatment using opioid agonist treatment is adequate dosage—most patients are prescribed suboptimal dosages [18,19]. Duration of treatment for this chronic condition can vary; 1 year is considered an absolute minimum for maintenance, but typical duration of treatment is several years, and can even be a lifetime [17].

Barriers to opioid use disorder treatment

The current opioid crisis in the United States has unveiled shortcomings in our ability to provide treatment. Despite documented efficacy of pharmacotherapy, only

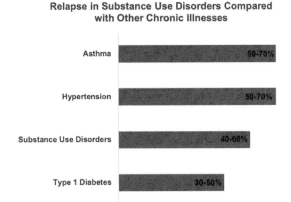

Relapse in Substance Use Disorders Compared with Other Chronic Illnesses

- Asthma: 50-70%
- Hypertension: 50-70%
- Substance Use Disorders: 40-60%
- Type 1 Diabetes: 30-50%

FIGURE 9.1

Relapse rates for substance use disorders are similar to other chronic conditions with pharmacologic and behavioral management [17].

10% of people with OUD in the United States who are eligible for treatment receive it [20]. Barriers to treatment are multilevel and include those at the patient, clinician, and structural levels. Patients are often not ready to stop using [21], have inaccurate beliefs about the availability and effectiveness of pharmacotherapies [22–24], have preference for counseling and abstinence-based programs despite evidence favoring medication [25], experience stigma against both OUD itself and its treatment [26–28], and are overly optimistic about their risk of avoiding relapse [29]. Clinician-level barriers to treatment expansion include perceived time constraints, concerns about diversion, unwillingness to prescribe, not perceiving patient need, and low confidence in their ability to prescribe pharmacotherapy. This may rise from inadequate training and stigma against patients with OUD (see Table 9.1) [30,31]. Structural barriers limiting treatment access include shortage of trained providers, reimbursement models that do not adequately compensate for care coordination and psychosocial services, stigma, geographical barriers (extensive travel to treatment in rural areas) [6], long waitlists for treatment entry [32], restrictions on the number of patients that can be treated, and lack of Medicaid expansion in some states [33].

Scale-up of opioid use disorder treatment is a critical public health priority: an overview of expansion strategies

OUD can be treated in a number of nonaddiction clinical settings. One of the key challenges in addressing the opioid crisis is ensuring that OUD treatment scale-up in these settings is prioritized and supported. An expansion strategy focusing only on specialty addiction treatment settings will be inadequate to overcome existing

Table 9.1 Common barriers cited for prescribing OUD and potential solutions suggested by clinicians who provide OUD treatment in their practice.[30] [119,120].

Barriers	Potential solutions to ease the burden
Getting started as an OUD pharmacotherapy provider may be daunting	1. Find a mentor to answer questions and provide support (other locally waivered providers or requested through SAMHSA-sponsored site PCSS.org) 2. Enroll in a Project ECHO tele-education program that focuses on treating addiction 3. Obtaining a waiver can be done online or as hybrid half-day courses, such as through SAMHSA and ASAM websites, many of which are free, and count toward Continued Medical Education (CME) requirements 4. Start with only a few patients 5. In the beginning, set aside a discrete time for services (e.g., 1 day a month or several days a week)
Maintaining patients with OUD in long-term pharmacotherapy services may seem challenging	1. Use a treatment contract with patients (i.e., to make clear the expectations of both provider and patients) 2. Establish boundaries that hold both patient and provider accountable and clarify what is allowable in any given practice. Boundaries can be informed by a harm reduction approach, which is associated with better retention and decreases the likelihood of adverse consequences (e.g., overdose, unsafe injection, etc.) 3. Transfer treatment to a higher level of care for OUD if the patient not responding to treatment or the relationship is difficult 4. Hub and Spoke model, as described below, can provide increased practice support
Complying with legal requirements set forth by DEA	Follow the rules (on DEA and SAMHSA websites), keep detailed records, and be prepared for DEA visit https://www. deadiversion.usdoj.gov/pubs/docs/dwp_buprenorphine.htm
Clinic-based programs may be concerned about financial viability or that Medicaid or private insurance reimbursement may be too low for the time required to treat OUD	This can be challenging to address at the practice level rather than policy level, and is common to managing many chronic conditions, but some clinicians can accept cash, private insurance, and a sliding fee

Table 9.1 Common barriers cited for prescribing OUD and potential solutions suggested by clinicians who provide OUD treatment in their practice.[30] [119,120].—cont'd

Barriers	Potential solutions to ease the burden
	scale to ensure accessible treatment. Most State Medicaid programs provide some coverage for buprenorphine treatment.
Private and governmental insurance programs may limit or restrict the duration of treatment, or require considerable documentation	This is also an issue that needs attention at the policy level, though it is similar to the increasing paperwork burden required in many aspects of clinical care
Concerns for diversion and misuse	There is less diversion of buprenorphine than other opioids, and when it *is* diverted for street use, it is frequently used for self-treatment to reduce withdrawal symptoms, paradoxically reflecting shortage of medical treatment[121]. There is also low overdose risk. Most providers have found the benefit of OUD treatment outweighed the risk of diversion. Providers can monitor with random urine drug screens, pill counts, use of the state prescription drug monitoring programs, and local pharmacies
Ensuring access to ancillary counseling services	Despite recommendations to provide a minimum of monthly counseling (the specificity in terms of content or duration is not described), a randomized controlled trial of medical management (brief counseling when prescribing) versus regularly cognitive behavioral treatment found no difference in outcomes. Strategies include providing brief counseling during prescription, referring to offsite counseling, or engaging patients in group counseling either within the practice or offsite. Additionally, computer-based or online counseling services (e.g.,www.cbt4cbt.com) [122] are also available
Overcoming stigma or patient mistreatment from other clinicians, medical staff, or pharmacies	Have open and honest dialogues with colleagues and staff. Encourage them to shadow clinicians who are treating OUD, humanize patients, and cultivate relationships with local pharmacies to address problems quickly and directly
Justice system administrators (drug court judges, probation officers) may discourage or prohibit use of OUD pharmacotherapy	Patients with OUD have an increased risk for incarceration, and those involved have the highest risk for mortality. Clinicians may be able to serve as impactful advocates for individual patients who would benefit from

Continued

Table 9.1 Common barriers cited for prescribing OUD and potential solutions suggested by clinicians who provide OUD treatment in their practice.[30] [119,120].—*cont'd*

Barriers	Potential solutions to ease the burden
	medications. Establishing aftercare programs in partnership with drug courts, community-based corrections (probation or parole) or jails and prisons can effectively engage patients during this vulnerable time

Facilitators

Many clinicians report finding this work highly rewarding and fulfilling, especially in watching patients with OUD drastically improve their lives and seeing the impact on families and communities.

Clinicians feel they are part of a solution in addressing an important public health crisis.

barriers to treatment. Instead, increasing treatment access requires a multipronged strategy that includes treatment of OUD in multiple settings, like primary and IDs clinical care, the justice system, emergency departments, during hospitalization, and, eventually, in pharmacies. Expanding access and uptake in treatment is a national public health priority for addressing the opioid crisis [34,35].

Strategies for expanding access can begin with existing opioid treatment centers. Conventionally, specialty treatment centers utilize a high-threshold approach that limits patient access [36], such as highly selective intake criteria, long waiting lists, no primary care access, high cost of treatment, and exclusion of patients with comorbid conditions. Once in treatment, patients may face punitive discharge policies, lack of treatment individualization, no shared patient decision-making, and other barriers to retention. In contrast, innovative, low-threshold models that have decreased barriers and increase service capacity, as with an open-access system, have been shown to deliver care while preserving patient outcomes without increase in cost [32].

Access and capacity can be further expanded with nonspecialty sites that conduct intake and monitoring (i.e., clinics, emergency departments, hospitalization, pharmacies, and the justice system). This is exemplified in the Hub and Spoke model [37]. The hub is the existing opioid treatment specialty center with a board-certified addiction specialist, able to dispense methadone, buprenorphine, and other related treatments. Community and healthcare sites serve as spokes into the hub. Transfers between hubs and spokes are bidirectional. Hubs can do initial intake and evaluate appropriate treatment placement for more stabilized patients. Patients can thus be initiated on buprenorphine within the hub then transferred to primary care provider. Alternatively, patients may be initiated on buprenorphine at clinics, or during the crucial windows of acute crisis (nonfatal overdose, infections in hospitals, or transition from justice system to community). Patients can then be referred to the hub for further evaluation, or reevaluation if they are having inadequate response to treatment. This model is akin to the provision of medical care where a specialty hospital or academic medical center serves as a hub and smaller nearby hospitals and clinics serve as the spokes. This can be further expanded with telemedicine, which uses videoconferencing to conduct remote diagnosis and treatment. Evidence for telemedicine's effectiveness in mental health is well-established, though it is currently nascent in addiction treatment. Despite advocacy from the President's Commission on Combating Drug Addiction and Opioid Crisis [38] and the American Society of Addiction Medicine, several barriers exist to telemedicine expansion [39]. Even so, its use has increased and may be a promising means by which to overcome barriers to care in areas with low access to providers, such as in rural areas [40]. Additionally, telemedicine can be used for distance-based learning by providing tele-education to connect primary care providers with specialty care for facilitating case-based learning, as in Project ECHO (Extension for Community Healthcare Outcomes). This can expand access to specialized treatments in underserved areas, including in primary care, justice, and IDs clinical care settings [41]. Outside the United States, OUD treatment can additionally be provided in pharmacies and overseen by pharmacists, a strategy that has been used successfully in the United Kingdom [42,43].

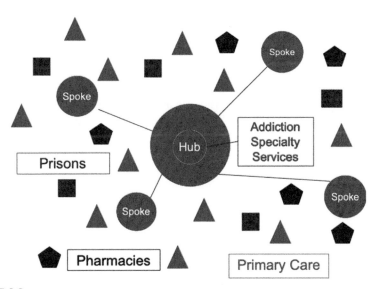

FIGURE 9.2

In addition to expanding existing specialty treatment capacity such as with an open-access model [32], the hub-and-spoke model can link specialty care with clinics, hospitals, and the criminal justice system to expand access to OUD treatment [37]. Pharmacy-based OUD treatment is not currently available in the United States but has been shown to be feasible and effective in the United Kingdom [42,43].

Expansion of opioid use disorder pharmacologic treatment in nonaddiction specialty clinics is a promising public health strategy

Primary care and other specialty ambulatory clinics (e.g., HIV clinical care settings, hepatology practices treating HCV) are a high priority and promising opportunity for treatment expansion [44] but have been underutilized [45]. Primary care is deeply essential, as treating OUD *without* comprehensive medical care is associated with an increased hazard of death [46]. In addition to being at the frontlines of care (especially for underserved and vulnerable populations), primary and ID physicians are especially expert at managing complex patients with multiple comorbidities requiring coordination of care with specialists [47,48]. The ambulatory clinic is therefore especially well-suited for serving as a medical home for OUD [49]. International guidelines [50], including those from the International Association of Physicians in AIDS Care (IAPAC), recommend integration of treatment for OUD as a key priority for optimizing HIV treatment outcomes [51].

Indeed, HIV providers have long called for integration of services to improve care for their patients [52,53], including for mental health, gynecological, hepatitis C, and other services, in addition to treating addiction. One of the earliest models for integrating OUD into multidisciplinary care was the BHIVES collaborative, which called for introducing buprenorphine into the HIV care setting. This 10-site demonstration project showed not only feasibility but that HIV patients initiated on buprenorphine were significantly more likely to initiate ART and to achieve viral suppression [54]. Additional models have emerged from the initiative, confirming that buprenorphine treatment could easily be delivered by both HIV and addiction medicine specialists. Such models do require a "glue" person—nurse, counselor, social workers, or other individual who was able to coordinate the activities—for successful implementation [55]. Several representative models of integrating OUD treatment into HIV clinical care settings have since been identified [53]. The primary care model posits that the primary clinician be responsible for managing OUD, only referring when patients become too complicated. The onsite addiction specialist places an expert within the clinic (colocation), providing addiction treatment onsite. A hybrid model allows for the addiction expert to induct patients and refer stable patients to all providers. An emerging model showing promise is group visit models, in which providers see many patients at once, which improves symptoms, retention, and provides a unique peer support [49,56]. All models include four central components: pharmacologic therapy, complementary psychosocial services, integration of care, and education and outreach [44].

Legislative history for expanding access to pharmacotherapy in the ambulatory setting

The Drug Abuse Treatment Act (DATA) of 2000 allowed FDA-approved schedule III-V opioid agonists for OUD treatment to be provided outside of specific federally approved treatment programs. The only opioid agonist meeting these criteria is buprenorphine, which was FDA-approved in 2002. Per DATA 2000, physicians can prescribe buprenorphine in settings other than licensed treatment centers if they complete an 8-hour training and apply to receive a waiver. Any physician is eligible to become a buprenorphine prescriber if they have an active state medical license, is registered with the Drug Enforcement Agency (DEA) to prescribe controlled substances, and is able to provide or refer patients to counseling and support services. The 8-hour training courses are available online, in person, or in combination formats. Popular courses are offered by the American Academy of Addiction Psychiatry, American Society of Addiction Medicine (ASAM), and Substance Abuse and Mental Health Services Administration (SAMHSA). The SAMHSA website also has a short online application for the waiver itself [1].

In 2016, with the Comprehensive Addiction and Recovery Act (CARA), the patient limit was expanded from 30 patients per practitioner and 100 patients after 1 year to additionally allow qualified waivered physicians to expand to 275 patients. CARA also broadened prescribing privileges to nurse practitioners and physician assistants [57]. Methadone, in contrast, is schedule II and available in the United States in licensed and accredited specialty treatment programs [6,45]. No waiver is required to administer extended-release naltrexone (XR-NTX), which is not a controlled substance.

Clinician-level barriers to prescribing treatment for opioid use disorder

Physicians reported several barriers in initiating and expanding OUD treatment in their practice [49]. Barriers such as government regulations, role of the justice system, and reimbursement need to be addressed at the policy and institutional level. At the provider level, clinicians have developed several strategies and facilitators for overcoming barriers to providing OUD treatment in their practice (Table 9.1). Additional resources for nonaddiction specialty clinicians for OUD pharmacotherapy can be found at the SAMHSA-sponsored Provider Clinical Support System (PCSSnow. org).

Screening for opioid use disorder, the benefit of treatment initiation, and additional work up

Screening is the first step for identifying patients with OUD who would benefit from treatment. All patients should be screened for problematic substance use. Patients with conditions closely associated with OUD or injection drug use, including chronic pain, HIV, Hepatitis C, and endocarditis, should especially prompt evaluation for OUD. Clinical observations such as signs of withdrawal, intoxication, or needle "track" marks should also prompt screening. "Drug seeking" behaviors such as repeated requests for refills of prescription pain medication or perseveration on need for opioids can be an indicator of OUD, but should be interpreted cautiously, as these signs may also reflect inadequate treatment of chronic pain (or both) [58]. Multiple screening tools exist (Table 9.2) [59]. Assessing whether patients are appropriate for pharmacotherapy involves evaluating patient interest and motivation, and ensuring they understand benefits, risks, and process (see Shared Decision-Making below).

Although SAMSHA supports the use of SBIRT (screening, brief intervention, and referral to treatment) [60] for substance use disorders, the single most important clinical step in caring for patients with OUD is initiating medication, as pharmacotherapy is stabilizing and initiation is associated with improved mortality [8,61]. A

Table 9.2 Screening tools available for substance use generally including OUD [58] [123,124]. All tools are positive if there are two or more affirmative answers, except for SSAQ, which is positive with single affirmative answer.

Tool	No. of questions	Population	Sensitivity	Specificity
CAGE-AID	4		Any substance use problem: 70%	Any substance use problem: 85%
DAST-10	10	Discriminates current and former users	Any substance use problem: 80% Substance use disorder: 85%	Any substance use problem: 88% Substance use disorder: 78%
CRAFFT	5	Useful for adolescents	Any substance use problem: 76% Any substance use disorder: 80% Drug dependence: 92%	Any substance use problem: 94% Any substance use disorder: 86% Drug dependence: 80%
SSAQ [125]	1		Substance use disorder: 100% Current substance use: 80%	Substance use disorder: 74% Current substance use: 94%
ASSIST [126]	8		Substance use disorder: 95% −100%	Substance use disorder: 79% −93%
SAMISS [127]	16	Patients with HIV	Substance use disorder: 86%	Substance use disorder: 75%

systematic review of SBIRT effectiveness in substance use disorders suggested this strategy is only effective in alcohol use disorder [62]. However, this study mostly included substances *without* available pharmacotherapy (e.g., cannabis, stimulants). In contrast, OUD *does* have effective medications available that *can* be initiated immediately after screening, without requiring specialty referral. These medications provide the opportunity to screen and *treat*, since nonmedication interventions with referrals to outside treatment have been found to be ineffective—the minute the patient leaves a comfortable clinical care setting, they are unlikely to follow-through due to problematic drug use and stigma, e.g., concerns for meeting unfamiliar clinicians and encountering discrimination. Furthermore, patients often encounter waiting lists, one of the leading barriers to specialty care for OUD. Being on such a waiting list and not receiving treatment is associated with a 10-fold higher mortality relative to patients who were admitted immediately to care [63,64]. When on waiting lists, patients often experience symptoms of opioid withdrawal, chaotic opioid (and other drug) use, and resultant death. Thus, identifying and expeditiously initiating treatment and connecting patients to care is critical.

The evaluation of OUD includes screening for important and common cooccurring conditions, such as infections, mental health status and psychiatric disorders, chronic pain, other substance use disorders, and pregnancy. Initiating buprenorphine or XR-NTX can potentially induce opioid withdrawal syndrome, which is contraindicated in pregnancy (women already on buprenorphine can safely continue it). A brief physical exam may include using a validated clinical scale for withdrawal symptoms such as the Clinical Opioid Withdrawal Scale (COWS) [65]. Evaluation of social and environmental barriers and facilitators to treatment should be completed. Initial lab testing generally includes urine toxicology screening, complete blood count, liver function tests, and serology testing for hepatitis C and HIV, if not already done. Tuberculosis and sexual transmitted infections should also be evaluated if indicated. Women who are able to get pregnant should be tested for such, and interviewed regarding interest in contraception, especially since effective treatment of OUD can result in increase in fertility (see Women with OUD below) [66].

Available pharmacotherapy options for treating opioid use disorder

There are a number of evidence-based pharmacotherapies for the treatment of OUD, including methadone, buprenorphine (various formulations), and extended-release naltrexone (XR-NTX). A description of the attribute of each treatment strategy is described below and summarized in Table 9.3.

Methadone

Overview: Methadone is a long-acting opioid agonist available in a daily liquid oral form that has been successfully used for OUD treatment since 1965 [1].

Table 9.3 FDA-approved pharmacotherapy formulations available for OUD treatment.

Name	Methadone	Sublingual buprenorphine or buprenorphine-naloxone	Implantable buprenorphine	Injectable buprenorphine	Extended-release naltrexone
Mechanism	Opioid agonist	Partial opioid agonist			Opioid antagonist
Dosing frequency	Daily	Usually daily	Every 6 months	Monthly, or weekly (approval pending)	Every month
Administrative route	Liquid, oral	Tablet or dissolvable tab, sublingual; prescription can be dispensed up to monthly	Implantable rod	Injected intramuscularly or subcutaneously	Injected intramuscularly
Induction process	None	6–48 h of opioid abstinence before first dose	6–48 days of supervised abstinence, period of stabilizing dose with sublingual buprenorphine	48 days of supervised abstinence, period of stabilizing dose with sublingual buprenorphine	7–10 days of supervised opioid withdrawal before injection
Location of administration	Only by supervision licensed, addiction specialty treatment centers	Specialty and nonspecialty clinical care settings (e.g., primary care, HIV clinics) by prescription and distributed from pharmacy, taken at home			Specialty and nonspecialty clinical care settings (e.g., primary care, HIV clinics) by monthly injection
Federal counseling requirements	Minimum once monthly	Required, frequency determined by patient need			No requirements
Pharmacological drug interactions	CYP3A4 metabolism, many potential interactions reported	Few interactions reported, e.g., saquinavir (QT prolongation) and serotonergic agents (serotonin syndrome)			Very few interactions

Maintenance treatment with methadone is associated with a 70% mortality reduction for all causes in OUD [67]. As a Schedule II controlled substance, it is generally available only in licensed treatment programs. Although not usually available to prescribe in the typical ambulatory setting, the clinician should be aware of methadone as an option for OUD treatment and refer if indicated. Methadone, when dosed appropriately at higher dosages, is associated with significantly better retention than buprenorphine [5] and may be preferable for some patients; however, lower dose methadone is associated with lower retention than buprenorphine. Most programs require highly structured and supervised medication administration, usually daily clinical presentation when starting treatment. Patients may, however, "earn" take-home dosing days over time as they adhere to treatment. The high demand characteristics and historical stigma [68] of methadone can be a barrier to many patients. While a subset of patients may prefer more structure, supervision, and the specialized programming that accompanies methadone [22], the majority of patients on opioid agonist treatment at this time are on methadone without much choice in determining the level of structure involved in their treatment.

Induction, dosing, monitoring, and medication administration: These are done in specialized OUD treatment centers, but there are some principles to keep in mind as an ID clinician comanaging a patient. Methadone is initiated and increased slowly, given its long half-life. An adequate dose for symptom relief and effectiveness usually ranges from 60 to 120 mg [66]. Common adverse effects include constipation, mild drowsiness, sweating, and similar to heroin, can impair sexual function, such as with erectile dysfunction. Less common but more serious effects include a significant (though weak) correlation between methadone and QTc prolongation at very high doses (300 mg), which in turn is a risk factor for cardiac arrhythmias, especially if there are additional arrhythmia risk factors (such as other QTc prolonging medications and cardiac comorbidities) [69]. Additionally, methadone is metabolized extensively by CYP3A4 with the potential for several drug-drug interactions [70]. Specific interactions of note for ID physicians include HIV antiretrovirals, in which NNRTIs such as efavirenz and PIs (combination lopinavir/ritonavir) have been reported to precipitate opiate withdrawal by inducing CYP 450 3A4 and reducing plasma levels of methadone. Rifampin is also known to induce opiate withdrawal symptoms and can be substituted with rifabutin. Fluconazole, voriconazole, and ciprofloxacin inhibit CYP 450 3A4 and increase plasma methadone, with case reports of life-threatening opioid toxicity. Antidepressants are another class of medication with variable interaction with methadone metabolism. Anxiolytics such as benzodiazepines can be synergistically sedating and contribute to respiratory depression and remain a major risk factor for overdose on methadone. Medication interactions should be reviewed with appropriate databases and pharmacists, with dose adjustments or substitutions as needed. It is also important to note that should patients self-cease methadone treatment and resume former opioid drug use behaviors, they are at higher risk for overdose than if they were to resume drug use while continuing on methadone.

Buprenorphine

Overview: Buprenorphine is a partial mu-opioid agonist and partial antagonist. It is available in oral form as either a tablet or sublingual/buccal soluble film strip in isolation and (more commonly) coformulated with naloxone. This coformulation is intended to discourage diversion as the naloxone is minimally bioavailable when administered sublingually, but when crushed for injection, is an active opioid antagonist that precipitates withdrawal. There are also more recently approved long-acting formulations that include implantable buprenorphine that lasts 6 months [71] available in 2016 and injectable long-acting buprenorphine lasting 1 month available in 2018. A newer anticipated formulation will have both 1 week and 1-month options. Dissemination of these long-acting formulations is currently limited but may be increasingly available over time. Buprenorphine is often better received by patients compared with methadone as there is less associated stigma [72], more access through low-threshold outpatient treatment, less stringent regulations, and a better safety profile.

Since DATA 2000, access to buprenorphine in the ambulatory setting has expanded, but remains limited [6,45]. More than half of waivered physicians were from nonaddiction specialties in 2006 and as of 2016, 32,240 physicians in the United States were waivered to provide treatment for up to 30 or 100 patients. However, only two-thirds of waivered physicians actually prescribed buprenorphine, maintaining patient panels much below their limit [73]. There are significant geographic disparities in access and use of buprenorphine treatment, especially in rural areas, with about half of US counties having no access to a waivered physician [6,74,75].

Induction: Because buprenorphine is a high-affinity, partial mu-opioid agonist, it can displace the full agonist opioids from the receptor, initiating opioid withdrawal. It is thus recommended that the patient be abstinent from opioids for an adequate duration, to the point of mild or moderate withdrawal. This duration depends on what opioid the patient has been using. Those using heroin can initiate 6–12 h after last use, those using methadone may need 24 h or more [66]. At that point, buprenorphine will provide relief from withdrawal symptoms.

While there are various induction strategies available, it is important to use strategies that are most suitable for the clinical practice. For example, some practices involve very close supervision over the induction process during the first day, while others have successfully inducted patients on buprenorphine using home induction protocols. Patient-centered home-based induction protocols have similar effectiveness as office-based induction, while overcoming some of the barriers of office-based induction [76,77]. Clinicians can use either effective method, depending on their comfort level.

Monitoring: Once on a stable regimen, patients should be monitored frequently in the beginning (weekly) until stable, then monthly to evaluate patient treatment response, ongoing stability, adverse effects, and to address patient concerns. Clinicians should utilize the prescription drug monitoring program (PDMP) and perform toxicology screens regularly and at random to assess treatment response. A positive screen for illicit drugs should *not* lead to treatment cessation; rather it should prompt reevaluation of treatment adequacy and whether escalation is indicated, such as dose increase, visit frequency increase, transition to a different medication such as methadone, or referral to specialty care [66].

Adverse effects and other considerations: Serious side effects are uncommon. Respiratory depression of oral and long-acting formulations is usually minimal given the partial antagonist mechanism of action that prevents complete activation of mu-opioid receptors. Cases of buprenorphine-related deaths have largely occurred in the setting of combination with other substances (benzodiazepines, alcohol) and with nonmedical high dose intravenous injection of buprenorphine. More common adverse effects include sedation, headache, nausea, constipation and insomnia. Long-acting formulations such as injection or implant may include irritation or skin and soft tissue infection at site of procedure [78]. In those with severe liver impairment, naloxone component is thought to have increased bioavailability, so coformulated buprenorphine-naloxone is not recommended in these patients.

Extended release naltrexone (XR-NTX)

Overview: Oral naltrexone should not be used for the treatment of OUD due to lack of demonstrated effectiveness [79]. In 2010, the FDA approved an extended-release formula for OUD treatment after randomized controlled studies confirmed its effectiveness relative to placebo [12]. As an opioid antagonist, there are no regulations that restrict treatment. Uptake in the ambulatory settings has been slow, though from 2014 to 2015, a substantial increase in the use of XR-NTX was observed [80]. Low uptake of XR-NTX is related to patient preferences and concerns regarding the necessary supervised withdrawal from opioids ("detox") before starting, the volume of injection (2cc), and cost. From a clinician perspective, low XR-NTX uptake may be due to the perception that it is not the best treatment for many patients, that there is less patient demand [6], and concern for overdose risk when patients discontinue treatment. There is a subset of patients who can do well on this medication, especially if they are provided extensive support with counseling, frequent meetings, and other resources [81]. It is important to evaluate XR-NTX readiness in patients and conduct shared decision-making (see below).

Induction, dosing, administration, monitoring, and adverse effects: Initiation can be done in the office or by referral to specialty center. If a patient has not had any opioid use within the previous 7 days, assess COWS. If score is greater than 4, treat with adjunctive medications and reevaluate in 1—2 days. Adjunctive medications include clonidine, clonazepam, ibuprofen, or trazadone. If COWS score is 4 or less and patient has urine toxicology that is negative for opioids, one option is to administer a naloxone or oral naltrexone challenge. If the patient does not go into withdrawal after the short-acting naltrexone challenge, they may be started on XR-NTX. If the patient has used opioids within the previous 7 days, the clinician can either support 7-day cessation of opioid use with adjunctive medication or conduct a buprenorphine-assisted withdrawal protocol.

XR-NTX must be refrigerated and removed from refrigeration at least 30 min prior to administration (it can be returned to refrigeration if not used). Some offices require patients first obtain the medication from a pharmacy before administration in the clinic. The medication is delivered intramuscularly (fat layer must allow muscular injection access, approximately correlated with BMI < 40). Instruction for administration is available in package insert or in videos developed by PCSS [82]. Injection should be dorsogluteal (upper outer quadrant). Observe patient for 10 min for any immediate reactions. Counsel patient to contact clinic if any subsequent adverse effects. Alternate buttocks with subsequent injections. Provide patient with a medication safety card (available online) [83] or bracelet to present in the setting of an emergency[84]. Patients should also be counseled on increased overdose risk should they relapse to opioid use as the XR-NTX antagonist effect wanes after 4 weeks, as they will have markedly reduced opioid tolerance.

The most common adverse effect is injection site reactions (65%), ranging from induration, pruritis, irritation, and less commonly, infection. Additional common reactions include nausea and headache. Less common but more serious effects include syncope, anxiety, and depression [85].

Special considerations in opioid use disorder pharmacologic treatment
Informed and shared decision-making

When access barriers are overcome, there are an unprecedented number of effective and evidence-based treatment paths and medication formulations for treating OUD (Table 9.3), making treatment decisions among multiple effective options a preference-sensitive decision [86]. Clinicians should evaluate the best fit for any given patient by evaluating the medical context and patient's preferences. Shared decision-making is recommended by the National Academy of Medicine as an ethical necessity [87] and decision aids that facilitate shared decision-making are supported by over 105 RCTs [88]. Transforming patient (and loved ones) beliefs that OUD medication will be efficacious is associated with treatment entry [89] and retention [90,91,91], which in turn improves mortality and outcomes. In shared decision-making, clinicians offer information on treatment options, and patients clarify their concerns and preferences that might affect their choices [88]. Shared decision-making confers agency and can elicit an endowment effect [92], meaning an individual "owns" a particular idea by engaging in the process, thus making the decision more meaningful and improving retention [93,94].

Supporting shared decision-making can be approached with three steps [95]. (1) Choice talk: involves eliciting what a patient already knows and ensuring the patient understands the choice to be made and that reasonable options are available. (2)

Option talk: is a more detailed discussion of options, outcomes, and paths to those outcomes. (3) Decision talk: involves supporting patients' consideration of their preferences and deciding. A decision aid is an efficient and systematic means to facilitate these steps and can be administered by one of the many lay and professional caregivers that a patient often encounters in the ambulatory setting, including counselors, nurses, and clinicians. While not yet widely available, there are online versions for patients to use on their own [96] and point-of-care tools that are currently being developed and validated [22].

Psychosocial treatment

The purpose of psychosocial interventions is to address the psychological and social context that contributes to OUD and that may contribute to barriers to treatment and/ or remission. DATA 2000 requires that brief counseling be offered along with buprenorphine, either by the physician or nonphysician staff, without additional specifications. Evidence-based interventions include cognitive-behavioral therapy; motivational enhancement therapy; and individual, group, or family counseling; peer-delivered recovery support; and coordination and management of medical and psychiatric comorbidities and needs, including for other substances use disorders, IDs, or pregnancy [97]. Studies comparing different modalities of adjunct counseling with pharmacology in the ambulatory setting, such as comparison between brief (20 min) medically focused sessions and in-depth counseling (45 min), found no difference in effectiveness. Other studies have also evaluated Internet-based reinforcement, contingency management, cognitive behavior counseling, network therapy, directly observed buprenorphine administration of varying frequency, guided drug counseling, physician and nurse counseling, and adherence management. The data are heterogeneous and difficult to compare, but in general, there are no apparent differences in effectiveness among these modalities [6].

Treating women with OUD

There are several unique considerations in caring for women with OUD [98]. While men are more likely to have OUD, the gap has been rapidly narrowing [99], and women constitute more than half of emergency department visits for prescription opioid overdose [100]. Women are more likely to have a history of childhood trauma, chronic pain, interpersonal violence, and mental health problems, all risk factors and complicators of OUD [101]. Among individuals with both OUD and HIV in treatment, women experienced more medication side effects, higher addiction severity, more psychiatric problems, and lower health-related quality of life than men [102], warranting careful consideration of unique needs and experiences.

Contraception: Reproductive health is an essential part of overall health. Women with OUD are twice as likely to have unplanned pregnancy compared with the general population [103]. Many desired delaying pregnancy but few were able to access contraceptives [104]. Counseling women on contraception options is an important part of OUD treatment. Providers should nonjudgmentally communicate risks of pregnancy, identify the patients' reproductive goals, and provide contraception options if desired by the patient or refer to specialty providers as needed.

Pregnancy: The prevalence of OUD among perinatal women has increased four-fold in 15 years and exceeds 3% in some regions such as West Virginia and Vermont [105]. Opioid detoxification is contraindicated in pregnancy. Pregnant women should be initiated or continued on pharmacotherapy to avoid the risks of both ongoing OUD and of precipitating withdrawal. In pregnant women, buprenorphine has been found to be equivalent or superior to methadone, improving both maternal and fetal outcomes [106]. Historically, there has been concern about initiating or continuing coformulated buprenorphine-naloxone in the setting of possible fetal exposure to naloxone, but emerging evidence has not found harm [107,108]; practitioners can review risks and benefits with patients. Patients stable on a given OUD medication generally should not be changed if they become pregnant.

Pregnancy in women with OUD can be associated with significant psychosocial and medical needs. In one cohort, half of the pregnant women had a history of incarceration, a third had current legal involvement, and 15% had unstable housing. Prevalence of hepatitis C was 70%, physical interpersonal violence 65% and sexual violence 57% [109]. Identifying multidisciplinary prenatal support services, optimally with gender-specific and trauma-informed care, is an important addition to prenatal care and OUD treatment [110]. Practitioners should be aware of neonatal withdrawal syndrome during the first 3–7 days of life, which can occur with active OUD, methadone, and buprenorphine (preliminary data indicate shorter hospital stay and treatment time with buprenorphine). This can be managed with observation and symptom management. Pharmacotherapy should not be decreased or stopped to prevent neonatal withdrawal symptom as stopping treatment is associated with more dangerous risk of withdrawal and relapse. Breastfeeding is safe and encouraged with OUD pharmacotherapy [111].

Several states have legally sanctioned pregnant women for using substances while pregnant, with criminal or civil prosecution, involuntary civil detainment, and threat of child separation and limited parental rights [112]. Women are keenly aware of how closely scrutinized their pregnancies are [113], and this scrutiny can be a significant barrier to accessing prenatal care, social services, and OUD treatment [114]. Providers should be familiar with government and clinic policies with regard to testing and reporting, partner with patients, and advocate on their behalf. The perinatal time and parenting are also profound motivators for treatment for most patients and, with adequate support, provide an opportunity for improving the health of patients and their families [115].

Chronic pain

There is a high prevalence of chronic pain among patients with OUD in treatment, ranging from 37% to 60% [116]. Chronic pain can be both a driver and complication of OUD and is usually interconnected to complex medical and psychiatric comorbidities. ID physicians often treat highly complex patients with interrelated comorbidities and the strategy is similar to approach the patient as a whole person, while systematically treating OUD, comorbidities, and chronic pain while minimizing polypharmacy, and partnering with other providers as needed. Chronic pain should be treated with an individualized plan with multidimensional approach, including education, behavioral and psychological treatment, mobilization, careful use of medication, and attention to influential psychological conditions like insomnia [117].

Other harm reduction

In addition to OUD pharmacotherapy, counseling for additional harm reduction methods is warranted. These include syringe exchange and safe injection practices; overdose prevention, including not using alone and naloxone prescription; and pre-exposure prophylaxis (PrEP) for those who inject drugs who share injection equipment [15,118].

Conclusion

The ID physician has often been at the forefront of identifying and addressing major public health challenges, and the opioid epidemic is no different. In treating the many infectious complications of OUD, ID physicians have the opportunity to treat the root cause, with the potential to radically improve health outcomes for our patients. Screening for OUD, becoming waivered to prescribe buprenorphine, rapidly initiating OUD treatment, and partnering with specialty care providers are critical ways in which to save lives.

References

[1] Westlake AA, Eisenberg MP. Infectious disease (ID) learning unit: what the ID clinician needs to know about buprenorphine treatment for opioid use disorder. Open Forum Infect Dis 2017;4(1):ofw251.
[2] Bahorik AL, Satre DD, Kline-Simon AH, Weisner CM, Campbell CI. Alcohol, cannabis, and opioid use disorders, and disease burden in an integrated health care system. J Addict Med 2017;11(1):3—9.
[3] Lawson PJ, Flocke SA. Teachable moments for health behavior change: a concept analysis. Patient Educ Couns 2009;76(1):25—30.
[4] Altice FL, Kamarulzaman A, Soriano VV, Schechter M, Friedland GH. Treatment of medical, psychiatric, and substance-use comorbidities in people infected with HIV who use drugs. Lancet 2010;376(9738):367—87.
[5] Mattick RP, Breen C, Kimber J, Davoli M. Buprenorphine maintenance versus placebo or methadone maintenance for opioid dependence. Cochrane Database Syst Rev 2014;(2):CD002207.

[6] Chou R, Korthuis PT, Weimer M, et al. Medication-assisted treatment models of care for opioid use disorder in primary care settings. Rockville, MD: Agency for Healthcare Research and Quality (US); 2016. Available from:http://www.ncbi.nlm.nih.gov/books/NBK402352/.

[7] Sordo L, Barrio G, Bravo MJ, et al. Mortality risk during and after opioid substitution treatment: systematic review and meta-analysis of cohort studies. BMJ 2017;357: j1550.

[8] Larochelle MR, Bernson D, Land T, et al. Medication for opioid use disorder after nonfatal opioid overdose and association with mortality: a cohort study. Ann Intern Med 2018;169(3):137–45.

[9] Rodger L, Glockler-Lauf S, Shojaei E, et al. Clinical characteristics and factors associated with mortality in first-episode infective endocarditis among persons who inject drugs. JAMA Netw Open 2018;1(7):e185220.

[10] Nielsen S, Larance B, D'egenhardt L, Gowing LR, Kehler C, Lintzeris N. Opioid agonist treatment for pharmaceutical opioid dependent people. Cochrane Database Syst Rev 2016;May 9:2016.

[11] Low AJ, Mburu G, Welton NJ, et al. Impact of opioid substitution therapy on antiretroviral therapy outcomes: a systematic review and meta-analysis. Clin Infect Dis 2016;63(8):1094–104.

[12] Krupitsky E, Nunes EV, Ling W, Illeperuma A, Gastfriend DR, Silverman BL. Injectable extended-release naltrexone for opioid dependence: a double-blind, placebo-controlled, multicentre randomised trial. Lancet 2011;377(9776):1506–13.

[13] Lee JD, Friedmann PD, Kinlock TW, et al. Extended-release naltrexone to prevent opioid relapse in criminal justice offenders. N Engl J Med 2016;374(13):1232–42.

[14] Springer SA, Di Paola A, Barbour R, Azar MM, Altice FL. Extended-release naltrexone improves viral suppression among incarcerated persons living with HIV and alcohol use disorders transitioning to the community: results from a double-blind, placebo-controlled trial. Acquir Immune Defic Syndr 2018;79(1):92–100.

[15] Brinkley-Rubinstein L, Cloud D, Drucker E, Zaller N. Opioid use among those who have criminal justice experience: harm reduction strategies to lessen HIV risk. Curr HIV/AIDS Rep 2018;15(3):255–8.

[16] Platt L, Minozzi S, Reed J, et al. Needle syringe programmes and opioid substitution therapy for preventing hepatitis C transmission in people who inject drugs. Cochrane Database Syst Rev 2017;9:Cd012021.

[17] Principles of drug addiction treatment: a research-based guide. 2018. Available from: https://www.drugabuse.gov/publications/principles-drug-addiction-treatment-research-based-guide-third-edition.

[18] Amiri S, Hirchak K, Lutz R, et al. Three-year retention in methadone opioid agonist treatment: a survival analysis of clients by dose, area deprivation, and availability of alcohol and cannabis outlets. Drug Alcohol Depend 2018;193:63–8.

[19] Dumchev K, Dvoryak S, Chernova O, Morozova O, Altice FL. Retention in medication-assisted treatment programs in Ukraine—identifying factors contributing to a continuing HIV epidemic. Int J Drug Policy 2017;48:44–53.

[20] Wu L-T, Zhu H, Swartz MS. Treatment utilization among persons with opioid use disorder in the United States. Drug Alcohol Depend 2016;169:117–27.

[21] Substance Abuse and Mental Health Services Administration. Center for behavioral health statistics and quality. Key substance use and mental health indicators in the United States: results from the 2015. National Survey on Drug Use and Health;

2016. Available from:https://www.samhsa.gov/data/sites/default/files/NSDUH-FFR1-2015/NSDUH-FFR1-2015/NSDUH-FFR1-2015.pdf.

[22] Muthulingam D, Bia J, Madden LM, Farnum SO, Barry DT, Altice FL. Using nominal group technique to identify barriers, facilitators, and preferences among patients seeking treatment for opioid use disorder: a needs assessment for decision making support. J Subst Abuse Treat 2019;100:18−28.

[23] Uebelacker LA, Bailey G, Herman D, Anderson B, Stein M. Patients' beliefs about medications are associated with stated preference for methadone, buprenorphine, naltrexone, or no medication-assisted therapy following inpatient opioid detoxification. J Subst Abuse Treat 2016;66:48−53.

[24] Pinto H, Rumball D, Holland R. Attitudes and knowledge of substance misusers regarding buprenorphine and methadone maintenance therapy. J Subst Use 2008; 13(3):143−53.

[25] Olsen Y, Sharfstein JM. Confronting the stigma of opioid use disorder-and its treatment. JAMA 2014;311(14):1393−4.

[26] Bagley SM, Hadland SE, Carney BL, Saitz R. Addressing stigma in medication treatment of adolescents with opioid use disorder. J Addict Med 2017;11(6):415−6.

[27] Gryczynski J, Kinlock TW, Kelly SM, O'Grady KE, Gordon MS, Schwartz RP. Opioid agonist maintenance for probationers: patient-level predictors of treatment retention, drug use, and crime. Subst Abuse 2012;33(1):30−9.

[28] Yarborough BJ, Stumbo SP, McCarty D, Mertens J, Weisner C, Green CA. Methadone, buprenorphine and preferences for opioid agonist treatment: a qualitative analysis. Drug Alcohol Depend 2016;160:112−8.

[29] Polonsky M, Rozanova J, Azbel L, et al. Attitudes toward addiction, methadone treatment, and recovery among HIV-infected Ukrainian prisoners who inject drugs: incarceration effects and exploration of mediators. AIDS Behav 2016;20(12): 2950−60.

[30] Andrilla C, Coulthard C, Larson EH. Barriers rural physicians face prescribing buprenorphine for opioid use disorder. Ann Fam Med 2017;15(4):359−62.

[31] D'Onofrio G, McCormack RP, Hawk K. Emergency departments — a 24/7/365 option for combating the opioid crisis. N Engl J Med 2018;379(26):2487−90.

[32] Madden LM, Farnum SO, Eggert KF, et al. An investigation of an open-access model for scaling up methadone maintenance treatment. Addiction 2018;113(8):1450−8.

[33] Venkataramani AS, Chatterjee P. Early Medicaid expansions and drug overdose mortality in the USA: a quasi-experimental analysis. J Gen Intern Med 2019; 34(1):23−5.

[34] Factsheet: President Obama proposes $1.1 billion in new funding to address the prescription opioid abuse and heroin use epidemic. whitehouse.gov; 2016. Available from:https://obamawhitehouse.archives.gov/the-press-office/2016/02/02/president-obama-proposes-11-billion-new-funding-address-prescription.

[35] Health Resources and Services Administration. Opioid Crisis | Official web site of the U.S. Health Resources & Services Administration. [cited 2019 Mar 11]; Available from:https://www.hrsa.gov/opioids.

[36] Kourounis G, Richards BD, Kyprianou E, Symeonidou E, Malliori MM, Samartzis L. Opioid substitution therapy: lowering the treatment thresholds. Drug Alcohol Depend 2016;161:1−8.

[37] Brooklyn JR, Sigmon SC. Vermont hub-and-spoke model of care for opioid use disorder: development, implementation, and impact. J Addict Med 2017;11(4):286−92.

[38] Christie C, Baker C, Cooper R, Kennedy CPJ, Madras B, Bondi P. The president's commission on combating drug addiction and the opioid crisis. Washington, DC: United States Government Printing Office; 2017.

[39] Huskamp HA, Busch AB, Souza J, et al. How is telemedicine being used in opioid and other substance use disorder treatment? Health Aff 2018;37(12):1940−7.

[40] Schranz AJ, Barrett J, Hurt CB, Malvestutto C, Miller WC. Challenges facing a rural opioid epidemic: treatment and prevention of HIV and hepatitis C. Curr HIV/AIDS Rep 2018;15(3):245−54.

[41] Komaromy M, Duhigg D, Metcalf A, et al. Project ECHO (Extension for Community Healthcare Outcomes): a new model for educating primary care providers about treatment of substance use disorders. Subst Abuse 2016;37(1):20−4.

[42] Mathers BM, Degenhardt L, Ali H, et al. HIV prevention, treatment, and care services for people who inject drugs: a systematic review of global, regional, and national coverage. Lancet 2010;375(9719):1014−28.

[43] Bachireddy C, Weisberg DF, Altice FL. Balancing access and safety in prescribing opioid agonist therapy to prevent HIV transmission. Addiction 2015;110(12):1869−71.

[44] Korthuis PT, McCarty D, Weimer M, et al. Primary care-based models for the treatment of opioid use disorder: a scoping review. Ann Intern Med 2017;166(4):268−78.

[45] Jones CM, Campopiano M, Baldwin G, McCance-Katz E. National and state treatment need and capacity for opioid agonist medication-assisted treatment. Am J Public Health 2015;105(8):e55−63.

[46] Dupouy J, Palmaro A, Fatséas M, et al. Mortality associated with time in and out of buprenorphine treatment in French office-based general practice: a 7-year cohort study. Ann Fam Med 2017;15(4):355−8.

[47] Saitz R, Daaleman TP. Now is the time to address substance use disorders in primary care. Ann Fam Med 2017;15(4):306−8.

[48] Tonelli M, Wiebe N, Manns BJ, et al. Comparison of the complexity of patients seen by different medical subspecialists in a universal health care system. JAMA Netw Open 2018;1(7):e184852.

[49] Edelman EJ, Oldfield BJ, Tetrault JM. Office-based addiction treatment in primary care: approaches that work. Med Clin North Am 2018;102(4):635−52.

[50] World Health Organization (WHO). Integrating collaborative TB and HIV services within a comprehensive package of care for people who inject drugs: consolidated Guidelines. Geneva, Switzerland. 2016. Available from:http://apps.who.int/iris/bitstream/10665/204484/204481/9789241510226_eng.pdf?ua=9789241510221.

[51] Thompson MA, Mugavero MJ, Amico KR, et al. Guidelines for improving entry into and retention in care and antiretroviral adherence for persons with HIV: evidence-based recommendations from an International Association of Physicians in AIDS Care panel. Ann Intern Med 2012;156(11):817−33. W-284, W-285, W-286, W-287, W-288, W-289, W-290, W-291, W-292, W-293, W-294.

[52] Bond G. Breaking the chain: STDs and HIV. WorldAIDS 1992;(22) [4] p.

[53] Basu S, Smith-Rohrberg D, Bruce RD, Altice FL. Models for integrating buprenorphine therapy into the primary HIV care setting. Clin Infect Dis 2006;42(5):716−21.

[54] Altice FL, Bruce RD, Lucas GM, et al. HIV treatment outcomes among HIV-infected, opioid-dependent patients receiving buprenorphine/naloxone treatment within HIV clinical care settings: results from a multisite study. J Acquir Immune Defic Syndr 2011;56(Suppl. 1):S22−32.

[55] Weiss L, Netherland J, Egan JE, et al. Integration of buprenorphine/naloxone treatment into HIV clinical care: lessons from the BHIVES collaborative. J Acquir Immune Defic Syndr 2011;56(Suppl. 1):S68−75.

[56] Sokol R, LaVertu AE, Morrill D, Albanese C, Schuman-Olivier Z. Group-based treatment of opioid use disorder with buprenorphine: a systematic review. J Subst Abuse Treat 2018;84:78−87.

[57] Jones CM, McCance-Katz EF. Characteristics and prescribing practices of clinicians recently waivered to prescribe buprenorphine for the treatment of opioid use disorder. Addiction 2018;114(3):471−82.

[58] Bowman S, Eiserman J, Beletsky L, Stancliff S, Bruce RD. Reducing the health consequences of opioid addiction in primary care. Am J Med 2013;126(7):565−71.

[59] Ferri FF. Opioid use disorder- ClinicalKey. In: Ferri's clinical advisor 2019. Elsevier; 2019. p. 977−9. e1. Available from:https://www.clinicalkey.com/#!/content/book/3-s2.0-B9780323530422005952?scrollTo=%23hl0000413.

[60] Substance Abuse and Mental Health Services Administration. SBIRT/SAMHSA-HRSA. 2019. Available from:https://www.integration.samhsa.gov/clinical-practice/sbirt.

[61] D'Onofrio G, O'Connor PG, Pantalon MV, et al. Emergency department-initiated buprenorphine/naloxone treatment for opioid dependence: a randomized clinical trial. JAMA 2015;313(16):1636−44.

[62] Barata IA, Shandro JR, Montgomery M, et al. Effectiveness of SBIRT for alcohol use disorders in the emergency department: a systematic review. West J Emerg Med 2017; 18(6):1143−52.

[63] Peles E, Schreiber S, Adelson M. Opiate-dependent patients on a waiting list for methadone maintenance treatment are at high risk for mortality until treatment entry. J Addict Med 2013;7(3):177−82.

[64] Sigmon SC. Interim treatment: bridging delays to opioid treatment access. Prev Med 2015;80:32−6.

[65] Wesson DR, Ling W. The clinical opiate withdrawal scale (COWS). J Psychoactive Drugs 2003;35(2):253−9.

[66] Cunningham C, Fishman M. The ASAM national practice guidelines for the use of medications in the treatment of addiction involving opioid use. Lake Mary, Florida: American Society of Addiction Medicine; 2015. Available from:https://www.asam.org/docs/default-source/practice-support/guidelines-and-consensus-docs/asam-national-practice-guideline-pocketguide.pdf?sfvrsn=35ee6fc2_0.

[67] Desmond DP, Maddux JF. Deaths among heroin users in and out of methadone treatment. J Maint Addict 2000;1(4):45−61.

[68] Earnshaw V, Smith L, Copenhaver M. Drug addiction stigma in the context of methadone maintenance therapy: an investigation into understudied sources of stigma. Int J Ment Health Addict 2013;11(1):110−22.

[69] Micromedex. Methadone: adverse effects. Greenwood Village, CO: Truven Health Analytics; 2019.

[70] McCance-Katz EF, Sullivan LE, Nallani S. Drug interactions of clinical importance among the opioids, methadone and buprenorphine, and other frequently prescribed medications: a review. Am J Addict 2010;19(1):4−16.

[71] Goodbar NH, Hanlon KE. Implantable buprenorphine (probuphine) for maintenance treatment of opioid use disorder. Am Fam Physician 2018;97(10):668−70.

[72] Gryczynski J, Jaffe JH, Schwartz RP, et al. Patient perspectives on choosing buprenorphine over methadone in an urban, equal-access system. Am J Addict 2013;22(3):285—91.

[73] Fiellin DA, Moore BA, Sullivan LE, et al. Long-term treatment with buprenorphine/naloxone in primary care: results at 2-5 years. Am J Addict 2008;17(2):116—20.

[74] Dick AW, Pacula RL, Gordon AJ, et al. Growth in buprenorphine waivers for physicians increased potential access to opioid agonist treatment, 2002-11. Health Aff 2015;34(6):1028—34.

[75] Stein BD, Gordon AJ, Dick AW, et al. Supply of buprenorphine waivered physicians: the influence of state policies. J Subst Abuse Treat 2015;48(1):104—11.

[76] Cunningham EB, Hajarizadeh B, Amin J, et al. Longitudinal injecting risk behaviours among people with a history of injecting drug use in an Australian prison setting: the HITS-p study. Int J Drug Policy 2018;54:18—25. Cunningham, Hajarizadeh, Amin, Bretana, Dore, Luciani, Lloyd, Grebely. The Kirby Institute, UNSW Sydney, Sydney, Australia.

[77] Kermack A, Flannery M, Tofighi B, McNeely J, Lee JD. Buprenorphine prescribing practice trends and attitudes among New York providers. J Subst Abuse Treat 2017; 74:1—6.

[78] Micromedex. Buprenorphine: adverse effects. Greenwood Village, CO: Truven Health Analytics; 2019.

[79] Minozzi S, Amato L, Vecchi S, Davoli M, Kirchmayer U, Verster A. Oral naltrexone maintenance treatment for opioid dependence. Cochrane Database Syst Rev 2011;(4): Cd001333.

[80] ASPE/HHS. Use of medication-assisted treatment for opioid use disorders in employer-sponsored health insurance. Office of the Assistant Secretary for Planning and Evaluation (ASPE), US Department of Health and Human Services; 2019.

[81] Jahagirdar D, Wright M-D. Naltrexone for opioid use disorders: a review of clinical effectiveness, cost-effectiveness, and guidelines. Ottawa, ON: Canadian Agency for Drugs and Technologies in Health; 2017. Available from:http://www.ncbi.nlm.nih.gov/books/NBK525041/.

[82] ColumbiaPsych. Vivitrol injection preparation. 2019. Available from:https://www.youtube.com/watch?v=lZBaDCIWSwg.

[83] Providers' Clinical Support System. Your patient safety card for emergency pain management. 2019. Available from:https://custom.cvent.com/10D3BAE39269457884C1D96DE1DF8D8D/files/2b4a51da47474de2a3b68ea131bbf45a.pdf.

[84] Providers' Clinical Support System. XR-naltrexone: a step-by-step. 2017. Available from:http://pcssnow.org/wp-content/uploads/2017/02/Naltrexone_Step-by-Step_Virtual_Brochure-1.pdf.

[85] Micromedex. Naltrexone: adverse effects. Greenwood Village, CO: Truven Health Analytics; 2019.

[86] Dehlendorf C, Fitzpatrick J, Steinauer J, et al. Development and field testing of a decision support tool to facilitate shared decision making in contraceptive counseling. Patient Edu Couns 2017;100(7):1374—81.

[87] Institute of Medicine Committee on Quality of Health Care in A.. In: Crossing the quality chasm: a new health system for the 21st century. Washington, DC: National Academies Press (US); 2001. Copyright 2001 by the National Academy of Sciences. All rights reserved.

[88] Stacey D, Legare F, Lewis K, et al. Decision aids for people facing health treatment or screening decisions. Cochrane Database Syst Rev 2017;4:Cd001431.

[89]   Millery M, Kleinman BP, Polissar NL, Millman RB, Scimeca M. Detoxification as a gateway to long-term treatment: assessing two interventions. J Subst Abuse Treat 2002;23(3):183–90.

[90]   Bentzley BS, Barth KS, Back SE, Book SW. Discontinuation of buprenorphine maintenance therapy: perspectives and outcomes. J Subst Abuse Treat 2015;52: 48–57.

[91]   Kayman DJ, Goldstein MF, Deren S, Rosenblum A. Predicting treatment retention with a brief "opinions about methadone" scale. J Psychoactive Drugs 2006;38(1): 93–100.

[92]   Thaler R. Toward a positive theory of consumer choice. J Econ Behav Organ 1980; 1(1):39–60.

[93]   Knetsch JL. The endowment effect and evidence of nonreversible indifference curves. Am Econ Rev 1989;79(5):1277–84.

[94]   Tversky A, Kahneman D. Advances in prospect theory: cumulative representation of uncertainty. J Risk Uncertain 1992;5(4):297–323.

[95]   Elwyn G, Frosch D, Thomson R, et al. Shared decision making: a model for clinical practice. J Gen Intern Med 2012;27(10):1361–7.

[96]   Substance Abuse and Mental Health Services Administration. Decisions in recover: treatment for opioid use disorder. 2018. Available from:www.samhsa.gov/brss-tacs/ shared-decision-making.

[97]   Center for Substance Abuse Treatment. Medication-assisted treatment for opioid, addiction in opioid treatment programs. SAMHSA/CSAT medication-assisted treatment for opioid addiction in opioid treatment programs. SAMHSA/CSAT treatment improvement protocol (TIP). Rockville, MD: U.S. Substance Abuse and Mental Health Services Administration; 2019. Available from:http://www.ncbi.nlm.nih.gov/ books/NBK64 164/pdf/Bookshelf_NBK64164.pdf.

[98]   Jacobs AA, Cangiano M. Medication-assisted treatment considerations for women with opiate addiction disorders. Prim Care 2018;45(4):731–42.

[99]   Marsh JC, Park K, Lin Y-A, Bersamira C. Gender differences in trends for heroin use and nonmedical prescription opioid use, 2007-2014. J Subst Abuse Treat 2018;87: 79–85.

[100] Tadros A, Layman SM, Davis SM, Bozeman R, Davidov DM. Emergency department visits by pediatric patients for poisoning by prescription opioids. Am J Drug Alcohol Abuse 2016;42(5):550–5.

[101] Lister JJ, Brown S, Greenwald MK, Ledgerwood DM. Gender-specific predictors of methadone treatment outcomes among African Americans at an urban clinic. Subst Abus 2019;1–9.

[102] Haug N, Sorensen J, Lollo N, Gruber V, Delucchi K, Hall S. Gender differences among HIV-positive methadone maintenance patients enrolled in a medication adherence trial. AIDS Care 2005;17(8):1022–9.

[103] Heil SH, Jones HE, Arria A, et al. Unintended pregnancy in opioid-abusing women. J Subst Abuse Treat 2011;40(2):199–202.

[104] Bornstein M, Gipson JD, Bleck R, Sridhar A, Berger A. Perceptions of pregnancy and contraceptive use: an in-depth study of women in Los Angeles methadone clinics. Wom Health Issues 2019;29(2):176–81.

[105] Haight SC. Opioid use disorder documented at delivery hospitalization — United States, 1999–2014. MMWR Morb Mortal Wkly Rep 2018;67. Available from: https://www.cdc.gov/mmwr/volumes/67/wr/mm6731a1.htm.

[106] Poon S, Pupco A, Koren G, Bozzo P. Safety of the newer class of opioid antagonists in pregnancy. Can Fam Physician 2014;60(7):631−2. e348−9.

[107] Dooley J, Gerber-Finn L, Antone I, et al. Buprenorphine-naloxone use in pregnancy for treatment of opioid dependence. Can Fam Physician 2016;62(4):e194−200.

[108] Substance Abuse and Mental Health Services Administration. Clinical guidance for treating pregnant and parenting women with opioid use disorder and their infants. Rockville, MD: Substance Abuse and Mental Health Services Administration; 2018. Available from:https://store.samhsa.gov/system/files/sma18-5054.pdf.

[109] Brogly SB, Saia KE, Werler MM, Regan E, Hernandez-Diaz S. Prenatal treatment and outcomes of women with opioid use disorder. Obstet Gynecol 2018;132(4):916−22.

[110] Patrick SW, Schiff DM, Ryan SA, Quigley J, Gonzalez PK, Walker LR. A public health response to opioid use in pregnancy. Pediatrics 2017;139(3). Available from:https://www.scopus.com/inward/record.uri?eid=2-s2.0-85016029675&doi=10.1542%2fpeds.2016-4070&partnerID=40&md5=e2c95980ca640b0a66485a090cfe7c23.

[111] Kremer ME, Arora KS. Clinical, ethical, and legal considerations in pregnant women with opioid Abuse. Obstet Gynecol 2015;126(3):474−8.

[112] Miranda L, Dixon V, Reyes C. How states handle drug use during pregnancy. 2015. Available from:http://projects.propublica.org/graphics/maternity-drug-policies-by-state.

[113] Ostrach B, Leiner C. "I didn't want to be on suboxone at first…"- ambivalence in perinatal substance use treatment. J Addict Med 2018;13(4):264−71.

[114] Roberts SCM, Nuru-Jeter A. Women's perspectives on screening for alcohol and drug use in prenatal care. Womens Health Issues 2010;20(3):193−200.

[115] Racine N, Motz M, Leslie M, Pepler D. Breaking the cycle pregnancy outreach program: reaching out to improve the health and well-being for pregnant substance-involved mothers. Racine, J Mother Initiative Res Community Involv J Assoc Res Mothering 2009;11(1). Available from:https://jarm.journals.yorku.ca/index.php/jarm/article/view/22525.

[116] Barry DT, Beitel M, Cutter CJ, et al. An evaluation of the feasibility, acceptability, and preliminary efficacy of cognitive-behavioral therapy for opioid use disorder and chronic pain. Drug Alcohol Depend 2019;194:460−7.

[117] Manhapra A, Becker WC. Pain and addiction: an integrative therapeutic approach. Med Clin North Am 2018;102(4):745−63.

[118] Center for Disease Control and Prevention. US public health service. Preexposure prophylaxis for the prevention of HIV infection in the United States-2017 update: a clinical practice guideline. 2018. Available from:https://www.cdc.gov/hiv/pdf/risk/prep/cdc-hiv-prep-guidelines-2017.pdf.

[119] D'Onofrio G, McCormack RP, Hawk K. Emergency Departments — A 24/7/365 Option for Combating the Opioid Crisis. N. Engl. J. Med. 2018;379(26):2487−90.

[120] Andraka-Christou B, Capone MJ. A qualitative study comparing physician-reported barriers to treating addiction using buprenorphine and extended-release naltrexone in U.S. office-based practices. Int J Drug Policy 2018;54:9−17.

[121] Mitchell SG, Gryczynski J, Schwartz RP. Commentary on "The More Things Change: Buprenorphine/Naloxone Diversion Continues While Treatment is Inaccessible." J Addict Med 2018;12(6):424−5.

[122] Shi JM, Henry SP, Dwy SL, Orazietti SA, Carroll KM. Randomized pilot trial of Web-based cognitive-behavioral therapy adapted for use in office-based buprenorphine maintenance. Subst Abus 2019:1−4.

[123] Yudko E, Lozhkina O, Fouts A. A comprehensive review of the psychometric properties of the Drug Abuse Screening Test. J Subst Abuse Treat 2007;32(2):189–98.

[124] Bowman S, Grau LE, Singer M, Scott G, Heimer R. Factors associated with hepatitis B vaccine series completion in a randomized trial for injection drug users reached through syringe exchange programs in three US cities. BMC Public Health [Internet] 2014;14(1). Available from: https://www.scopus.com/inward/record.uri?eid=2-s2.0-84908278410&doi=10.1186%2f1471-2458-14-820&partnerID=40&md5=364a6753c65a3874aa198b781db8eb3a.

[125] Smith PC, Schmidt SM, Allensworth-Davies D, Saitz R. A single-question screening test for drug use in primary care. Arch Intern Med 2010;170(13):1155–60.

[126] Gryczynski J, Kelly SM, Gwin Mitchell S, Kirk A, O'Grady KE, Schwartz RP. Validation and performance of the Alcohol, Smoking, and Substance Involvement Screening Test (ASSIST) among adolescent primary care patients. Addiction 2015; 110(2):240–7.

[127] Pence BW, Gaynes BN, Whetten K, Eron JJ, Ryder RW, Miller WC. Validation of a brief screening instrument for substance abuse and mental illness in HIV-positive patients. J Acquir Immune Defic Syndr 2005;40(4):434–44.

Inpatient opioid use disorder treatment for the infectious disease physician

10

Nikhil Seval, MD [1], Ellen Eaton, MD, MSPH [2], Sandra A. Springer, MD [3,4,5]

[1]*Instructor of Medicine, Department of Internal Medicine, Section of Infectious Diseases, AIDS Program, Yale School of Medicine, New Haven, CT, United States;* [2]*Assistant Professor, Department of Medicine, Division of Infectious Disease, University of Alabama at Birmingham, Birmingham, AL, United States;* [3]*Attending Physician, Internal Medicine, Infectious Disease, Veterans Administration Connecticut Healthcare System, West Haven, CT, United States;* [4]*Center for Interdisciplinary Research on AIDS, Yale University School of Public Health, New Haven, CT, United States;* [5]*Associate Professor of Medicine, Department of Internal Medicine, Section of Infectious Diseases, AIDS Program, Yale School of Medicine, New Haven, CT, United States*

Introduction

Infections are a common cause of hospitalization for patients with opioid use disorders (OUDs). In 2012, there were 530,000 OUD-related hospitalizations with a total estimated healthcare cost of $15 billion [1], approximately 6.500 of those admissions were related to infections, doubled from the previous decade, with an associated total cost of $700 million [1]. This is an underestimate in the context of the growing opioid crisis over the past decade in the United States. There is likely underreporting of infections related to OUD; chronic infections acquired via substance use are also not included in such estimates, such as Hepatitis C virus (HCV) or HIV infection and their downstream morbidities. Many receiving inpatient care for infectious issues do not have a diagnosis of OUD. Data from the 2016 National Survey on Drug Use and Health describe 11.8 million people age 12 and over as having misused opioids (IV or oral) in the past year with only 2.1 million of them having been diagnosed with OUD. This gap represents patients who are at high risk for developing OUD or potentially have undiagnosed disease.

For many patients with OUD, an inpatient hospital admission represents a "reachable moment" for life-saving interventions [2]. First, the patient can be identified and diagnosed with OUD and can be initiated on medications for treatment of OUD (MOUD): methadone, buprenorphine, or extended-release naltrexone. Second, comorbid conditions such as psychiatric comorbidities can be identified. The hospital setting can be a venue where OUD is reframed as a chronic relapsing medical disorder for the patient and managed as such, in a person-centric manner. Integrating

The Opioid Epidemic and Infectious Diseases. https://doi.org/10.1016/B978-0-323-68328-9.00010-2

treatment in a multidisciplinary manner is essential. With MOUD-based therapy and integrated medical team-based care, treatment outcomes can be optimized with a reduction in interrupted care and hospital discharges against medical advice (AMA). The infectious disease (ID) physician can and should play an integral role in these missions.

Pathophysiology of infections related to OUD

The vast majority of infections related to OUD are bacterial complications related to needle-associated pathogen entry [3]. Most of these infections are from the patient's own skin flora at time of needle puncture during injection drug use (IDU), and consequently streptococcal species and *Staphylococcus aureus* are the most common [4]. Site of injection informs the commensal flora involved; gram negative and anaerobic infections are more common in those who use groin access for injection [5]. Practices of general hygiene and skin decontamination with alcohol swabbing prior to injection may reduce abscess formation [6]. Although people who inject drugs (PWID) may think their drugs are contaminated [7], it is uncommon for infections to result from contamination of drug supply or paraphernalia [8,9].

Drug preparation and injection techniques play a large role in the microbiology of injection-related infections. Water used as heroin solvent can contain environmental gram-negative organisms, especially if sourced from clearly nonsterile sites (i.e., toilet water). Needle licking predisposes to infections with oral streptococcal and anaerobic species. Such practices are performed with the misconception that licking can clean the needle and a desire to "not waste" residual heroin on the syringe [10]. Acidification of opioids with nonsterile ascorbic acid sources such as citrus juices and fruit can be a source of *Candidal* exposure [11].

Needle reuse dulls the bevel of the instrument and increases the likelihood of trauma and venous damage during injection, predisposing to a skin or soft tissue infection (SSTI). Needle and syringe sharing is the key mode of transmission for viral infections such as HIV and HCV. The original case-control studies for HCV risk in the United States showed a 49-fold higher risk of seropositivity in IDU [12]. HIV and HBV both have an increased prevalence in PWID though the association is more nonspecific given transmission via sex. It is estimated that roughly 15%–20% of PWID are HIV positive globally but there are vast differences from country to country [13]. Improper decontamination of reused paraphernalia is common, such as lack of awareness of need for bleach products, or decontamination of the needle portion and not the syringe. Clonal analysis of bacteremias caused by *S. aureus* in clustered drug networks suggests that it can be transmissible by drug paraphernalia as well [14].

OUD not related to IDU (i.e., via smoking, snorting, or prescription pill use) technically should not have the same associated infectious risk factors, although any lifetime history of previous IDU could confer similar risk. Growing evidence supports epidemiological associations of oral opioid use with other conditions such as invasive pneumococcal disease [15]. Transactional sex and survival sex in exchange for opioids can also elevate transmission of STIs including HBV and HIV.

Inpatient OUD screening in the infectious disease consultation

Screening for OUD

A cross-sectional evaluation performed in 2009 of a large inpatient urban center found a substance use disorder incidence of approximately 11% (excluding alcohol, tobacco, and patients already stabilized on MOUD) [16]. The United States Preventative Services Task Force in 2008 found insufficient evidence for universal screening in the general medical setting for drug use. These guidelines are currently being revised to respond to the national OUD crisis, and other organizational bodies such as the National Institute for Drug Abuse (NIDA) recommend universal OUD screening [17]. We recommend consideration of OUD screening for all ID consultations, especially in those that may be IDU related. Optimally, initial ID consultation will occur early so as to potentially link to MOUD treatment and improve inpatient outcomes.

Certain infections and conditions elevate the pretest probability of having OUD. As mentioned above, HCV, HIV, and HBV infections all increase the likelihood of IDU-associated OUD. Bloodstream infections without a clear source such as *Staphylococcus* bacteremia or Candidiasis merit further OUD screening. Other conditions related to bacteremia or contiguous spread such as infectious endocarditis, osteomyelitis, or endophthalmitis could be injection related. Numerous noninfectious risk factors for OUD also exist. For the patient with prescribed oral opioids, four behavior patterns have been associated with illicit use: early refills, intoxication with the prescribed drug, dose increase of the patient's own volition, and oversedation [18]. Relevant state Prescription Monitoring Program review can display patterns of medication seeking. Finally, patients with frank opioid withdrawal or intoxication can be misdiagnosed without clinical suspicion for OUD.

The *NIDA Quick Screen* is a single screening question for past year use of alcohol, tobacco, nonmedical prescription drug, and illegal drug use [17]. It is meant for use by general medical practitioners and is an effective screen for OUD and other SUD. The doctor-patient discussion on screening is best prefaced by ensuring confidentiality and appropriate medical care. A positive screen reflexes to the NIDA-Modified Alcohol, Smoking, and Substance Involvement Screening Test (*NM-ASSIST*), which assesses for severity for a variety of illicit substances. The screening process is typically interpreted in tandem with a brief intervention (referred to as SBI) with a goal to frame a discussion and support deeper diagnostic evaluation. The discussion has been framed as the "5 As" *of SBI: Ask, Advise, Assess, Assist, and Arrange*. The provider begins by asking permission to discuss screening results, and then advises on drug use. Assessment regards the patient's readiness to quit—both readiness to start MOUD and/or harm reduction services (e.g., naloxone proficiency, needle syringe exchange) should be queried. Subsequently assistance is given in making behavioral changes, and "arrange" refers to creating follow-up care. The 5A framework should be tailored to the patient interview—if screening and OUD diagnosis occur at the same time, the intervention portion can be tailored to a discussion on MOUD initiation.

Urine toxicology screening is best used as an additional data point with a given sensitivity and specificity to be interpreted in a clinical context. Most clinical drug screening is a urine immunoassay in which an antibody panel binds against drugs or metabolites. Its major drawback is cross-reactivity, which can be assay-dependent, and includes cross reactions with naloxone (false positive for oxycodone) and both fluoroquinolones and rifampicin (false positives for opiates) [19]. Poppy seeds are known to have minute but detectable concentrations of morphine derivative that can trigger positivity. Confirmatory testing using liquid chromatography or mass spectrometry is typically not performed in clinical labs. Positivity duration depends on opioid type: codeine, heroin, and morphine can be detected for up to 2 days and methadone can be detected for up to 3 days using specific methadone assays. The general "opiate" immunoassay will *not* detect oxycodone, fentanyl, or methadone, although specific screens that will check for a broader panel of opioids and metabolites are now available.

Establishing the OUD diagnosis

For those that screen positive, a full assessment of severity is merited, with the goal of establishing whether OUD is present or not. If inpatient Addiction Medicine consultation is present, this role can be referred or shared. However, part of the movement for broader MOUD prescribing involves additional providers such as ID consultants to have competency with establishing a use disorder diagnosis.

Per the DSM-5 criteria depicted in Table 10.1, an OUD constitutes a problematic pattern of opioid use resulting in clinically significant impairment. The three broad criteria categories are (1) loss of control, (2) adverse consequences, including health, legal, etc., and (3) physiology of tolerance demonstrated in the past 12 months.

Presence of two or more criteria is consistent with a diagnosis of OUD. Severity is determined by total number of criteria, though frequency and amount of opioid use is used in conjunction with diagnostic severity for a more holistic understanding of drug-related dysfunction.

There are a variety of diagnostic assessment tools to be used for establishing the diagnosis of OUD. The use of a particular assessment tool depends in part in clinical role (addiction specialist/psychiatrist vs. generalist; researcher vs. clinician) and whether there is motive for in-depth diagnosis of other substance use disorders. The *SCID, or structured clinical interview* for DSM-V, is the gold standard for in-depth psychiatric or research-based evaluation [20]. It is a semistructured clinical interview based off of the DSM criteria. The *Mini-International Neuropsychiatric Review, or MINI*, is shorter and has been validated in relation to the SCID [21]. All are designed to maximize diagnostic performance and interprovider reliability.

Table 10.1 DSM-5 criteria for opioid use disorder.

1. Opioids are often taken in larger amounts or over a longer period than was intended.
2. There is a persistent desire or unsuccessful efforts to cut down or control opioid use.
3. A great deal of time is spent in activities necessary to obtain the opioid, use the opioid, or recover from its effects.
4. Craving, or a strong desire or urge to use opioids.
5. Recurrent opioid use resulting in a failure to fulfill major role obligations at work, school, or home.
6. Continued opioid use despite having persistent or recurrent social or interpersonal problems caused or exacerbated by the effects of opioids.
7. Important social, occupational, or recreational activities are given up or reduced because of opioid use.
8. Recurrent opioid use in situations in which it is physically hazardous.
9. Continued opioid use despite knowledge of having a persistent or recurrent physical or psychological problem that is likely to have been caused or exacerbated by the substance.
10. Exhibition of tolerance.
11. Exhibition of withdrawal.

Mild: two to three symptoms; moderate: four to five symptoms; severe: >6 symptoms.
Adapted from Diagnostic and statistical manual of mental disorders (fifth ed.), American Psychiatric Association, 2013.

For the targeted diagnosis and rapid treatment of OUD, direct use of the DSM-5 criteria serves an important role, especially in decentralized OUD treatment for non-addiction specialty providers. The *Rapid Opioid Dependence Screen (RODS)*, developed by co-author S. Springer, is an eight question brief assessment tool validated against the MINI specifically for rapid diagnosis of OUD in incarcerated populations with HIV and could be used more broadly with subsequent scale validation [22,23].

Clarifying OUD for the infectious disease physician

Following diagnosis of OUD, there are two main goals: to detail the patient's opioid use with particular attention paid to infection-related risk practices and to discuss initiation of MOUD. The clarification of OUD component can be woven into the framework of an ID consult history and physical and will guide the consultation.

Type, route, and frequency of opioid will greatly affect infection risk. Often patients will have a combination of different opioid use routes (e.g., injection, snorting, oral, and/or smoked) and types (e.g., both injection-based heroin/fentanyl and oral prescription illicit opioids). Site of injection can span from low-risk sites such as the antecubital fossa or hand to more central sites with higher commensal flora burden like the groin. Very high-risk injecting such as arterial or carotid ("shooting for big red") injection has an elevated risk for aneurysm formation and life-threatening bleeding. Skin decontamination practices should be queried especially if the patient's chief diagnosis is SSTI. Harm reduction requires hand hygiene and decontamination with proper equipment such as alcohol-based wipes. Skin-popping and muscle popping, which are subcutaneous and intramuscular injections, respectively, carry higher rates of abscess formation and spore forming bacterial infections. There is a wide spectrum of water sterility used among PWID. In ideal harm reduction settings, sterile water should be used, but sources including toilet water have been reported, often in the throes of withdrawal with limited alternative sources. This is fueled by misconceptions that the cooking of product will fully sterilize any infectious material. Paraphernalia sharing should be queried, with specific questions toward which pieces of equipment were shared and how—even if a syringe tip is replaced and a plunger is retained, residual body fluids could be reservoirs for HIV or HCV. Finally, there are a variety of real-world practices that PWID employ in attempts to sterilize paraphernalia. The most advisable form of decontamination is with undiluted household bleach retained for at least 2 min [24]. Local availability of other harm reduction strategies such as needle and syringe exchange programs and overdose education and naloxone distribution will guide subsequent counseling.

Expanding on past substance use history is informative in anticipation of initiating MOUD treatment. A detailed history will include past use of MOUD, response, and information on relapse. History of overdose, hospitalization, and rehabilitation therapy is also relevant. The Prescription Monitoring Program database will provide historical data in regard to prescribed opioid use—methadone will not be reported here and, if prescribed, the relevant opioid treatment program (OTP) should be contacted. There is a significant heritability to substance use disorder that should be explored for family history. Social support and living situation contributes to psychosocial risk factors for use but also assistance networks for treatment. A history of legal issues regarding substances assesses adverse consequences of drug use.

Comorbid psychiatric disease can have a major impact on treatment outcomes if left undiagnosed or unmanaged. The introductory *Patient Health Questionnaire (PHQ)-2* screen is a well-validated, brief screen for depression that can lead to further assessment of major depressive disorder with the *PHQ-9* [25]. Positive screening for suicidal or homicidal ideation requires psychiatric referral and stabilization. The NM-ASSIST, introduced above, can serve as a screen for other substance use disorders if performed to completion. Screening for chronic infectious diseases associated with IVDU such as HIV, HCV, and HBV should occur.

Withdrawal treatment with transition to medication maintenance

Opioid withdrawal treatment includes the patient-centered and evidence-based management of withdrawal symptoms using pharmacotherapy ideally with the use of opioid agonist therapy. Hospitalized patients with OUD may exhibit symptoms along the spectrum of acute intoxication to opioid withdrawal based on the timing of their opioid use. Goals of therapy for withdrawal treatment regard (1) humane care and relief of withdrawal symptoms, (2) forging of a therapeutic alliance, (3) retention in care, and (4) transitioning to maintenance use of MOUD (agonist vs. nonagonist therapy). Notably, there is no role of withdrawal (or the older stigmatizing terminology of "detoxification") for achieving sustained abstinence from opioids [26]. When a patient is in withdrawal, it is an ideal time to start an MOUD such as buprenorphine such that the withdrawal ceases, the patient remains in care, and is then able to be linked to outpatient care with a prescription upon release from the hospital.

Opioid withdrawal is a physiologic response to cessation of opioids after administration at dependence-inducing doses. Signs of withdrawal include insomnia, dysphoria, nausea/vomiting, lacrimation/rhinorrhea, pupillary dilation, yawning, diarrhea, tachycardia, and muscle aches. Temperature dysregulation and fever can occur. The physiology of opioid withdrawal is based on two main loci of neurotransmitter disruption: norepinephrine activity in the reticular activating system and dopamine activity in the mesolimbic pathway [27]. Increased norepinephrine levels in withdrawal lead to symptoms of tachycardia, piloerection, myalgias, and irritability. The mesolimbic pathway, also colloquially understood as the "reward" pathway, has low levels of dopamine transmission in withdrawal, associated with dysphoria, craving, and depression. The Clinical Opioid Withdrawal Scale (COWS) has high sensitivity and interuser reliability and allows quantification of symptoms in the clinical setting [28]. Pharmacologic treatments for withdrawal are based on targeting these specific pathways and are listed in Tables 10.2.

Alpha-2 adrenergic agonists relieve the autonomic symptoms of opioid withdrawal. Both clonidine and lofexidine, the latter of which was FDA approved in the United States in 2018, are superior to placebo in treatment completion. Opioid agonist-based therapy treats both autonomic and dopaminergic (craving based) symptoms and is superior to alpha-2 adrenergic therapy for treatment completion [29,30]. These nonopioid agonist therapies are now used for adjunctive support or in institutional settings in which MOUD are not available.

Table 10.2 Pharmacotherapy for medically supervised withdrawal.

Agonist
- Methadone, buprenorphine

Nonagonist

- Benzodiazepines: Anxiolysis
  • Alprazolam, diazepam, lorazepam
  • Lorazepam 0.5 mg po q8h prn for irritability/anxiety
- α-2 agonists: Reduction in centrally mediated adrenergic response
  • Clonidine: 0.1−0.3 mg po q4-q6h prn for diaphoresis, lacrimation, rhinorrhea
  • Lofexidine: 0.54 mg q4-q6h prn for diaphoresis, lacrimation, rhinorrhea
- Antidiarrheals
  • Loperamide: 4 mg po prn for diarrhea (2 mg po prn afterward), not to exceed 16 mg/24hr
- NSAIDs and acetaminophen: Antiinflammatory/antipyretics
  • PRN for myalgias/arthralgias
- Antiemetics
  • Prochlorperazine or ondansetron po/IV for nausea/vomiting

Medications for OUD

Methadone

Methadone was FDA approved for OUD in the 1970s making it the oldest and most well-studied MOUD. Methadone is a weak opioid agonist, meaning it mimics the effects of opioids such as heroin and reduces withdrawal symptoms without causing euphoria [31]. Because of its long half-life, daily methadone in the form of methadone maintenance treatment (MMT) can curb withdrawal symptoms for 24—36 h. Doses above 60 mg have consistently shown improved outcomes compared with lower doses [32]. By preventing withdrawal, MMT reduces illicit drug use and subsequently reduces complications of nonprescription opioids: overdose, death, injection, and additional criminalized behaviors such as drug seeking [33]. Methadone prevents the euphoria of heroin when used concurrently due to its effect on the opioid receptor, discouraging illicit drug use and promoting recovery.

In a clinical trial setting, methadone was significantly more effective than nonpharmacological interventions in its ability to retain patients in treatment and reduce heroin use [34]. In a review of three randomized controlled trials (RCTs) comparing methadone to nonpharmacological approaches, methadone was unable to significantly reduce criminal activity or mortality, though subsequent large-scale cohort studies have established reductions in all cause and overdose mortality with treatment [34—36]. Compared with buprenorphine, methadone is more effective at both low and flexible doses in retaining patients in treatment. At fixed medium and high doses, buprenorphine may be as effective as medium and high dose methadone, respectively, at retaining patients and suppressing illicit opioid use [37]. However, fixed doses are impractical as part of routine care. MMT has also been shown to improve drug-related HIV risk behaviors, criminal behaviors, and mortality in addition to maternal and fetal outcomes.

Though methadone is a sufficient medication for treatment of inpatient opioid withdrawal, there can be dose and duration restrictions on inpatient prescribing which vary state by state, often making buprenorphine a more practical choice.

Clinicians and patients should appreciate the risks associated with MMT, including death, respiratory depression, and QT prolongation. For this reason, methadone dose should be slowly increased, and MMT should be avoided altogether in patients with a long QT. Patients receiving MMT should avoid additional respiratory suppressants including alcohol and benzodiazepines and medications that might increase the QT interval [32]. Both methadone and buprenorphine are extensively metabolized by the CYP450 system (see Table 10.3).

Buprenorphine

Buprenorphine is a semisynthetic derivative of thebaine with both partial agonist effect at the mu opioid receptor and antagonistic effect at kappa receptors [38]. Due to these partial agonist properties, it exhibits a dose response curve with limited additional analgesia and euphoria, giving it a functional ceiling effect [39].

Table 10.3 Antiretroviral-related medication interactions with MOUD.

Medication	Buprenorphine	Methadone
NRTIs	*None*	ABC—decreased methadone levels. may need increased methadone dose
	None	AZT—glucuronidation and renal clearance of AZT affected, monitor for zidovudine toxicity
NNRTIs	EFV—PK effect (decreased), dose adjustments unlikely to be needed	EFV—decreased methadone levels, typically 30% dose increase needed
	RPV—no adjustment	RPV—decreased methadone levels, may need increased methadone dose
PIs	ATZ—Inc bup levels w/clinical correlate (oversedation, etc). Dose reduction or slower titration recommended	ATZ—mild increase in methadone levels, typically no dose change necessary
	DRV/r—some PK effect (increased bup levels), dose adjustments unlikely to be needed	DRV/r—decreased methadone levels, may need increased methadone dose
Integrase inhibitors	EVG/cobi—some PK effect (increased), dose adjustments unlikely to be needed	EVG—no effect w/cobicistat boosting, potential decrease of methadone levels with ritonavir, may need increased dose

Buprenorphine is highly potent and adherent to mu opioid receptors, and at moderate doses reduces cravings of illicit opioids through cross-tolerance and high-level receptor occupancy. This high-level occupancy, however, functions to displace other mu agonists which can lead to precipitated withdrawal.

Buprenorphine is ineffective via an oral route but is absorbed well via sublingual (i.e., transmucosal) and transdermal formulations. Naloxone has poor oral and sublingual bioavailability and as such plays no role in buprenorphine coformulated regimens (e.g., Suboxone) except to dissuade from snorting or injection of the medication. The four current formulations of buprenorphine are daily sublingual (tablet/film) or buccal (film), 6-month implantable (Probuphine), and monthly subcutaneous (Sublocade).

Drug allergies to buprenorphine are relatively rare, and it is advisable to educate patients on the difference between allergy and precipitated withdrawal symptoms. While the overdose potential is certainly lower than other full agonist opioids, it still exists—the risk of respiratory depression is increased when coadministered with benzodiazepines or alcohol [40]. Buprenorphine can be used in situations of liver disease. Combination naloxone products are not recommended in severe hepatic impairment (Childs B or C); even the negligible amount of sublingual naloxone absorbed can become clinically significant given impaired hepatic metabolism and can cause precipitated withdrawal [41]. Buprenorphine monotherapy can be used with dose reduction and caution for signs and symptoms of opioid toxicity. Hepatitis with fulminant hepatic failure has occurred in rare cases, typically in those with underlying liver disease such as underlying HBV and HCV. Unless there is known acute hepatitis, it is reasonable to prescribe and monitor closely without assessing LFTs prior to initiation [42]. Notably, additional concurrent substance use disorders such as stimulant use are not contraindications to starting therapy. Buprenorphine is metabolized via the CYP3A4 hepatic system and as such is affected by other medications that either inhibit or induce this system as depicted in Tables 10.3.

An abstinence period between last full mu opioid dose and initiation is required to avoid precipitated withdrawal. The abstinence period varies from approximately 12–16 h for short-acting opioids, 16–24 h for intermediate-acting opioids, and up to 48 h for high dose methadone dependence. In particular for the inpatient setting, it should be ensured that the patient is not receiving short-acting opioids for pain control. Typically at least mild withdrawal as noted by a COWS score of 5 or greater is sufficient to start treatment; however, some sources recommend a COWS score >12 as the goal prior to the first dose. An advantage to inpatient initiation of buprenorphine is the availability of a broad array of oral and IV medications to minimize withdrawal symptoms in the abstinence period; these should be liberally used. See Chart 10.1 for a depiction of initiating buprenorphine in the inpatient setting.

Patients should be informed not to swallow the sublingual medication and to allow for up to 10 min for it to fully dissolve before swallowing. The majority of patients stabilize on a maintenance dose of 8–16 mg, and the data for doses above 24 mg is currently limited [43].

Two additional buprenorphine formulations of consideration are the subdermal implant, brand name Probuphine®, and extended-release buprenorphine, brand name Sublocade®. The implantable formulation deploys a steady state of 8 mg or less of buprenorphine over the course of 6 months. The extended-release formulation medication is administered monthly (300 and 100 mg doses) and designed for patients who have already been stabilized on at least 7 days of transmucosal buprenorphine at a dose of at least 8 mg [44]. The inpatient setting may be an ideal time for transition to subdermal implantation or the extended-release buprenorphine formulation. Some patients will still require typically small doses of additional transmucosal agonist therapy to achieve resolution of cravings.

There is a subset of patients, particularly those with concurrent chronic pain, for which a period of opioid abstinence prior to induction might be infeasible. Transdermal buprenorphine (trade name Butrans®) appears to produce a more gradual exposure of opioid receptors to drug and is not associated with precipitated withdrawal when short-acting opioids are added. Regimens with initial transdermal buprenorphine with subsequent maintenance transition to sublingual dosing have been successfully reported and should be considered for those with chronic pain [45].

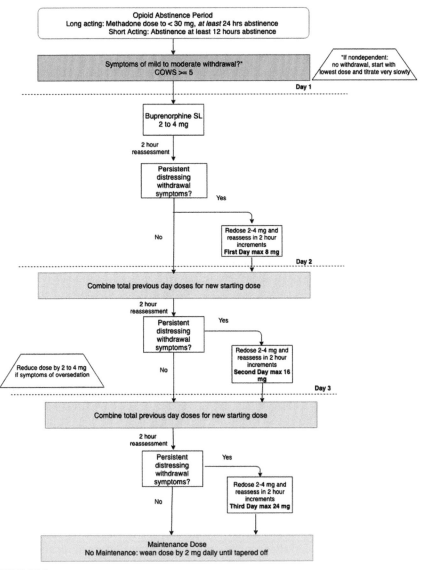

CHART 10.1

Flow diagram for sublingual buprenorphine induction in persons with active opioid addiction.

Extended-release naltrexone (XR-NTX)

Naltrexone was created in the 1960s and first FDA approved for opioid blockade in 1984 as an oral formulation. The extended-release formulation (XR-NTX) was formulated much later and ultimately FDA approved in 2010 for maintenance treatment of OUD. Naltrexone is a competitive mu opioid receptor antagonist with no agonist properties; as such, it requires no waiver or regulatory requirements for inpatient or outpatient prescribing. The oral formulation is noneffective for OUD with no reduction in illicit opioid use relative to placebo, largely secondary to poor adherence [46]. The extended-release formulation is a suspension of naltrexone embedded in biodegradable microsphere polymers meant for IM injection—dosing is 380 mg given every 4 weeks. Naltrexone is metabolized in the kidneys and liver (though not CYP450 mediated) and is excreted through the urine [47].

Despite initial concerns of drug-related hepatitis, clinically significant elevations of transaminases with XR-NTX appear to be relatively uncommon, and advanced cirrhosis (Child-Pugh Class C) is the only true hepatic contraindication [48–51]. Given its clearance via the kidneys, caution is advised when initiating in patients with moderate to severe renal impairment. The intramuscular route of entry is contraindicated in patients with severe coagulopathy. Naltrexone has not been studied thoroughly in pregnancy and hence its use is not recommended.

An appreciable period of opioid abstinence is required prior to XR-NTX initiation to prevent precipitated withdrawal. This is typically 7 days after last opioid use. This can be difficult in the outpatient setting, but can be manageable in the inpatient setting. There are some situations where this can be difficult, however, such as during surgical care requiring opioid analgesia. Patients should be counseled on the unique medication profile of naltrexone. The long abstinence initiation period might also be a barrier for some patients. Shared decision-making must be employed when selecting the ideal MOUD.

As naltrexone is not metabolized by the CYP450 system, there are relatively few drug-drug interactions. Injection site soreness is the most common side effect. More involved reactions such as hematoma, abscess, and cellulitis have been reported. At times it can be difficult to assess whether a patient has been adequately abstinent in order to initiate naltrexone. A naloxone challenge test can be considered prior to naltrexone initiation to avoid prolonged and unnecessary withdrawal. Though it can be useful, a negative naloxone challenge does not fully exclude in all cases that the patient will experience precipitated withdrawal [52].

For patients who arrive to the hospital with withdrawal symptoms and opt for agonist-assisted withdrawal but naltrexone-based maintenance, timing can be a significant barrier. With up to 7 days of agonist-assisted withdrawal needed plus seven additional days of abstinence, this could add up to 14 days of inpatient hospitalization. In these cases, rapid naltrexone induction can be considered. The agonist-based withdrawal portion of therapy is shortened by administering single dose buprenorphine on arrival to sate craving and symptoms, followed by oral naltrexone the next day with nonopioid medications such as clonidine to ease the transition. This regimen increased recruitment onto XR-NTX and the likelihood to receive a second injection at week 5 (50% vs. 26.9%) when compared with full buprenorphine-based agonist withdrawal therapy followed by abstinence and XR-NTX in a clinical trial [53].

Additional MOUD initiation considerations and therapy choice

One of the most impactful interventions for a patient admitted with OUD is initiation of FDA-approved MOUD. The main roles of inpatient initiation of MOUD are (1) agonist-based therapy for withdrawal treatment with taper (if per patient preference or in case of lack of outpatient MOUD), (2) withdrawal treatment with initiation of nonagonist-based therapy (i.e., XR-NTX) prior to discharge, or (3) continued agonist therapy as an outpatient. Of these options, continued outpatient MOUD therapy has the clearest and broadest benefit.

Choosing between MOUD therapies is based on a variety of factors including comorbidities, availability, medication profile, and patient preference. The patient's motivation for long-term treatment is essential to this decision. Other considerations are future site of outpatient treatment, be it OTP versus office-based treatment; side effects or drug interactions; and the overall decision for agonist versus nonagonist-based therapy.

There is a preponderance of evidence for agonist-based therapy (i.e., methadone, buprenorphine) for treatment of OUD in order to achieve retention in treatment, reduction in illicit opioid use, and mortality reduction [37,54]. The benefits extend to numerous ID-related outcomes as well such as improved retention in ART, improved CD4, and viral suppression for HIV [49,50,55–57]. Agonist therapies have been linked to increased retention in care for the HCV cascade and reductions of newly acquired HCV in PWID [58]. There is currently no guideline recommendation to endorse one MOUD over the other. Both buprenorphine and methadone have a similar evidenced mortality benefit when used at adequate doses [59]. Methadone in particular can only be prescribed and dispensed at a federally regulated OTP upon discharge. There are particular benefits for either continuing or initiating MOUD during the inpatient stay as well. Antagonist therapy, i.e., XR-NTX, is relatively newer and is associated with reduction in return to illicit opioid use and in treatment retention [60–62]. XR-NTX has also been found to improve HIV viral suppression in persons living with HIV (PLWH) released from prison or jail with comorbid OUD [49]. Additionally two large RCTs comparing buprenorphine to XR-NTX found similar opioid abstinence and retention outcomes when persons could successfully be inducted on XR-NTX [60,63].

Patients are often motivated to start pharmacotherapy when they are hospitalized and dealing with the direct sequelae of their use disorder. In a survey of 29 hospitalized patients with IDU-related endocarditis who were offered an addiction psychiatry consultation, the majority (62%) accepted and initiated buprenorphine or methadone during the hospital admission [64]. The inpatient setting has been validated as a feasible setting of MOUD as well. In a trial with randomization between inpatient buprenorphine administrations versus tapered withdrawal treatment with referral to an OTP, retention rates on buprenorphine at the 6-month mark were 16.7% versus 3% [65]. The data show that MOUD is not a panacea for OUD that is a chronic relapsing disease, but given the known mortality of continued use, MOUD plays an important role. As it currently stands, less than a quarter of patients with opioid-related hospitalizations are offered MOUD upon discharge [66]. This is suboptimal, and the disparity is particularly vast in patients with high morbidity infectious diseases such as infective endocarditis [67]. It is poorly understood that inpatient providers without a DEA-waiver can prescribe agonist therapies such as buprenorphine and methadone. The Drug Addiction Treatment Act of 2000 was created as an exception to Controlled Substance Act to permit FDA Schedule III, IV, and V medications for OUD treatment to be prescribed as an outpatient outside OTPs. Buprenorphine of note is a schedule III drug. Outpatient prescribing does require a waiver to be obtained for buprenorphine, and, in contrast, XR-NTX requires no waiver for inpatient or outpatient prescribing. Federal law states that inpatient providers are exempt from waiver requirements for maintenance or withdrawal treatment if the patient is admitted for reasons that are not directly related to withdrawal (administering or dispensing of narcotic drugs, 21 CFR § 1306.07). In a significant amount of cases, these patients are hospitalized for infectious complications and the law allows for ID physicians to potentially be said prescribers.

Inpatient infections

More detail on SSTIs (Chapter 8), Hepatitis C (Chapter 5), Hepatitis B (Chapter 6), HIV (Chapter 4), and endocarditis (Chapter 9) is located elsewhere in this text.

Pulmonary infections

Older epidemiologic studies found that PWID had a 10-fold higher rate of pneumonia than the general population, independent of HIV status [68]. A recent nested case control showed that opioid use itself (as measured from prescription refills) was associated with a 67% increase in invasive pneumococcal disease [15]. These factors are likely from a combination of associated conditions, such as concurrent smoking affecting ciliary function and other potential substance use disorders such as crack-cocaine, together with an increased susceptibility for aspiration [69]. Noninfectious insults can also cause underlying lung disease in heroin users such as emphysema, impairments in diffusion, and pulmonary hypertension at least partially from adulterants such as cotton and filler pieces depositing into lung tissue [70]. PWID with community-acquired pneumonia are at higher risk for multiple complications such as parapneumonic effusion, empyema, and bacteremia [71]. Notably, the syndrome of septic pulmonary emboli from endocarditis must be ruled out given significant change in management. IDU in particular is an independent risk factor for both latent TB infection (LTBI) and TB disease in low and high prevalence areas. Concurrent social determinants of health such as homelessness or incarceration contribute to the disparity, together with the increased prevalence of HIV. Notably the tuberculin skin test cutoff for LTBI treatment in PWID is 10 mm given the higher pretest probability in this population. One should consider drug-drug interactions for patients needing active tuberculosis treatment, as rifampin agents will have drug interactions with MOUD such as methadone and buprenorphine.

Bloodstream infections

Bloodstream infections result from either direct injection of bacteria from shared or dirty drug paraphernalia or inoculation of commensal flora. Invasive spread from a local SSTI may or may not also be apparent. It is key to have high suspicion and diagnostic rigor for infective endocarditis which would change medical medically management and potentially involve surgery. One cohort of 180 PWID hospitalized with bacteremia found that 74 patients, or 41%, had IE [72]. The most common organisms involved are *S. aureus*, including community-acquired MRSA, and streptococcus. Injection drug users have higher rates of nasal *S. aureus* carriage than the general population. A cohort of urban poor in San Francisco had a carriage rate of 22.8%, and 12% of all assessed had community-acquired MRSA carriage. Other injection risk behaviors inform the microbiology involved. Use of contaminated water predisposes to environmental gram negatives including *Pseudomonas aeruginosa*, *Sphingomonas*, and *Burkholderia* species. Needle licking can introduce oral streptococcal species and anaerobes including *Eikenella corrodens*. Injection site in the lower half of the body such as groin injection will increase the likelihood of gram-negative involvement. Candidemia is relatively common among PWID, and a similar obligation exists to exclude IE. In addition, patients should be screened for visual symptoms and have an ophthalmologic examination to assess for chorioretinitis. Acidification of the injected drug to increase solubility with fruit or fruit juice is an established risk factor for Candida [11]. Bacteremia with spore-forming bacteria such as *Bacillus cereus* or Clostridial spp. can occur in the presence or absence or an associated SSTI [73]. Less common considerations include other gram-positive skin flora such as *Corynebacteria* spp. and coagulase negative *Staphylococcus*. Cotton fever is a self-limited febrile illness that occurs after heroin injection with reused cotton fiber. Typically fever occurs about 30 min after injecting, with leukocytosis and appearance of sepsis but with negative blood cultures. It results from a process of reheating and extracting used cotton filters, a process known as "shooting the cotton" [74]. The pathophysiology is of presumed colonization of the cotton filter by *Enterobacter agglomerans* with subsequent endotoxin release.

Osteoarticular infections

Hematogenous seeding or local extension from SSTI can result in osteoarticular infections in PWID. Site of disease is informed by vasculature for hematogenous seeding and site of injection for local extension, and in some cases, both. Batson's venous plexus is the network of veins draining visceral organs and extremities along the spine that, by virtue of their location and valveless nature, predispose to infective spread to the vertebrae. PWID are more likely to have cervical vertebral involvement in particular [75]. Septic arthritis is more common on left-sided joints than the right, likely secondary to more right-handed persons injecting. As with other syndromes, ruling out infective endocarditis as a metastatic event is paramount. Providers should have a high index of suspicion for osteoarticular infections in drug use, as fever can be absent in up to one-third of cases, particularly in vertebral osteomyelitis with diskitis [76]. Pyogenic organisms are the most common, with *S. aureus* being the most common followed by pyogenic streptococcal species (A, G). Anaerobes, particularly *Eikenella corrodens*, can cause what has been termed "needle lickers osteomyelitis" in patients with the relevant exposure. Tuberculosis should be considered in undifferentiated vertebral osteomyelitis and diskitis. Rare cases of atypical mycobacteria and molds such as *Aspergillus* have been reported to cause osteomyelitis as well. Candida can cause a particular constellation of costochondral lesions, folliculitis, and chorioretinitis in people injecting brown heroin [77]. Infective spinal disease without source control or adequate treatment can result in contiguous spread and development of conditions such as psoas abscesses or spinal epidural abscesses. In the case of associated neurologic symptoms, urgent neurosurgical intervention is needed. Diagnosis should involve sampling of the affected site and bone biopsy, with 4−6 weeks of culture-directed antimicrobial therapy. Providers should be cognizant of acute pain management in this population as underlying opioid dependence may require higher doses of acute opioids to relieve patient symptoms and carry through with standard of care such as lying flat for MRIs or invasive procedures.

Endophthalmitis

Endophthalmitis is a potentially vision-threatening complication of intravenous drug use. Hematogenous spread, termed endogenous endophthalmitis, results in seeding to the highly vascular choroid plexus which can then progress through the retina and into the vitreous chamber. The aqueous chamber can be involved as well in severe cases. The bacteremia or fungemia associated with this dissemination is typically transient, and the majority of cases have negative blood cultures and are without fever; a vitreal tap with culture has a better yield for organism isolation [78]. As such, providers should have a high degree of clinical suspicion in patients who use IV drugs with acute unilateral visual complaints. Common symptoms are eye pain, decrease in visual acuity, and visualization of floaters. Candida has long been known to be associated with endophthalmitis in patients with intravenous heroin and buprenorphine use. The incidence is likely increasing as the opioid crisis in the United States worsens [79]. Treatment depends on the clinical syndrome and level of involvement of eye structures, as well as issues of ocular penetration. For those with solely chorioretinitis, azole-based therapy can be used based on susceptibility. Systemic amphotericin B with or without flucytosine is employed in azole-resistant isolates. Notably, because of suboptimal penetration into the retina and deeper vitreous, there is insufficient data for echinocandin use in chorioretinitis and it is not recommended in vitritis. If there is sight-threatening macular involvement or an element of vitritis, intravitreal antifungals (typically voriconazole or amphotericin B) are recommended in conjunction with systemic antifungals [80]. In patients with nonresolving or worsening vitritis, there should be consideration in conjunction with ophthalmology of vitrectomy, of which there is growing evidence for improved outcomes with early intervention [81]. Duration of therapy is at least 4—6 weeks or until resolution on ophthalmologic exam. Aspergillus is a less common cause of fungal endophthalmitis but can also be seen in PWID. Endogenous bacterial endophthalmitis is rare but has a distinctly rapid and site-threatening natural history. *S. aureus* is the most common organism, followed by *B. cereus*, the latter of which is likely introduced via contamination of drug product or paraphernalia. Progression from inoculation via transient bacteremia to eye pain with decreased visual acuity to vision loss can occur over the course of hours. Mainstay of therapy is culture-targeted intravitreous antibiotic; the role of adjunctive systemic antibiotics is a matter of debate but could potentially be useful.

Mycotic aneurysm and septic thrombophlebitis

Repeated suboptimal vascular access and endothelial damage from injection can cause sclerosis, fibrosis, thrombus formation, and aneurysms [82]. The incidence of venous thromboembolism (VTE) in PWID is higher than the general population; a cross-sectional analysis of people with OUD in the United Kingdom reported an annual incidence of 3.2% and a lifetime prevalence of 14% [83]. Septic thrombophlebitis should be suspected in clinical situations with bacteremia and underlying VTE. The femoral vein is the most common site of disease. *S. aureus* is the most common etiologic organism, followed by strep, with candida and gram-negative bacilli being identified less commonly. There is no clear prospective data to guide therapy—patients are often treated for 4—6 weeks with at least partial courses of parenteral antibiotics. Guidelines are extrapolated from recommendations for catheter-related thrombophlebitis and based on expert opinion [84]. The use of anticoagulation similarly has limited data and is based on expert opinion, with recommendations for its use in great central veins and not peripheral veins.

The mycotic aneurysm was originally described by Osler as a mushroom-shaped vascular lesion seen as an embolic complication of infective endocarditis. In current day, the terminology can be confusing as it is sometimes used as an all-encompassing term for three distinct categories of infected aneurysms: (1) IE-related (classically mycotic) aneurysms, (2) secondary hematogenous seeding of preexisting sterile aneurysms, and (3) direct trauma and inoculation of vessels leading to an infected pseudoaneurysm. Mycotic aneurysms that are sequelae of IE are discussed elsewhere (Chapter 9). In PWID, the direct arterial damage occurs from erroneous arterial venipuncture or contiguous spread from SSTI into the arterial vascular wall creating a pseudoaneurysm. They are epidemiologically relatively rare, with an estimated prevalence of 0.03% among PWID; however, they are surgical emergencies [85]. The common femoral artery is the most frequently affected site, with the majority of patients having swelling, pain, and erythema [86]. Resection with autologous vein implantation was the most common surgical strategy, though in general there is high associated morbidity. CT angiography has become the diagnostic modality of choice. *S. aureus* is the most common causative organism, and adjunctive medical treatment involves IV antibiotics for 4—6 weeks.

Patient-centered care

Providing acute medical care to persons with OUD is challenging but essential to reducing the associated morbidity and mortality. Persons with OUD infrequently access medical care due to stigma, criminalization of substance use disorder, and social determinants like poverty and rurality that are associated with OUD [2]. Those who do seek care may be reluctant to disclose nonprescription and illicit opioid use for similar reasons leaving OUD undiagnosed despite frequent interactions with the healthcare system.

When hospitalized people who use drugs (PWUD) receive inappropriate treatment for cravings, withdrawal, and pain, patients may experience an exacerbation of substance use disorders leading to illicit drug use in the hospital and mistrust of providers and care teams [87]. Without patient-centered treatment for OUD and related conditions, many fail to engage in their treatment plan, and elopement and discharges against medical conditions are a common challenge to inpatient treatment of OUD [87—89]. A growing body of evidence suggests that a lack of patient-centered care contributes to adverse hospital outcomes such as untreated pain, illicit drug use, discharges AMA, and readmissions [90,91]. Furthermore, stigma, inadequate treatment of addiction (e.g., withdrawal), and attitudes and behaviors of nurses and physicians may create an unsafe environment for many with OUD [87,92]. To provide comprehensive, inpatient care for persons with substance use disorder, it is important to recognize and appropriately manage the following conditions.

Acute pain

Because OUD is associated with trauma, violence, and injection-related infections, persons with OUD are at a high risk for pain [93—95]. Unfortunately, those with OUD are also at risk for inadequate treatment of acute pain. Providing analgesia in patients with OUD, especially in the context of MOUD, is challenging. Yet adequate treatment of acute pain is essential to patient care [96]. Furthermore, pain is a risk factor for substance abuse and may trigger a relapse for those in recovery [97]. In the context of the opioid epidemic, many clinicians have restricted opioid prescriptions for most of their patients, yet it is important for clinicians to appreciate that those with OUD are at greatest risk for untreated and/or inadequately treated acute pain.

Acute pain must be appropriately managed in order to support treatment of addiction and painful comorbidities such as bacterial infections. This will include continuation of MOUD and aggressive pain management incorporating both nonopioid therapies and nonpharmacologic interventions [96]. Some medications to consider include nonsteroidal antiinflammatory agents and acetaminophen. Treatment of comorbid anxiety, depression, and withdrawal symptoms is imperative [96]. When possible, an expert in pain management should be involved in the treatment plan. Anesthesia consultation can be useful for localized pain that can be alleviated by nerve block. Buprenorphine itself provides potent pain relief but its analgesic effects only last for 4—8 h—doses can be split three times a day for improved pain control.

Opioid-related medical conditions
Opioid-induced bowel syndrome

Chronic opioid use is associated with opioid-induced bowel dysfunction (OIBD), a spectrum of conditions including constipation, nausea, vomiting, delayed gastric emptying, and gastroesophageal reflux disease. Of the many manifestations of OIBD, pain is the most debilitating feature [98]. Opioid-induced constipation (OIC) affects up to 57% of patients with chronic, noncancer pain using opioids [99]. OIC is the result of opioids on the peripheral mu opioid receptors leading to impaired bowel motility, reduced stool frequency/straining, incomplete evacuation, and harder stool. A subset of patients may develop narcotic bowel syndrome (NBS), a paradoxical increase in abdominal pain which only partially responds to escalating opioids and is likely related to central hyperalgesia [100]. Diagnosis of OIC and/or NBS both require exclusion of alternate diagnoses, which may be contributing.

First and foremost, treatment of OIBD requires empathy and communication to engage and educate patients on the link between their symptoms and opioids. Many pharmacologic options are available for OIC. Laxatives are often the first-line therapy and may improve stool frequency although there are no RCTs supporting their use. Through chloride channel activation, Lubiprostone improves nonmethadone OIC in noncancer pain patients and is superior to placebo in time to bowel movement [99]. Prucalopride, a selective 5-HT4 agonist, has been shown to effectively treat OIC, but it is FDA-approved in the United States only for chronic idiopathic constipation, rather than OIC [99].

Some opioid receptor antagonists have the potential to act peripherally and centrally, but their central effects have been attenuated to target OIC in the bowel. Oral naloxone acts predominantly on local mu opioid receptors in the gastrointestinal tract and has been shown to reduce laxative use with only mild withdrawal symptoms (e.g., yawning, shivering) [101]. When used with oxycodone per rectum, Naloxone per rectum reduces colonic transit time [101]. Naloxegol, a polyethylene glycol derivative (PEGylated) of naloxone, has limited ability to cross the blood-brain barrier and therefore targets the gastrointestinal tract to reduce transit time [101]. Similarly, oral methylnaltrexone acts on peripheral mu opioid receptors to safely and effectively relieve OIC in those with chronic noncancer pain [102].

Peripherally active mu opioid receptors antagonist (PAMORAs) alleviate OIC symptoms without antagonizing the central opioid receptors, which provide analgesia. Subcutaneous methylnaltrexone is a PAMORA approved for OIC in those receiving palliative care with an inadequate response to laxatives. Many novel therapeutics are under development and are expected to change the treatment paradigm for OIC in coming years.

NBS is unique in its association with central opioid receptor manipulation, and, as a result, treatment with peripherally acting medications will be ineffective. For most, treatment will require reduction in opioid dosage and/or cessation. Although this is controversial, when used for patients with presumed NBS, opioid cessation has been shown to significantly improve abdominal and nonabdominal pain [103]. According to the protocol used by Drossman et al., approximately 90% successfully stopped using opioids and 60% experienced improvement in symptoms. However, half who successfully ceased opioid usage resumed opioid use at 3 months, highlighting the challenges to treating opioid-related conditions [103]. Several antidepressants and glutaminergic agents show promise in the treatment NBS but have not been thoroughly studied.

Hyperalgesia

Paradoxically, exposure to opioids can sensitize pain receptors leading to heightened pain responses, also known as opioid-induced hyperalgesia (OIH). By increasing pain perception in those on chronic opioid therapy, this phenomenon may lead to loss of opioid efficacy and/or the need for opioid dose escalation. OIH is not entirely understood but is thought to result from alterations in the peripheral and central nervous system (CNS) that sensitize pronociceptive pathways [104]. While tolerance can be overcome by increasing doses of opioids, OIH cannot because it is a pain sensitization, which occurs in the CNS and peripheral nervous system [105]. The resulting OIH pain may be the same as or distinct from the original pain. OIH is associated with a higher morphine dose and duration of therapy [106,107].

The diagnosis of OIH is challenging because the differential diagnosis includes opioid tolerance, exacerbation, or progression of an underlying disease process, and acute injury because the treatments are distinct [105]. OIH is often diffuse and poorly defined in character and location, extending to areas beyond the primary pain process. OIH will not respond or will worsen with increasing opioid doses, whereas tolerance and an inadequately treated pain process will usually improve with dose escalation [105].

OIH treatment should be managed by an expert in pain management and may include initial dose escalation to evaluate for tolerance. Subsequently, reducing or eliminating opioids, rotating opioids (buprenorphine, methadone), and adding opioid-sparing treatments may be considered [105]. These adjunctive medications may include NMDA receptor antagonists and COX-2 inhibitors. Regardless of the approach, treatment of OIH is time and resource-intensive and will require frequent clinic visits, patient engagement, communication, and education in the outpatient setting.

Illicit and unprescribed opioid use in the hospital

Due to the nature of addiction, patients may continue to use illicit and unprescribed controlled substances while hospitalized. This may be related to withdrawal symptoms, emotional stress including anxiety, and/or pain. In one study, patients reported using drugs during hospitalization to manage pain and withdrawal symptoms and that these symptoms, when not managed medically, interfered with their treatment [87].

Because illicit drug use is criminalized, many hospitalized patients may inject or swallow illicit drugs quickly and privately behind locked bathroom doors. This scenario is not conducive to harm reduction strategies and puts patients at risk of overdose and infection. IDU in the hospital also increases the risk of leaving AMA [90,91]. To prevent adverse outcomes associated with inpatient illicit drug use, providers must focus on treating the aforementioned symptoms related to abstinence (withdrawal, cravings) while managing comorbid mood disorders, anxiety, and pain [89]. Although there are little data examining the impact of MOUD on inpatient illicit drug use, it is likely that timely initiation will reduce these high-risk behaviors.

Unplanned disposition and discharge against medical advice

Hospitalization has been described as a "reachable" moment for persons with substance use disorders because the inpatient setting allows access to social services, case management, and medical care for addiction and related complications [2]. But persons with OUD and specifically PWID are more likely to disengage from medical care and leave the hospital prematurely [90,91]. As many as 30% of PWID leave the hospital AMA [88]. Not only does this abbreviate inpatient services, such as antibiotics for injection-related infections, but also it precludes linkage to necessary outpatient services for substance use disorder and is associated with hospital readmissions and mortality [90,91]. One Canadian study found a threefold higher risk of death in the year following AMA discharge [90]. There are, however, limited data on the frequency of these events in the United States in the context of the opioid epidemic and their impact on long-term morbidity and mortality. By focusing on the patients themselves and not the health system, we have missed an opportunity to restructure and align our healthcare models with the values and preferences of those with OUD, and specifically those who inject opioids. Even the term "against medical advice" is an adversarial term placing fault on patients rather than the health system that failed to engage them.

Ideally, patients at risk for AMA and other adverse hospital outcomes would be identified early in their hospitalization and receive frequent counseling, treatment of withdrawal and cravings by clinicians with expertise in Addiction Medicine, and MOUD, if indicated. In the absence of such services, the hospital serves as a "risk environment" for PWID [87]. Preliminary data suggest that a patient-oriented treatment approach, including MOUD and adequate pain control, may reduce AMA, illicit drug usage, and other hospital risk behaviors allowing patients to engage in their care [108].

Outpatient parenteral antibiotic treatment

Providing safe, effective outpatient parenteral antibiotic treatment (OPAT) for PWID is national priority due to rising rates of bacterial complications of injection drug usage. Because a peripherally inserted central catheter (PICC) provides durable venous access, PICC lines are critical to an effective OPAT plan. Guideline committees have previously discouraged the use of OPATs for PWID due to concerns of PICC misuse and diversion for illicit drug usage, and recent updates have accommodated case-by-case use [109,110]. But, in the context of the opioid epidemic and rising rates of injection drug usage, more providers and health systems are looking for alternatives to prolonged hospitalizations for completion of antibiotics. In a recent study conducted by the Infectious Diseases Society of America, a majority of the physician respondents (78%) reported caring for patients with infectious complications of injection drug usage [95]. Respondents indicated a need for guidelines related to the safe, frequent provision of parenteral antibiotics for community-based treatment of infections.

Available data on OPAT protocols for PWID are limited in size and rigor [110,111]. Yet, according to a recent review by Suzuki et al., results are reassuring including reported OPAT completions rates of 72%—100% over the course of OPAT treatment, which may range from approximately 18 to 42 days [111]. In some cases, OPAT participants with a history of IDU had a high mortality (up to 10%) and readmission rate (up to 41%). In at least two studies, PWID had favorable outcomes relative to other OPAT participants: one study found lower complication rates and another reported similar rates of readmissions, treatment failure, and death [112,113]. Because there are no RCT studies of OPAT in PWID, it remains unclear if these associations are due to the comorbidities of PWID, the OPAT protocol, or both.

Peripherally inserted central catheter

Several studies evaluating OPAT in PWID have documented adverse events related to PICC access. PICC complications occur in 3%—9% of patients [110,112—114]. Adverse events include deliberate misuse of a PICC line, which occurred in 2% in one population and as many as 11% left their medical respite facility with their intravenous access in place [114]. Many unconventional methods have been used to deter and detect PICC tampering including the use of tape and/or dressing on valves and tubing of PICC catheters and daily PICC inspection. But it is worth noting that at least two studies have demonstrated that the rate of PICC-related infection in PWID is similar to those who do not [112].

Models of care

As it currently stands, the majority of US healthcare systems are not adequately equipped to treat OUD and associated infections in an integrated manner [115]. In some settings, especially in community and rural hospitals, specialty services such as addiction medicine or ID might be minimal. The most common situation is the lack of multidisciplinary integration between existing specialties and a lack of structural support to do so. Recently, there has been increasing recognition for the benefit of team-based specialty management for infections related to addiction, and unique models of care are now emerging.

For decades practitioners have understood the need for addiction medicine as a distinct medical field. After incremental and structural change throughout the latter half of the 20th century, it was relatively recently that the American Board of Addiction Medicine was created, in 2007, with the goal of establishing a board certified subspecialty. In 2015, the American Board of Medical Specialties (ABMS) approved this and the certification process is now open to any of the primary ABMS specialties. A strong relationship between ID and addiction medicine providers is essential for multidisciplinary treatment of patients with OUD and infections. Inpatient addiction consultation has been shown to reduce composite scores of SUD severity and number of days abstinence 1 month after discharge [117]. Addiction treatment teams themselves can contain members of different backgrounds and skills. One model, termed the Improving Addiction Care Team (IMPACT) model, formed a team of addiction medicine providers together with social workers and peers with lived experience in recovery [118]. The protocol included screening and diagnosis of SUD (including OUD), pharmacotherapy by physicians, CBT and mindfulness therapy by social workers, and group-based training with other healthcare workers such as nurses. The training groups included the creation of a Patient Safety Care Plan for patients with risk for illicit inpatient substance use or AMA risk, and another for PICC Community Safety Assessment to make a team-based informed decision on ability for discharge with an indwelling line. ID providers themselves can train and apply for buprenorphine waivers for inpatient and outpatient prescribing of MOUD. A survey of ID physician beliefs regarding OUD showed that a slim but significant majority believed that their field should be involved in MOUD prescribing [95].

For those patients who do not require admission, the emergency room is an important point of contact for patients with OUD and infections. Similar to inpatient trends, OUD-related ER visits nearly doubled from 2005 to 2014 [119]. Many patients who present with infections related to IV substance use have conditions such as minor abscesses and mild cellulitis that are routinely managed in the ER then discharged. A recent RCT evaluated the feasibility of buprenorphine initiation in the ER setting and found that retention in addiction care at 1 month was significantly higher for those either initiated on site or given medications for home induction [120]. Follow-up data showed that the three groups appeared similar at the 2 month mark, though with methodological issues—all patients in the ED-initiated buprenorphine arm had to switch from primary care-based treatment to an OTP, perhaps affecting retention of care [121]. Further study is required to assess generalizability and optimal implementation strategies.

Transitioning to the outpatient setting

As previously noted, there is no consensus on the appropriate timing of discharge for hospitalized persons given the aforementioned concerns about OPAT, and specifically PICC line use, for this population. In fact, when surveyed, as many as 41% ID physicians "frequently" manage the entire course of intravenous antibiotics for

PWID in the inpatient setting, which may be 6 weeks or longer [95]. And, following discharge, there are no best practices for patient care related to the delivery of antibiotics or the frequency of monitoring via a home health nurse or provider. For this reason, several health systems have implemented protocols aimed at reducing prolonged admissions for PWID at low risk for complication.

One academic hospital developed a risk assessment tool to determine if and when to transition patient care to OPAT. This study tool stratified PWID according to their risk of continued IDU [122]. Patients deemed "low risk" were discharged to OPAT, while all others received the entire course of parenteral antibiotics in the hospital. By transitioning low-risk patients (27%) to OPAT, this hospital was able to reduce length of stay and direct hospital costs and create capacity for additional acutely ill PWID without increasing 30 day readmissions [122]. Englander et al. developed the medically enhanced residential treatment (MERT), a hybrid residential treatment model integrating treatment for substance use disorder and parenteral antibiotics for patients requiring two or more weeks of antibiotics [123]. Although this model was viewed as overall positive by key informants, few eligible patients enrolled in the MERT model of care. Among the barriers to MERT were concerns about restrictive policies in residential treatment and stigma from staff [123]. This is consistent with findings by Fanucchi and colleagues that hospitalized persons with substance use disorders are unlikely to want residential treatment although many are interested in pharmacotherapy for addiction [124].

Prevention

Although some areas of patient care related to OUD are uncertain, many opportunities for infection prevention are evidence based. In 2015, approximately 9% of new HIV infections were attributed, at least in part, to IDU [125]. Fortunately, HIV preexposure prophylaxis (PrEP) is an effective HIV prevention option for adult PWID at substantial risk for HIV. HIV PrEP should be offered to persons who are injecting drugs regardless of recent treatment for addiction.

Because infectious diseases disproportionately affect PWUD, vaccination is an additional public health strategy to improve health outcomes for this population. Hepatitis B and C are acquired through sharing of needles and drug preparation equipment, but only Hepatitis B can be prevented through vaccination. Hepatitis B vaccination is, therefore, recommended for all current or recent injection drug users. Recently, there has been an increase in Hepatitis A outbreaks among PWID through both fecal-oral and percutaneous transmission. Because Hepatitis A vaccination is highly effective in preventing and abating such outbreaks, all PWID and all persons with homelessness should receive Hepatitis A vaccination [126]. Due to poor hygiene and close living quarters, other vaccine preventable infections such as influenza can be devastating for PWID. For this reason, all PWID should receive evidence-based vaccination according to the Advisory Committee on Immunization Practices guidelines [126].

Future directions

Research on optimizing care for OUD and its downstream infections is burgeoning. This is in part derived from need in the context of the ever-worsening opioid crisis in the United States. Novel treatment strategies could one day preclude the need, in certain infections, for intravenous therapy and its attendant challenges of requiring a PICC line for administration. Two major trials have been recently been published regarding use of oral antibiotics traditionally treated for long courses with intravenous antibiotics: one for a variety of bone and joint infections and another for partial oral treatment of infective endocarditis [127,128]. Both were pragmatic studies that demonstrated noninferiority of their primary endpoints using a variety of oral antibiotic regimens with and without rifampin use. However there were very few participants with IDU in either trial affecting their generalizability, and this will be crucial to be studied further. Long-acting injectable lipoglycopeptides have demonstrated noninferiority for SSTI treatment, at times with single dose treatment [129]. Preliminary clinical data suggest its potential effectiveness in treatment of osteoarticular infections with randomized trial data needed [130].

There is a profound gap between the patient need and the availability of prescribing providers for MOUD—in 2012, it was estimated that this gap was approximately one million people, and it has potentially widened in the context of the worsening opioid crisis [131]. Providers of all specialties that have contact with people with OUD should apply for buprenorphine waivers for outpatient prescribing. Midlevel providers will play an important role in addressing the current need as well. All physicians with a primary ABMS specialty are permitted to sit for Addiction Medicine subspecialty boarding, for those who would like to pursue expertise in the field. Current study of the benefit of MOUD prescribing on inpatient ID consult services is promising and could serve to provide unified continuity for subacute infectious treatment and addiction treatment for patients with conditions such as infective endocarditis. Ultimately, full multidisciplinary integration of health systems in the inpatient setting for the treatment of addiction and infection will be the best modality for improving care.

References

[1] Ronan MV, Herzig SJ. Hospitalizations related to opioid abuse/dependence and associated serious infections increased sharply, 2002-12. Health Aff 2016;35(5):832−7.
[2] Velez CM, Nicolaidis C, Korthuis PT, Englander H. "It's been an experience, a life learning experience": aqualitative study of hospitalized patients with substance use disorders. J Gen Intern Med 2017;32(3):296−303.
[3] Gordon RJ, Lowy FD. Bacterial infections in drug users. N Engl J Med 2005;353(18): 1945−54.
[4] Louria DB, Hensle T, Rose J. The major medical complications of heroin addiction. Ann Intern Med 1967;67(1):1−22.

214 **CHAPTER 10** Inpatient opioid use disorder treatment

[5] Binswanger IA, Kral AH, Bluthenthal RN, Rybold DJ, Edlin BR. High prevalence of abscesses and cellulitis among community-recruited injection drug users in San Francisco. Clin Infect Dis 2000;30(3):579–81.

[6] Vlahov D, Sullivan M, Astemborski J, Nelson KE. Bacterial infections and skin cleaning prior to injection among intravenous drug users. Public Health Rep 1992;107(5):595–8.

[7] Dunleavy K, Hope V, Roy K, Taylor A. People who inject drugs' experiences of skin and soft tissue infections and harm reduction: a qualitative study. Int J Drug Policy 2019;65:65–72.

[8] Abbara A, Brooks T, Taylor GP, et al. Lessons for control of heroin-associated anthrax in Europe from 2009-2010 outbreak case studies, London, UK. Emerg Infect Dis 2014;20(7):1115–22.

[9] Passaro DJ, Werner SB, McGee J, Mac Kenzie WR, Vugia DJ. Wound botulism associated with black tar heroin among injecting drug users. JAMA 1998;279(11):859–63.

[10] Deutscher M, Perlman DC. Why some injection drug users lick their needles: a preliminary survey. Int J Drug Policy 2008;19(4):342–5.

[11] Scheidegger C, Pietrzak J, Frei R. Methadone diluted with contaminated orange juice or raspberry syrup as a potential source of disseminated candidiasis in drug abusers. Eur J Clin Microbiol Infect Dis 1993;12(3):229–31.

[12] Murphy EL, Bryzman SM, Glynn SA, et al. Risk factors for hepatitis C virus infection in United States blood donors. NHLBI Retrovirus Epidemiology Donor Study (REDS). Hepatology 2000;31(3):756–62.

[13] Mathers BM, Degenhardt L, Phillips B, et al. Global epidemiology of injecting drug use and HIV among people who inject drugs: a systematic review. Lancet 2008;372(9651):1733–45.

[14] Craven DE, Rixinger AI, Goularte TA, McCabe WR. Methicillin-resistant *Staphylococcus aureus* bacteremia linked to intravenous drug abusers using a "shooting gallery". Am J Med 1986;80(5):770–6.

[15] Wiese AD, Griffin MR, Schaffner W, et al. Opioid analgesic use and risk for invasive pneumococcal diseases: anested case-control study. Ann Intern Med 2018;168(6):396–404.

[16] Holt SR, Ramos J, Harma MA, et al. Prevalence of unhealthy substance use on teaching and hospitalist medical services: implications for education. Am J Addict 2012;21(2):111–9.

[17] NIDA. Resource guide: screening for drug use in general medical settings. March 1, 2012. Retrieved from: https://www.drugabuse.gov/publications/resource-guide-screening-drug-use-in-general-medical-settings.

[18] Fleming MF, Balousek SL, Klessig CL, Mundt MP, Brown DD. Substance use disorders in a primary care sample receiving daily opioid therapy. J Pain 2007;8(7):573–82.

[19] Jenkins AJ, Poirier 3rd JG, Juhascik MP. Cross-reactivity of naloxone with oxycodone immunoassays: implications for individuals taking Suboxone. Clin Chem 2009;55(7):1434–6.

[20] First MBWJ, Karg RS, Spitzer RL. Structured clinical interview for DSM-5 disorders, clinician version (SCID-5-CV), Arlington, VA. 2016.

[21] Sheehan DV, Lecrubier Y, Sheehan KH, et al. The Mini-International Neuropsychiatric Interview (M.I.N.I.): the development and validation of a structured diagnostic psychiatric interview for DSM-IV and ICD-10. J Clin Psychiatry 1998;59(Suppl. 20):22–33. quiz 34–57.

[22] Wickersham JA, Azar MM, Cannon CM, Altice FL, Springer SA. Validation of a brief measure of opioid dependence: the rapid opioid dependence screen (RODS). J Correct Health Care 2015;21(1):12−26.

[23] Erratum to validation of a brief measure of opioid dependence: The rapid opioid dependence screen (RODS). J Correct Health Care 2020 [e pub ahead of print].

[24] Binka M, Paintsil E, Patel A, Lindenbach BD, Heimer R. Disinfection of syringes contaminated with hepatitis C virus by rinsing with household products. Open Forum Infect Dis 2015;2(1). ofv017.

[25] Kroenke K, Spitzer RL, Williams JB. The patient health questionnaire-2: validity of a two-item depression screener. Med Care 2003;41(11):1284−92.

[26] Mattick RP, Hall W. Are detoxification programmes effective? Lancet 1996; 347(8994):97−100.

[27] Kaye AD, Vadivelu N, Urman RD. Substance abuse: inpatient and outpatient management for every clinician. Springer; 2014.

[28] Wesson DR, Ling W. The clinical opiate withdrawal scale (COWS). J Psychoactive Drugs 2003;35(2):253−9.

[29] Gowing L, Ali R, White JM, Mbewe D. Buprenorphine for managing opioid withdrawal. Cochrane Database Syst Rev 2017;2:Cd002025.

[30] Meader N. A comparison of methadone, buprenorphine and alpha(2) adrenergic agonists for opioid detoxification: a mixed treatment comparison meta-analysis. Drug Alcohol Depend 2010;108(1−2):110−4.

[31] Jaffe J. Drug addiction and drug abuse. In: Goodman LS, Gilman A, editors. The pharmacological basis of therapeutics a textbook of pharmacology, toxicology, and therapeutics for physicians and medical students. 8th ed. New York: New York Macmillan; 1990.

[32] Medication-assisted treatment with methadone: assessing the evidence. Psychiatr Serv 2014;65(2):146−57.

[33] Dole VP, Robinson JW, Orraca J, Towns E, Searcy P, Caine E. Methadone treatment of randomly selected criminal addicts. N Engl J Med 1969;280(25):1372−5.

[34] Mattick RP, Breen C, Kimber J, Davoli M. Methadone maintenance therapy versus no opioid replacement therapy for opioid dependence. Cochrane Database Syst Rev 2009; (3):Cd002209.

[35] Larochelle MR, Bernson D, Land T, et al. Medication for opioid use disorder after nonfatal opioid overdose and association with mortality: acohort study. Ann Intern Med 2018;169(3):137−45.

[36] Sordo L, Barrio G, Bravo MJ, et al. Mortality risk during and after opioid substitution treatment: systematic review and meta-analysis of cohort studies. BMJ 2017;357: j1550.

[37] Mattick RP, Breen C, Kimber J, Davoli M. Buprenorphine maintenance versus placebo or methadone maintenance for opioid dependence. Cochrane Database Syst Rev 2014; (2):Cd002207.

[38] Lewis JW. Ring C-bridged derivatives of thebaine and oripavine. Adv Biochem Psychopharmacol 1973;8:123−36. 0.

[39] Cowan A, Lewis JW, Macfarlane IR. Agonist and antagonist properties of buprenorphine, a new antinociceptive agent. Br J Pharmacol 1977;60(4):537−45.

[40] Lofwall MR, Walsh SL. A review of buprenorphine diversion and misuse: the current evidence base and experiences from around the world. J Addict Med 2014;8(5): 315−26.

[41] Nasser AF, Heidbreder C, Liu Y, Fudala PJ. Pharmacokinetics of sublingual buprenorphine and naloxone in subjects with mild to severe hepatic impairment (child-pugh classes A, B, and C), in hepatitis C virus-seropositive subjects, and in healthy volunteers. Clin Pharmacokinet 2015;54(8):837−49.

[42] Saxon AJ, Ling W, Hillhouse M, et al. Buprenorphine/naloxone and methadone effects on laboratory indices of liver health: a randomized trial. Drug Alcohol Depend 2013; 128(1−2):71−6.

[43] Hser YI, Saxon AJ, Huang D, et al. Treatment retention among patients randomized to buprenorphine/naloxone compared to methadone in a multi-site trial. Addiction 2014; 109(1):79−87.

[44] Haight BR, Learned SM, Laffont CM, et al. Efficacy and safety of a monthly buprenorphine depot injection for opioid use disorder: a multicentre, randomised, double-blind, placebo-controlled, phase 3 trial. Lancet 2019;393(10173):778−90.

[45] Kornfeld H, Reetz H. Transdermal buprenorphine, opioid rotation to sublingual buprenorphine, and the avoidance of precipitated withdrawal: a review of the literature and demonstration in three chronic pain patients treated with butrans. Am J Ther 2015; 22(3):199−205.

[46] Minozzi S, Amato L, Vecchi S, Davoli M, Kirchmayer U, Verster A. Oral naltrexone maintenance treatment for opioid dependence. Cochrane Database Syst Rev 2011;(4): Cd001333.

[47] Vivitrol (naltrexone for extended release injectable suspension) 380 mg/vial. Press release; 2015.

[48] Mitchell MC, Memisoglu A, Silverman BL. Hepatic safety of injectable extended-release naltrexone in patients with chronic hepatitis C and HIV infection. J Stud Alcohol Drugs 2012;73(6):991−7.

[49] Springer SA, Di Paola A, Azar MM, et al. Extended-release naltrexone improves viral suppression among incarcerated persons living with HIV with opioid use disorders transitioning to the community: results of a double-blind, placebo-controlled randomized trial. J Acquir Immune Defic Syndr 2018;78(1):43−53.

[50] Springer SA, Di Paola A, Barbour R, Azar MM, Altice FL. Extended-release naltrexone improves viral suppression among incarcerated persons living with HIV and alcohol use disorders transitioning to the community: results from a double-blind, placebo-controlled trial. J Acquir Immune Defic Syndr 2018;79(1):92−100.

[51] Vagenas P, Di Paola A, Herme M, et al. An evaluation of hepatic enzyme elevations among HIV-infected released prisoners enrolled in two randomized placebo-controlled trials of extended release naltrexone. J Subst Abuse Treat 2014;47(1): 35−40.

[52] Services SAaMH, Administration, editor. Clinical use of extended-release injectable naltrexone in the treatment of opioid use disorder: a brief guide; 2015. Rockville, MD.

[53] Sullivan M, Bisaga A, Pavlicova M, et al. Long-acting injectable naltrexone induction: arandomized trial of outpatient opioid detoxification with naltrexone versus buprenorphine. Am J Psychiatry 2017;174(5):459−67.

[54] Gibson A, Degenhardt L, Mattick RP, Ali R, White J, O'Brien S. Exposure to opioid maintenance treatment reduces long-term mortality. Addiction 2008;103(3):462−8.

[55] Low AJ, Mburu G, Welton NJ, et al. Impact of opioid substitution therapy on antiretroviral therapy outcomes: asystematic review and meta-analysis. Clin Infect Dis 2016; 63(8):1094−104.

[56] Altice FL, Bruce RD, Lucas GM, et al. HIV treatment outcomes among HIV-infected, opioid-dependent patients receiving buprenorphine/naloxone treatment within HIV clinical care settings: results from a multisite study. J Acquir Immune Defic Syndr 2011;56(Suppl. 1):S22−32.

[57] Springer SA, Qiu J, Saber-Tehrani AS, Altice FL. Retention on buprenorphine is associated with high levels of maximal viral suppression among HIV-infected opioid dependent released prisoners. PLoS One 2012;7(5):e38335.

[58] Hagan H, Pouget ER, Des Jarlais DC. A systematic review and meta-analysis of interventions to prevent hepatitis C virus infection in people who inject drugs. J Infect Dis 2011;204(1):74−83.

[59] Potter JS, Marino EN, Hillhouse MP, et al. Buprenorphine/naloxone and methadone maintenance treatment outcomes for opioid analgesic, heroin, and combined users: findings from starting treatment with agonist replacement therapies (START). J Stud Alcohol Drugs 2013;74(4):605−13.

[60] Tanum L, Solli KK, Latif ZE, et al. Effectiveness of injectable extended-release naltrexone vs daily buprenorphine-naloxone for opioid dependence: arandomized clinical noninferiority trial. JAMA Psychiatry 2017;74(12):1197−205.

[61] Krupitsky E, Nunes EV, Ling W, Illeperuma A, Gastfriend DR, Silverman BL. Injectable extended-release naltrexone for opioid dependence: a double-blind, placebo-controlled, multicentre randomised trial. Lancet 2011;377(9776):1506−13.

[62] Lee JD, Friedmann PD, Kinlock TW, et al. Extended-release naltrexone to prevent opioid relapse in criminal justice offenders. N Engl J Med 2016;374(13):1232−42.

[63] Lee JD, Nunes Jr EV, Novo P, et al. Comparative effectiveness of extended-release naltrexone versus buprenorphine-naloxone for opioid relapse prevention (X:BOT): a multicentre, open-label, randomised controlled trial. Lancet 2018;391(10118):309−18.

[64] Suzuki J. Medication-assisted treatment for hospitalized patients with intravenous-drug-use related infective endocarditis. Am J Addict 2016;25(3):191−4.

[65] Liebschutz JM, Crooks D, Herman D, et al. Buprenorphine treatment for hospitalized, opioid-dependent patients: a randomized clinical trial. JAMA Intern Med 2014;174(8):1369−76.

[66] Naeger S, Mutter R, Ali MM, Mark T, Hughey L. Post-discharge treatment engagement among patients with an opioid-use disorder. J Subst Abuse Treat 2016;69:64−71.

[67] Rosenthal ES, Karchmer AW, Theisen-Toupal J, Castillo RA, Rowley CF. Suboptimal addiction interventions for patients hospitalized with injection drug use-associated infective endocarditis. Am J Med 2016;129(5):481−5.

[68] Hind CR. Pulmonary complications of intravenous drug misuse. 2. Infective and HIV related complications. Thorax 1990;45(12):957−61.

[69] Boschini A, Smacchia C, Di Fine M, et al. Community-acquired pneumonia in a cohort of former injection drug users with and without human immunodeficiency virus infection: incidence, etiologies, and clinical aspects. Clin Infect Dis 1996;23(1):107−13.

[70] Wolff AJ, O'Donnell AE. Pulmonary effects of illicit drug use. Clin Chest Med 2004;25(1):203−16.

[71] Chalmers JD, Singanayagam A, Murray MP, Scally C, Fawzi A, Hill AT. Risk factors for complicated parapneumonic effusion and empyema on presentation to hospital with community-acquired pneumonia. Thorax 2009;64(7):592−7.

[72] Levine DP, Crane LR, Zervos MJ. Bacteremia in narcotic addicts at the Detroit Medical Center. II. Infectious endocarditis: a prospective comparative study. Rev Infect Dis 1986;8(3):374–96.

[73] Dancer SJ, McNair D, Finn P, Kolsto AB. Bacillus cereus cellulitis from contaminated heroin. J Med Microbiol 2002;51(3):278–81.

[74] Wurcel AG, Merchant EA, Clark RP, Stone DR. Emerging and underrecognized complications of illicit drug use. Clin Infect Dis 2015;61(12):1840–9.

[75] Wang Z, Lenehan B, Itshayek E, et al. Primary pyogenic infection of the spine in intravenous drug users: a prospective observational study. Spine 2012;37(8):685–92.

[76] Chandrasekar PH, Narula AP. Bone and joint infections in intravenous drug abusers. Rev Infect Dis 1986;8(6):904–11.

[77] Bisbe J, Miro JM, Latorre X, et al. Disseminated candidiasis in addicts who use brown heroin: report of 83 cases and review. Clin Infect Dis 1992;15(6):910–23.

[78] Aguilar GL, Blumenkrantz MS, Egbert PR, McCulley JP. Candida endophthalmitis after intravenous drug abuse. Arch Ophthalmol 1979;97(1):96–100.

[79] Tirpack AR, Duker JS, Baumal CR. An outbreak of endogenous fungal endophthalmitis among intravenous drug abusers in New England. Endogenousfungal endophthalmitis among intravenous drug abusers. Endogenous fungal endophthalmitis among intravenous drug abusers. JAMA Ophthalmol 2017;135(6):534–40.

[80] Riddell J, Comer GM, Kauffman CA. Treatment of endogenous fungal endophthalmitis: focus on new antifungal agents. Clin Infect Dis 2011;52(5):648–53.

[81] Kim DY, Moon HI, Joe SG, Kim JG, Yoon YH, Lee JY. Recent clinical manifestation and prognosis of fungal endophthalmitis: a 7-year experience at a tertiary referral center in Korea. J Korean Med Sci 2015;30(7):960–4.

[82] Yeager RA, Hobson 2nd RW, Padberg FT, Lynch TG, Chakravarty M. Vascular complications related to drug abuse. J Trauma 1987;27(3):305–8.

[83] Cornford CS, Mason JM, Inns F. Deep vein thromboses in users of opioid drugs: incidence, prevalence, and risk factors. Br J Gen Pract 2011;61(593):e781–786.

[84] Mermel LA, Farr BM, Sherertz RJ, et al. Guidelines for the management of intravascular catheter-related infections. Clin Infect Dis 2001;32(9):1249–72.

[85] Tsao JW, Marder SR, Goldstone J, Bloom AI. Presentation, diagnosis, and management of arterial mycotic pseudoaneurysms in injection drug users. Ann Vasc Surg 2002;16(5):652–62.

[86] Jayaraman S, Richardson D, Conrad M, Eichler C, Schecter W. Mycotic pseudoaneurysms due to injection drug use: a ten-year experience. Ann Vasc Surg 2012;26(6):819–24.

[87] McNeil R, Small W, Wood E, Kerr T. Hospitals as a 'risk environment': an ethno-epidemiological study of voluntary and involuntary discharge from hospital against medical advice among people who inject drugs. Soc Sci Med 2014;105:59–66.

[88] Ti L, Ti L. Leaving the hospital against medical advice among people who use illicit drugs: asystematic review. Am J Public Health 2015;105(12):e53–59.

[89] Summers PJ, Hellman JL, MacLean MR, Rees VW, Wilkes MS. Negative experiences of pain and withdrawal create barriers to abscess care for people who inject heroin. A mixed methods analysis. Drug Alcohol Depend 2018;190:200–8.

[90] Choi M, Kim H, Qian H, Palepu A. Readmission rates of patients discharged against medical advice: a matched cohort study. PLoS One 2011;6(9):e24459.

[91]   Yong TY, Fok JS, Hakendorf P, Ben-Tovim D, Thompson CH, Li JY. Characteristics and outcomes of discharges against medical advice among hospitalised patients. Intern Med J 2013;43(7):798−802.

[92]   Edlin BR, Carden MR, Gourevitch MN, et al. Overcoming barriers to prevention, care, and treatment of hepatitis C in illicit drug users. Clin Infect Dis 2005;40(Suppl. 5): S276−85.

[93]   Gomes T, Redelmeier DA, Juurlink DN, Dhalla IA, Camacho X, Mamdani MM. Opioid dose and risk of road trauma in Canada: apopulation-based study opioid dose and risk of road trauma. JAMA Intern Med 2013;173(3):196−201.

[94]   Seal KH, Shi Y, Cohen G, et al. Association of mental health disorders with prescription opioids and high-risk opioid use in US Veterans of Iraq and Afghanistan. JAMA 2012;307(9):940−7.

[95]   Rapoport AB, Fischer LS, Santibanez S, Beekmann SE, Polgreen PM, Rowley CF. Infectious diseases physicians' perspectives regarding injection drug use and related infections, United States, 2017. Open Forum Infect Dis 2018;5(7). ofy132.

[96]   Alford DP, Compton P, Samet JH. Acute pain management for patients receiving maintenance methadone or buprenorphine therapy acute pain management for patients receiving OAT. Ann Intern Med 2006;144(2):127−34.

[97]   Voon P, Greer AM, Amlani A, Newman C, Burmeister C, Buxton JA. Pain as a risk factor for substance use: a qualitative study of people who use drugs in British Columbia, Canada. Harm Reduct J 2018;15(1):35.

[98]   Tuteja AK, Biskupiak J, Stoddard GJ, Lipman AG. Opioid-induced bowel disorders and narcotic bowel syndrome in patients with chronic non-cancer pain. Neurogastroenterol Motil 2010;22(4):424−e496.

[99]   Camilleri M, Drossman DA, Becker G, Webster LR, Davies AN, Mawe GM. Emerging treatments in neurogastroenterology: a multidisciplinary working group consensus statement on opioid-induced constipation. Neurogastroenterol Motil 2014;26(10): 1386−95.

[100]   Szigethy E, Schwartz M, Drossman D. Narcotic bowel syndrome and opioid-induced constipation. Curr Gastroenterol Rep 2014;16(10):410.

[101]   Nelson AD, Camilleri M. Opioid-induced constipation: advances and clinical guidance. Ther Adv Chronic Dis 2016;7(2):121−34.

[102]   Rauck R, Slatkin NE, Stambler N, Harper JR, Israel RJ. Randomized, double-blind trial of oral methylnaltrexone for the treatment of opioid-induced constipation in patients with chronic noncancer pain. Pain Pract 2017;17(6):820−8.

[103]   Drossman DA, Morris CB, Edwards H, et al. Diagnosis, characterization, and 3-month outcome after detoxification of 39 patients with narcotic bowel syndrome. Am J Gastroenterol 2012;107(9):1426−40.

[104]   Yang DZ, Sin B, Beckhusen J, Xia D, Khaimova R, Iliev I. Opioid-induced hyperalgesia in the nonsurgical setting: asystematic review. Am J Ther 2019;26(3):e397−405.

[105]   Lee M, Silverman S, Hansen H, Patel V, Manchikanti L. A comprehensive review of opioid-induced hyperalgesia. Pain Physician 2011;14(2):145−61.

[106]   Hooten WM, Mantilla CB, Sandroni P, Townsend CO. Associations between heat pain perception and opioid dose among patients with chronic pain undergoing opioid tapering. Pain Med 2010;11(11):1587−98.

[107]   Cohen SP, Christo PJ, Wang S, et al. The effect of opioid dose and treatment duration on the perception of a painful standardized clinical stimulus. Reg Anesth Pain Med 2008;33(3):199−206.

[108] Chan AC, Palepu A, Guh DP, et al. HIV-positive injection drug users who leave the hospital against medical advice: the mitigating role of methadone and social support. J Acquir Immune Defic Syndr 2004;35(1):56−9.

[109] Tice AD, Rehm SJ, Dalovisio JR, et al. Practice guidelines for outpatient parenteral antimicrobial therapy. IDSA guidelines. Clin Infect Dis 2004;38(12):1651−72.

[110] Norris AH, Shrestha NK, Allison GM, et al. 2018. Infectious diseases society of America clinical practice guideline for the management of outpatient parenteral antimicrobial therapy. Clinical Infectious Diseases: An Official Publication of the Infectious Diseases Society of America 2019;68(1):e1−35.

[111] Ho J, Archuleta S, Sulaiman Z, Fisher D. Safe and successful treatment of intravenous drug users with a peripherally inserted central catheter in an outpatient parenteral antibiotic treatment service. J Antimicrob Chemother 2010;65(12):2641−4.

[112] Suzuki J, Johnson J, Montgomery M, Hayden M, Price C. Outpatient parenteral antimicrobial therapy among people who inject drugs: areview of the literature. Open Forum Infect Dis 2018;5(9):ofy194.

[113] Vazirian M, Jerry JM, Shrestha NK, Gordon SM. Outcomes of outpatient parenteral antimicrobial therapy in patients with injection drug use. Psychosomatics 2018; 59(5):490−5.

[114] Dobson PM, Loewenthal MR, Schneider K, Lai K. Comparing injecting drug users with others receiving outpatient parenteral antibiotic therapy. Open Forum Infect Dis 2017;4(4):ofx183.

[115] Beieler AM, Dellit TH, Chan JD, et al. Successful implementation of outpatient parenteral antimicrobial therapy at a medical respite facility for homeless patients. J Hosp Med 2016;11(8):531−5.

[116] Fanucchi L, Lofwall MR. Putting parity into practice - integrating opioid-use disorder treatment into the hospital setting. N Engl J Med 2016;375(9):811−3.

[117] Wakeman SE, Metlay JP, Chang Y, Herman GE, Rigotti NA. Inpatient addiction consultation for hospitalized patients increases post-discharge abstinence and reduces addiction severity. J Gen Intern Med 2017;32(8):909−16.

[118] Englander H, Mahoney S, Brandt K, et al. Tools to support hospital-based addiction care: core components, values, and activities of the improving addiction care team. J Addict Med 2019;13(2):85−9.

[119] Weiss AJ, Elixhauser A, Barrett ML, Steiner CA, Bailey MK, O'Malley L. Opioid-related inpatient stays and emergency department visits by state, 2009-2014: statistical brief #219. Healthcare Cost and Utilization Project (HCUP) statistical briefs. Rockville, MD: Agency for Healthcare Research and Quality (US); 2006.

[120] D'Onofrio G, O'Connor PG, Pantalon MV, et al. Emergency department-initiated buprenorphine/naloxone treatment for opioid dependence: a randomized clinical trial. JAMA 2015;313(16):1636−44.

[121] D'Onofrio G, Chawarski MC, O'Connor PG, et al. Emergency department-initiated buprenorphine for opioid dependence with continuation in primary care: outcomes during and after intervention. J Gen Intern Med 2017;32(6):660−6.

[122] Eaton EF, Lee RA. 9-Item risk assessment for hospitalized persons who inject drugs. In: Paper presented at: ID week; October 5, 2018, San Francisco, CA; 2018.

[123] Wilson T, Collins D, Phoutrides E, et al. Lessons learned from the implementation of a medically enhanced residential treatment (MERT) model integrating intravenous antibiotics and residential addiction treatment AU - Englander, Honora. Subst Abuse 2018;39(2):225−32.

[124] Fanucchi LC, Lofwall MR, Nuzzo PA, Walsh SL. In-hospital illicit drug use, substance use disorders, and acceptance of residential treatment in a prospective pilot needs assessment of hospitalized adults with severe infections from injecting drugs. J Subst Abuse Treat 2018;92:64—9.

[125] Centers for Disease Control and Prevention. Preexposure prophylaxis for the prevention of HIV infection in the United States-2017 Update. 2017. https://www.cdc.gov/hiv/pdf/risk/prep/cdc-hiv-prep-guidelines-2017.pdf.

[126] Kim DK, Hunter P. Advisory committee on immunization practices recommended immunization schedule for adults aged 19 years or older - United States, 2019. MMWR Morb Mortal Wkly Rep 2019;68(5):115—8.

[127] Li HK, Rombach I, Zambellas R, et al. Oral versus intravenous antibiotics for bone and joint infection. N Engl J Med 2019;380(5):425—36.

[128] Iversen K, Ihlemann N, Gill SU, et al. Partial oral versus intravenous antibiotic treatment of endocarditis. N Engl J Med 2019;380(5):415—24.

[129] Boucher HW, Wilcox M, Talbot GH, Puttagunta S, Das AF, Dunne MW. Once-weekly dalbavancin versus daily conventional therapy for skin infection. N Engl J Med 2014;370(23):2169—79.

[130] Almangour TA, Perry GK, Terriff CM, Alhifany AA, Kaye KS. Dalbavancin for the management of gram-positive osteomyelitis: effectiveness and potential utility. Diagn Microbiol Infect Dis 2019;93(3):213—8.

[131] Jones CM, Campopiano M, Baldwin G, McCance-Katz E. National and state treatment need and capacity for opioid agonist medication-assisted treatment. Am J Public Health 2015;105(8):e55—63.

HIV pre-exposure prophylaxis for people who inject drugs

11

Roman Shrestha, PhD [1], Benjamin McCoy-Redd, BS [2], Jaimie P. Meyer, MD, MS, FACP [3]

[1]*Associate Research Scientist, Yale School of Medicine, Section of Infectious Disease, AIDS Program, New Haven, CT, United States;* [2]*Predoctoral Fellow, Yale School of Medicine, Section of Infectious Disease, AIDS Program, New Haven, CT, United States;* [3]*Associate Professor of Medicine, Yale School of Medicine, Section of Infectious Disease, AIDS Program, New Haven, CT, United States*

HIV prevention in people who inject drugs

According to the CDC, 9% of incident HIV cases in the United States are directly attributable to injection drug use [1]. Among people who inject drugs (PWID), the risk for HIV and other blood-borne pathogens is primarily related to injecting behaviors, including sharing needles, syringes, and other injecting and drug preparation equipment. Data from the National HIV Behavioral Surveillance System reflects that approximately 34% of PWID share syringes and 58% share other injection paraphernalia [2]. In the setting of ongoing and untreated substance use, PWID also experience heightened risk for HIV related to sex because of (1) sex in the context of intoxication with associated disinhibition, (2) high-risk sex networks, and/or (3) sexual bartering (i.e., exchanging sex for drugs, money, goods, or other services). Women who inject drugs experience "double risk" for HIV because of overlapping sex and drug use networks [3]. HIV risk among PWID is compounded by concomitant infections with hepatitis B and C that are more prevalent in PWID (a topic addressed more completely in Chapter 6 and 2).

PWID not only experience inordinate risk for HIV but also face numerous barriers to engaging with effective prevention and treatment services for HIV. Despite the high HIV risk, PWID often have less access to prevention innovations because of stigmatization, underinsurance, poor socioeconomic status, homelessness, criminal justice involvement, and other challenges navigating systems of care and support. In the setting of the current opioid epidemic, in which there are increasing numbers of PWID, particularly in nonurban settings, access to harm reduction and HIV prevention resources is often limited. As multiple recent hepatitis C virus and HIV outbreaks in the United States illustrate, PWID experience a high burden of HIV risk, particularly when resources are not available or accessible to reduce harms associated with injecting [4,5].

The Opioid Epidemic and Infectious Diseases. https://doi.org/10.1016/B978-0-323-68328-9.00011-4

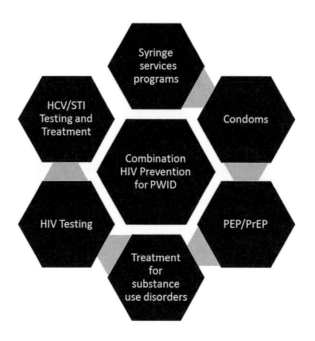

FIGURE 11.1

Combination HIV prevention for people who inject drugs (PWID).

HCV, *hepatitis C virus*; PEP, *postexposure prophylaxis*; PrEP, *preexposure prophylaxis*; STI, *sexually transmitted infection*.

PWID are a key target population for HIV prevention in the global and US national strategies [6,7]. A number of evidence-based HIV prevention approaches are available for PWID, including treatment for opioid use disorder with medication-assisted therapy (MAT), syringe services programs (SSPs) for harm reduction, frequent testing for HIV and sexually transmitted infections, and barrier protection (i.e., condoms) to reduce HIV risk associated with sex. Outcomes are optimized when these approaches are used together, known as "combination prevention" (Fig. 11.1).

In light of the US opioid crisis, multiple methods of HIV prevention are needed for PWID. HIV preexposure prophylaxis (PrEP) is an important addition to the HIV prevention armamentarium for PWID. PrEP is grounded in the principle that giving antiretrovirals to people without HIV (but who are at high risk for acquiring HIV) is effective in preventing infection in spite of exposure, as is the case of prevention of maternal to child transmission of HIV. At present, the only FDA-approved medications for PrEP are tenofovir diphosphate (tenofovir disoproxil fumarate [TDF]) or tenofovir alafenamide fumarate (TAF) given in combination with emtricitabine (FTC). Co-formulated TDF/FTC (manufactured by Gilead and sold as Truvada) or TAF/FTC (manufactured by Gilead and sold as Descovy) are available as single-tablet daily medication. Other dosing strategies (e.g., "on-demand" pericoital dosing) and formulations (e.g., TDF 1% vaginal gel) are investigational in select populations or not yet widely used in the United States. In a meta-analysis, TDF alone was shown to be equally effective as TDF/FTC. Other medications for

PrEP, including injectable cabotegravir and a dapivirine vaginal ring are currently in development and testing. In multiple large randomized clinical trials of men who have sex with men (MSM) and serodiscordant heterosexual couples, PrEP was significantly effective at preventing HIV when it was taken consistently [8]. In this chapter, we review the evidence and indications for PrEP in PWID and discuss strategies to address key challenges to scale-up.

Evidence of efficacy of preexposure prophylaxis in people who inject drugs

To date, there has been a single large randomized clinical trial for PrEP in PWID, known as the Bangkok Tenofovir Study (BTS) [9]. The BTS was a phase III randomized, double-blind, placebo-controlled trial conducted in Thailand. The study population was recruited from 17 Bangkok Metropolitan Administration drug treatment clinics and composed of 1924 men and 489 women who had injected drugs in the past year, excluding pregnant women, people with chronic hepatitis B, and people already diagnosed with HIV-1. About 22% of participants were receiving methadone at study baseline. Participants were randomly assigned to receive either TDF 300 mg ($n = 1204$) or placebo ($n = 1209$) and participants could choose to receive study drug as a 28-day supply for self-administration or as daily directly observed therapy. Adherence was determined by direct observation (for those opting for this delivery strategy) or by dried blood spot testing for TDF levels. Risk behavior was repeatedly analyzed to look for evidence of possible risk compensation. Over 9665 person-years of follow-up, there were 17 new HIV infections in the TDF group and 33 new infections in the placebo group. Thus compared with placebo, TDF was associated with a relative risk reduction of HIV infection of 48.9% (95% confidence interval [CI], 9.6% −72.2%; $P = .01$). Participants with high adherence, categorized as taking the medication at least 71% of prescribed days (approximately 5 days per week), had a 73.5% (95% CI, 16.6−94.0; $P = .03$) risk reduction. In other subgroup analyses, TDF had higher efficacy in women than men (78.6%; 95% CI, 16.8%−96.7%; $P = .03$) and in participants aged 40 years or more compared with those aged <40 years (88.9%; 95% CI, 41.1%−99.4%; $P = .01$). Reported sexual and injecting risk behavior decreased significantly overall during the trial. Side effects were minimal, with the treatment arm experiencing nausea and/or vomiting at a higher rate than the control.

The BTS established the efficacy of TDF in a high-risk population of PWID but has not been replicated to date. There are a number of possible reasons why additional large-scale randomized controlled trials of PrEP have not been conducted among PWID. One is the concern about the ethics of providing PrEP to PWID in settings where other harm reduction tools, such as MAT for opioid use disorder or SSPs, are not available, including in global regions where HIV incidence is rising and is primarily attributable to injection drug use [10]. The other concern about a randomized controlled trial of PrEP among PWID is that study recruitment would require people to disclose their ongoing injecting behaviors, which is not only highly stigmatized but also criminalized, including in the United States [11].

Preexposure prophylaxis effectiveness in the "real world"

In the absence of other clinical trials for PrEP efficacy, data from demonstration projects support PrEP effectiveness in the "real world" and can provide guidance on PrEP implementation. For example, in the open-label extension of the BTS, known as BTS-OLE, 798 (60%) of originally enrolled participants chose to continue on PrEP. Those who were aged 30 years or more, injected heroin, or had been incarcerated in prison during the trial more often chose to continue on PrEP, suggesting PrEP might be acceptable to PWID at the highest risk of HIV who would benefit from it the most [12]. In preliminary outcome data, the HIV incidence rate in participants not on PrEP was 0.7 per 100 person-years compared with 0.5 per 100 person-years in the group on PrEP, yielding a significant protective benefit of PrEP in this high-risk population of PWID [8]. Although not exhaustive, an updated list of large-scale PrEP demonstration and implementation projects in United States and international settings is maintained online [13] and on ClinicalTrials.gov for federally funded studies.

Additional evidence for PrEP in PWID is derived from mathematic modeling studies. Published data support the cost-effectiveness of PrEP for PWID, particularly when it is combined with expanded HIV screening strategies and early treatment for those found to have HIV, averting up to 26,700 new infections and reducing HIV prevalence by up to 14% among PWID in the United States [14]. Another modeling study found that the most cost-effective approach to HIV prevention for PWID combines PrEP for HIV prevention with naloxone for overdose prevention and linkage to addiction treatment [15]. Sustainable cost-effectiveness of PrEP for PWID depends on pharmaceutical drug pricing and enrollment strategies [16].

Indications for preexposure prophylaxis in people who inject drugs

Since the FDA approval of TDF/FTC in 2012 and based on data from the BTS, the CDC has developed clinical guidance on PrEP indications for PWID [17]. Because PWID may experience HIV risk not only from injecting but also related to high-risk sex, PWID may meet PrEP eligibility criteria in one or more categories of risk (Box 11.1).

To assess people for PrEP, healthcare providers need to be prepared to accurately and comprehensively evaluate risk. This requires a nonjudgmental approach to screening in order to foster trust, encourage disclosure, and prevent further stigmatization of PWID. Although the US Preventive Services Task Force does not currently recommend universal screening for PrEP eligibility or HIV, they do recommend that providers prescribe PrEP if they deem patients to be at sufficiently high risk for HIV [18]. To assess HIV risk, providers should inquire whether patients

1. have injected any drugs not prescribed to them in the past 6 months;
2. have shared needles, syringes, or other injecting or preparation equipment (e.g., cotton, "cookers," syringes for splitting or sharing drugs, etc.);
3. are on MAT (e.g., methadone, buprenorphine, or naltrexone);

Box 11.1 Preexposure prophylaxis indications for PWID.

An adult person or adolescent weighing $\geq$35 kg without established HIV infection meets at least one of the following sets of HIV risk criteria:

Risk from injection drug use	Risk from MSM	Risk from heterosexual sex
Injecting of any nonprescribed substance in the past 6 months	A man with any male sex partners in the past 6 months	A man or woman with any opposite sex partners in the past 6 months
AND shared injecting or preparation equipment	Not monogamous with an HIV− man	Not monogamous with an HIV− partner
At high risk for relapse, including among people on MAT	AND any anal sex (receptive or insertive) without condoms in the past 6 months	AND infrequently uses condoms with a partner of unknown HIV status, who is HIV+, or who is at high risk of HIV (PWID, MSM)
	Recent bacterial STI	Recent bacterial STI
	Any transactional sex	Any transactional sex

---

4. are at short-term risk of relapse to injection or noninjection drug use;
5. engage in condomless sex with high-risk partners (MSM, PWID, transactional sex, unknown HIV status, HIV+, and not virally suppressed);
6. have had a recent bacterial sexually transmitted infection (e.g., chlamydia, gonorrhea, or syphilis).

If in the course of a behavioral risk assessment, patients disclose ongoing injection drug use, they should be offered access to harm reduction services (including SSPs and overdose prevention with naloxone) and treatment for opioid use disorder (including MAT if indicated). Per clinical care guidelines, in addition to conducting a behavioral risk assessment, providers should perform baseline HIV testing and phlebotomy for renal function testing. Because PWID often experience housing instability, underinsurance, partner violence, unemployment, and criminal justice involvement, wraparound services need to be in place to address these issues in addition to PrEP provision. PrEP is a program not a drug.

The HIV prevention or preexposure prophylaxis care continuum

The current prevailing model of PrEP delivery parallels the HIV care continuum [19,20]. In this model, patients must first be identified as being "at risk" for HIV infection. This requires an accurate self-perception of personal risk and disclosure of risk behaviors to a possible PrEP provider or referral source. Patients must also test negative for HIV. If patients and their providers are aware of PrEP, they can be linked to PrEP care. Although PrEP services have traditionally been the domain

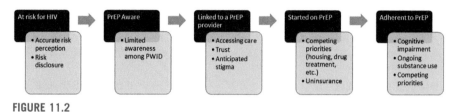

FIGURE 11.2

Preexposure prophylaxis (PrEP) care continuum and key challenges for people who inject drugs (PWID).

of infectious disease clinicians (who have experience prescribing TDF/FTC as part of a treatment regimen for HIV), PrEP scale-up demands expansion of the pool of potential providers, including to primary care [21]. A limited pool of potential PrEP providers is especially limiting for PWID [22]. Because the PrEP care continuum is predicated on patients actively engaging with healthcare providers and traditional systems of care, PWID face several challenges at every step (Fig. 11.2).

Major challenges to PrEP care engagement for PWID in the prevailing model of care include competing priorities, such as co-occurring medical conditions (hepatitis C, sexually transmitted infections), psychiatric conditions, substance use disorders, and social conditions that each require treatment and intervention. If left undiagnosed and/or undermanaged, these conditions can interfere with the ability of PWID to access and be retained on PrEP. Although ideally care for these co-occurring conditions is integrated into PrEP delivery programs, at a minimum, PrEP providers can screen, briefly intervene, and refer to treatment (SBIRT). Perhaps in part because of these barriers to engagement in the PrEP care continuum for PWID, there is a translational efficacy-effectiveness gap in PrEP among PWID. Although an estimated 72,000–115,000 PWID would qualify for PrEP based on current clinical criteria [23], <1% have actually received it since TDF/FTC was approved as PrEP in 2012 [24].

Challenges facing scale-up and widespread adoption
Individual barriers

At the individual level, an increasing number of studies have identified low knowledge of the existence of PrEP among PWID [25–31]. For example, a study conducted by Stein et al. [27] among PWID in Massachusetts found that only 7% of PWID were aware of PrEP, yet once informed, 47% were willing to take it to reduce their chances of HIV acquisition. Likewise, research among opioid-dependent patients enrolled in a methadone maintenance program in Connecticut found awareness of PrEP to be low (18%) but nearly two-thirds (62.7%) were willing to initiate PrEP once the PrEP-related information deficit was corrected [32]. A study has further explored individual-level cognitive barriers, including beliefs about PrEP, concerns about taking PrEP and its side effects, and PrEP perception [33]. Many PWID consider themselves at low risk for HIV infection despite reporting risk behaviors (e.g., sharing of injection equipment, condomless sex, multiple sex partners) [31,32]. Additional concerns about PrEP side effects and health consequences, including how PrEP might reduce the efficacy of other medications (e.g., antidepressants, methadone), has negatively impacted overall PrEP scale-up for PWID. Moreover, the significance of competing priorities in the lives of PWID, including the demands imposed by physical dependence and withdrawal symptoms, has been a challenge for PrEP utilization [33].

Interpersonal-level barriers

Interpersonal-level barriers to PrEP utilization and widespread scale-up include negative experiences from interacting with healthcare providers and HIV-related stigma within social networks. PWID also report anticipated stigma within their social, sexual, and drug networks, worrying that others would think they were HIV infected if they were seen using PrEP [31,33]. For example, Shrestha and Copenhaver [33] reported a similar concern among PWID that taking PrEP could lead others to believe they are HIV infected and are on antiretroviral therapy (ART), which would negatively influence their uptake and adherence to PrEP. Other studies have noted the potential social risks (e.g., discrimination, exclusion, loss of trust) of taking PrEP as evidenced by experienced and enacted stigma, which contribute to low PrEP uptake among PWID. For example, Biello et al. [31] found negative experiences from interacting with healthcare providers as an important interpersonal-level barrier to PrEP utilization. Interactions of PWID with healthcare providers were overwhelmingly negative, and several described experiencing stigma or mistreatment that made them reluctant to disclose their drug use or other risk behaviors when seeking PrEP care. Furthermore, distrust from healthcare providers because of unsubstantiated concerns about poor adherence has led to poor PrEP access for PWID [31,33].

Clinic- and structural-level barriers

Studies have indicated various important barriers to PrEP scale-up at the clinic and broader structural levels. Lack of access to and utilization of healthcare contribute to the slow PrEP uptake observed among PWID. Previous studies have established a widespread lack of prescribing providers and poor infrastructure for PrEP delivery, and clinicians have been shown to lack knowledge on PrEP or willingness to provide PrEP to PWID [33–35]. Even when PWID are able to access healthcare, their providers may not have the training or resources to facilitate PrEP education or uptake. For example, in a qualitative study, some providers shared their reluctance to prescribe PrEP to PWID because of concerns of risk compensation and suboptimal adherence [33]. Barriers at the broader structural level include issues related to lack of money or identification to fill prescriptions, homelessness, criminal justice system involvement, and transportation difficulties [31]. Although the majority of PWID have some form of health insurance, many private insurance plans have high monthly deductibles that can impact the ability of individuals to afford treatment. Furthermore, the drug assistance program (offered by Gilead, who produced Truvada) for people without insurance does not cover additional costs, including copays and cost of laboratory tests and doctor visits. Therefore in states without Medicaid expansion, these costs associated with PrEP are an important disincentive to uptake. Even if they successfully start PrEP, PWID may encounter challenges related to action planning and medication logistics, such as having to take a pill every day and seeing a provider regularly, as well as counseling support to stay on PrEP.

Strategies for preexposure prophylaxis scale-up among people who inject drugs

Low-threshold access to preexposure prophylaxis

The traditional PrEP care model is a multistep process that requires long waits and multiple clinic visits before PrEP is prescribed. This complex process, along with other patient-specific factors, discourages individuals from returning to the clinic to receive PrEP prescription. One potential strategy to address this barrier would be to encourage earlier linkage to care by utilizing rapid linkage to care protocols. In the case of HIV treatment, several randomized clinical trials [36–38] have demonstrated the feasibility, acceptability, safety, and efficacy of same-day ART initiation (also known as "test and treat") [39]. Same-day access to PrEP is a safe and feasible strategy to initiate PrEP care among patients attending sexual health clinics [40,41]. Rapid PrEP initiation may be particularly important for PWID, as they remain a hard-to-reach group and are more likely to lose to follow-up before treatment initiation.

mHealth-based approaches

mHealth, which refers to the use of mobile and wireless technologies to improve health, holds significant promise for PrEP scale-up, given the widespread mobile phone ownership among PWID. Several studies have evaluated the use of mHealth interventions (e.g., text messaging, phone calls, web-based, or app-based) to optimize PrEP uptake among key populations. It is a promising and cost-effective strategy to increase access to PrEP services. It also helps promote prevention and treatment behaviors by allowing for private communication and incorporating flexible reminders and content [42–46]. Particularly for PWID, leveraging mHealth-based approaches will help reduce individuals' discomfort and distrust of disclosing their sexual behavior to providers, will address the low cultural competency of providers for working with individuals of diverse sexual identities, and will circumvent challenging compliance with rigid clinic scheduling.

Using nonphysician prescribers for preexposure prophylaxis scale-up

One crucial consideration to facilitate wide-scale PrEP implementation in PWID is the way in which healthcare professionals can be organized to optimize its delivery and management. Nonphysician prescribers, such as nurse practitioners (NPs), are the most common points of contact for individuals accessing healthcare and are specially trained to improve the health of vulnerable populations through a unique, holistic approach that emphasizes community health, health education and prevention, and social well-being [47]. Research suggests that NPs can manage 80%−90% of care provided by primary care physicians [48] and that they are more likely than physicians to practice with vulnerable populations, including in rural areas where the opioid epidemic is currently focused [49]. Importantly, a growing body of evidence has demonstrated that NPs tend to provide more information to patients and that NPs are equivalent to physicians in terms of patient satisfaction, safety, and health outcomes [50−56]. Given this evidence, leveraging NP assets in the delivery of PrEP care is a step toward closing the gap in the adoption of PrEP as a prevention practice among key populations, including PWID [57].

Integrating preexposure prophylaxis with other treatment services

Clinics and programs that only or mainly offer PrEP and fail to provide other services to make long-term engagement desirable are more likely to experience high drop-off. Prior research suggests that providing PrEP in the context of a wide range of programs and clinical services is crucial to adherence and retention [58]. For example, substance abuse treatment settings (e.g., methadone clinic) are fundamental to the adoption and delivery of PrEP and the implementation of PrEP research, through their roles in counseling and coordination of care with clients' primary care providers [34,59,60]. Likewise, SSPs have great potential to engage their at-risk clients in PrEP through counseling and referrals and may also effectively promote adherence to PrEP through counseling and monitoring.

Patient education and empowerment

As noted earlier, lack of awareness of PrEP can be a critical barrier to PrEP uptake. Limited PrEP knowledge among PWID may reflect that PrEP marketing and, to a lesser extent, public health information campaigns have intensively targeted other populations, especially MSM, leading to misperceptions about the appropriateness of PrEP for PWID [28]. Information that is accessible and acceptable to this population is needed to increase the knowledge of PrEP availability and specific aspects of daily adherence, side effects, and the protections that are and are not provided. This information should be available in key areas that high-risk PWID frequent (e.g., SSPs and other community-based organizations, homeless shelters, and public transportation). In particular, SSPs and community-based organizations that work with this population and employ trusted staff and mobile outreach teams could help with the diffusion of PrEP information into PWID networks [28]. Furthermore, strategies that align HIV risk perceptions and actual behaviors may also be needed to increase PrEP interest in some high-risk individuals [32,61]. For example, counseling involving motivational interviewing could help individuals recognize and discuss their HIV risks, increase their motivation for HIV risk reduction, and improve their knowledge of PrEP. Interventions involving motivational interviewing could also help develop self-efficacy for PrEP use and other behavioral skills [29,62].

Advances in preexposure prophylaxis modalities and the future of preexposure prophylaxis for people who inject drugs

Although a daily oral TDF/FTC or TAF/FTC pill are the only approved and recommended forms of PrEP, there is growing interest in developing new methods for administering antiretroviral drugs as prevention. The past several years have witnessed a surge of research in the development of additional modalities of PrEP [63], which could be important to fill the HIV prevention gap in PWID. In order to minimize potential adherence barriers associated with taking daily oral PrEP, particularly forgetting due to competing priorities, cognitive impairment (associated with chronic substance use), and anticipated stigma related to inadvertent disclosure, new PrEP modalities are being developed and tested. Specifically, with the safety and acceptability of cabotegravir for long-acting injectable PrEP now established [64], large-scale clinical trials are underway to test its efficacy when given once every 2 months. Additional advances, such as parenteral formulations of injectable antiretrovirals and infusible antibodies, may increase the simplicity of PrEP delivery, potentially requiring injections or infusions every few months [65–68]. These approaches, as well as the advent of generic TDF/FTC, could decrease some of the costs associated with PrEP compared with daily regimens and make it more scalable for PWID.

References

[1] Centers for Disease Control and Prevention. HIV among people who inject drugs. 2019. Available from: https://www.cdc.gov/hiv/group/hiv-idu.html.

[2] Centers for Disease Control and Prevention. HIV surveillance report: HIV infection, risk, prevention, and testing behaviors among persons who inject drugs—national HIV behavioral surveillance: injection drug use, 20 U.S. Cities, 2015. May 2018. Report No.: Contract No.: HIV Surveillance Special Report 18.

[3] El-Bassel N, Terlikbaeva A, Pinkham S. HIV and women who use drugs: double neglect, double risk. Lancet 2010;376(9738):312–4.

[4] Gonsalves GS, Crawford FW. Dynamics of the HIV outbreak and response in Scott County, IN, USA, 2011-15: a modelling study. Lancet HIV 2018;5(10):e569–77.

[5] Des Jarlais DC, Kerr T, Carrieri P, Feelemyer J, Arasteh K. HIV infection among persons who inject drugs: ending old epidemics and addressing new outbreaks. AIDS 2016; 30(6):815−26.

[6] National HIV/AIDS strategy for the United States. 2010.

[7] World Health Organization. Consolidated guidelines on HIV prevention, diagnosis, treatment, and care for key populations. Geneva, Switzerland, ISBN 978 92 4 150743 1.

[8] Fonner VA, Dalglish SL, Kennedy CE, Baggaley R, O'Reilly KR, Koechlin FM, et al. Effectiveness and safety of oral HIV preexposure prophylaxis for all populations. AIDS 2016;30(12):1973−83.

[9] Choopanya K, Martin M, Suntharasamai P, Sangkum U, Mock PA, Leethochawalit M, et al. Antiretroviral prophylaxis for HIV infection in injecting drug users in Bangkok, Thailand (the Bangkok Tenofovir Study): a randomised, double-blind, placebo-controlled phase 3 trial. Lancet 2013;381(9883):2083−90.

[10] Guise A, Albers ER, Strathdee SA. 'PrEP is not ready for our community, and our community is not ready for PrEP': pre-exposure prophylaxis for HIV for people who inject drugs and limits to the HIV prevention response. Addiction 2017;112(4):572−8.

[11] DeBeck K, Cheng T, Montaner JS, Beyrer C, Elliott R, Sherman S, et al. HIV and the criminalisation of drug use among people who inject drugs: a systematic review. Lancet HIV 2017;4(8):e357−74.

[12] Martin M, Vanichseni S, Suntharasamai P, Sangkum U, Mock PA, Chaipung B, et al. Factors associated with the uptake of and adherence to HIV pre-exposure prophylaxis in people who have injected drugs: an observational, open-label extension of the Bangkok Tenofovir Study. Lancet HIV 2017;4(2):e59−66.

[13] AVAC. Ongoing and planned PrEP open label, demonstration and implementation projects. 2019. Available from: https://www.avac.org/sites/default/files/resource-files/ongoing_planned_oralPrEP_studies_jan2019.pdf.

[14] Bernard CL, Brandeau ML, Humphreys K, Bendavid E, Holodniy M, Weyant C, et al. Cost-effectiveness of HIV preexposure prophylaxis for people who inject drugs in the United States. Ann Intern Med 2016;165(1):10−9.

[15] Uyei J, Fiellin DA, Buchelli M, Rodriguez-Santana R, Braithwaite RS. Effects of naloxone distribution alone or in combination with addiction treatment with or without pre-exposure prophylaxis for HIV prevention in people who inject drugs: a cost-effectiveness modelling study. Lancet Public Health 2017;2(3):e133−40.

[16] Fu R, Owens DK, Brandeau ML. Cost-effectiveness of alternative strategies for provision of HIV preexposure prophylaxis for people who inject drugs. AIDS 2018;32(5):663−72.

[17] Centers for Disease Control and Prevention. Preexposure prophylaxis for the prevention of HIV infection in the United States- 2017 update, a Clinical practice guideline. 2018. Available from: https://www.cdc.gov/hiv/pdf/risk/prep/cdc-hiv-prep-guidelines-2017.pdf.

[18] U.S. Preventive Services Task Force. Draft recommendation statement: prevention of human immunodeficiency virus infection: pre-exposure prophylaxis. 2018. Available from: https://www.uspreventiveservicestaskforce.org/Page/Document/RecommendationStatementDraft/prevention-of-human-immunodeficiency-virus-hiv-infection-pre-exposure-prophylaxis#consider.

[19] Gardner EM, McLees MP, Steiner JF, Del Rio C, Burman WJ. The spectrum of engagement in HIV care and its relevance to test-and-treat strategies for prevention of HIV infection. Clin Infect Dis 2011;52(6):793−800.

[20] Nunn AS, Brinkley-Rubinstein L, Oldenburg CE, Mayer KH, Mimiaga M, Patel R, et al. Defining the HIV pre-exposure prophylaxis care continuum. AIDS 2017;31(5):731–4.

[21] Petroll AE, Walsh JL, Owczarzak JL, McAuliffe TL, Bogart LM, Kelly JA. PrEP awareness, familiarity, comfort, and prescribing experience among US primary care providers and HIV specialists. AIDS Behav 2017;21(5):1256–67.

[22] Edelman EJ, Moore BA, Calabrese SK, Berkenblit G, Cunningham C, Patel V, et al. Primary care physicians' willingness to prescribe HIV pre-exposure prophylaxis for people who inject drugs. AIDS Behav 2017;21(4):1025–33.

[23] Smith DK, Van Handel M, Wolitski RJ, Stryker JE, Hall HI, Prejean J, et al. Vital signs: estimated percentages and numbers of adults with indications for preexposure prophylaxis to prevent HIV acquisition-United States, 2015. MMWR Morb Mortal Wkly Rep 2015;64(46):1291–5.

[24] Garner W, Wilson BM, Beste L, Maier M, Ohl ME, Van Epps P. Gaps in preexposure prophylaxis uptake for HIV prevention in the veterans health administration. Am J Public Health 2018;108(S4):S305–10.

[25] Kuo I, Olsen H, Patrick R, Phillips II G, Magnus M, Opoku J, et al. Willingness to use HIV pre-exposure prophylaxis among community-recruited, older people who inject drugs in Washington, DC. Drug Alcohol Depend 2016;164:8–13.

[26] Escudero DJ, Kerr T, Wood E, Nguyen P, Lurie MN, Sued O, et al. Acceptability of HIV pre-exposure prophylaxis (PrEP) among people who inject drugs (PWID) in a Canadian setting. AIDS Behav 2015;19(5):752–7.

[27] Stein M, Thurmond P, Bailey G. Willingness to use HIV pre-exposure prophylaxis among opiate users. AIDS Behav 2014;18(9):1694–700.

[28] Walters SM, Reilly KH, Neaigus A, Braunstein S. Awareness of pre-exposure prophylaxis (PrEP) among women who inject drugs in NYC: the importance of networks and syringe exchange programs for HIV prevention. Harm Reduct J 2017;14(1):40.

[29] Shrestha R, Altice FL, Huedo-Medina TB, Karki P, Copenhaver M. Willingness to use pre-exposure prophylaxis (PrEP): an empirical test of the information-motivation-behavioral skills (IMB) model among high-risk drug users in treatment. AIDS Behav 2017;21(5):1299–308.

[30] Bazzi AR, Biancarelli DL, Childs E, Drainoni ML, Edeza A, Salhaney P, et al. Limited knowledge and mixed interest in pre-exposure prophylaxis for HIV prevention among people who inject drugs. AIDS Patient Care STDS 2018;32(12):529–37.

[31] Biello KB, Bazzi AR, Mimiaga MJ, Biancarelli DL, Edeza A, Salhaney P, et al. Perspectives on HIV pre-exposure prophylaxis (PrEP) utilization and related intervention needs among people who inject drugs. Harm Reduct J 2018;15(1):55.

[32] Shrestha R, Karki P, Altice FL, Huedo-Medina TB, Meyer JP, Madden L, et al. Correlates of willingness to initiate pre-exposure prophylaxis and anticipation of practicing safer drug- and sex-related behaviors among high-risk drug users on methadone treatment. Drug Alcohol Depend 2017;173:107–16.

[33] Shrestha R, Copenhaver M. Exploring the use of pre-exposure prophylaxis (PrEP) for HIV prevention among high-risk people who use drugs in treatment. Front Public Health 2018;6(195).

[34] Shrestha R, Altice F, Karki P, Copenhaver M. Developing an integrated, brief biobehavioral HIV prevention intervention for high-risk drug users in treatment: the process and outcome of formative research. Front Immunol 2017;8(561).

[35] Spector AY, Remien RH, Tross S. PrEP in substance abuse treatment: a qualitative study of treatment provider perspectives. Subst Abuse Treat Prev Policy 2015;10:1.

[36] Fatti G, Grimwood A, Meehan S, Nachega JB, Nelson J, LaSorda K, et al. Better virological outcomes when initiating early ART in the HPTN 071 (PoPART) trial. In: Conference on retroviruses and opportunistic infections (CROI). Seattle, Washington: Conference on Retroviruses and Opportunistic Infections (CROI); 2019.

[37] Labhardt ND, Ringera I, Lejone TI, Klimkait T, Muhairwe J, Amstutz A, et al. Effect of offering same-day ART vs usual health facility referral during home-based HIV testing on linkage to care and viral suppression among adults with HIV in Lesotho: the cascade randomized clinical trial. JAMA 2018;319(11):1103−12.

[38] Rosen S, Maskew M, Fox MP, Nyoni C, Mongwenyana C, Malete G, et al. Initiating antiretroviral therapy for HIV at a patient's first clinic visit: the RapIT randomized controlled trial. PLoS Med 2016;13(5):e1002015.

[39] Stevens B, Max B. Test and treat: a new model for better patient outcomes Washington, D.C. The American Academy of HIV Medicine (AAHIVM); 2018. Available from: https://aahivm.org/wp-content/uploads/2018/04/HIVspecialist_April2018_Output.pdf.

[40] Kamis K, Scott K, Gardner E, Wendel K, Marx G, Scott M, et al. Same-day HIV pre-exposure prophylaxis (PrEP) initiation during drop-in STD clinic appointments is a safe, feasible, and effective method to engage patients at risk for HIV in PrEP care. Open Forum Infect Dis 2018;5(Suppl. 1):S20−.

[41] Mikati T, Jamison K, Daskalakis DC. Immediate PrEP initiation at New York sexual health clinics. In: Conference on retroviruses and opportunistic infections (CROI) 2019; Seattle, Washington; 2019.

[42] WHO. mHealth: new horizons for health through mobile technologies: second global survey on eHealth. 2011. Geneva, Switzerland.

[43] Free C, Phillips G, Watson L, Galli L, Felix L, Edwards P, et al. The effectiveness of mobile-health technologies to improve health care service delivery processes: a systematic review and meta-analysis. PLoS Med 2013;10(1):e1001363.

[44] Lester RT, Ritvo P, Mills EJ, Kariri A, Karanja S, Chung MH, et al. Effects of a mobile phone short message service on antiretroviral treatment adherence in Kenya (WelTel Kenya1): a randomised trial. Lancet 2010;376(9755):1838−45.

[45] Milward J, Lynskey M, Strang J. Solving the problem of non-attendance in substance abuse services. Drug Alcohol Rev 2014;33(6):625−36.

[46] Mbuagbaw L, Mursleen S, Lytvyn L, Smieja M, Dolovich L, Thabane L. Mobile phone text messaging interventions for HIV and other chronic diseases: an overview of systematic reviews and framework for evidence transfer. BMC Health Serv Res 2015;15(1):33.

[47] Henry L. Physician assistants, nurse practitioners, and community health centers under the Affordable Care Act. Hum Org 2015;74(1):42.

[48] Mundinger MO. Advanced-practice nursing - good medicine for physicians? N Engl J Med 1994;330(3):211−4.

[49] Buerhaus PI, DesRoches CM, Dittus R, Donelan K. Practice characteristics of primary care nurse practitioners and physicians. Nurs Outlook 2015;63(2):144−53.

[50] Naylor MD, Kurtzman ET. The role of nurse practitioners in reinventing primary care. Health Aff 2010;29(5):893−9.

[51] Laurant M, Reeves D, Hermens R, Braspenning J, Grol R, Sibbald B. Substitution of doctors by nurses in primary care. Cochrane Database Syst Rev 2005;(2).

[52] Horrocks S, Anderson E, Salisbury C. Systematic review of whether nurse practitioners working in primary care can provide equivalent care to doctors. BMJ 2002;324(7341): 819−23.

[53] Prescott PA, Driscoll L. Evaluating nurse practitioner performance. Nurse Pract 1980; 5(4):28–32.

[54] Mundinger MO, Kane RL, Lenz ER, Totten AM, Tsai W-Y, Cleary PD, et al. Primary care outcomes in patients treated by nurse practitioners or physicians: a randomized trial. JAMA 2000;283(1):59–68.

[55] Kurtzman ET, Barnow BS. A comparison of nurse practitioners, physician assistants, and primary care physicians' patterns of practice and quality of care in health centers. Med Care 2017;55(6):615–22.

[56] Jiao S, Murimi IB, Stafford RS, Mojtabai R, Alexander GC. Quality of prescribing by physicians, nurse practitioners, and physician assistants in the United States. Pharmacotherapy 2018;38(4):417–27.

[57] Nelson LE, McMahon JM, Leblanc NM, Braksmajer A, Crean HF, Smith K, et al. Advancing the case for nurse practitioner-based models to accelerate scale-up of HIV pre-exposure prophylaxis. J Clin Nurs 2019;28(1–2):351–61.

[58] Rivet Amico K, Bekker L-G. Global PrEP roll-out: recommendations for programmatic success. Lancet HIV 2019;6(2):e137–40.

[59] Marshall BD, Milloy MJ. Improving the effectiveness and delivery of pre-exposure prophylaxis (PrEP) to people who inject drugs. Addiction 2017;112(4):580–2.

[60] Alistar SS, Owens DK, Brandeau ML. Effectiveness and cost effectiveness of oral pre-exposure prophylaxis in a portfolio of prevention programs for injection drug users in mixed HIV epidemics. PLoS One 2014;9(1):e86584.

[61] Ojikutu BO, Bogart LM, Higgins-Biddle M, Dale SK, Allen W, Dominique T, et al. Facilitators and barriers to pre-exposure prophylaxis (PrEP) use among black individuals in the United States: results from the national survey on HIV in the black community (NSHBC). AIDS Behav 2018;22(11):3576–87.

[62] Dubov A, Altice FL, Fraenkel L. An information-motivation-behavioral skills model of PrEP uptake. AIDS Behav 2018;22(11):3603–16.

[63] Riddell IV J, Amico KR, Mayer KH. HIV preexposure prophylaxis: a review. JAMA 2018;319(12):1261–8.

[64] Markowitz M, Frank I, Grant RM, Mayer KH, Elion R, Goldstein D, et al. Safety and tolerability of long-acting cabotegravir injections in HIV-uninfected men (ECLAIR): a multicentre, double-blind, randomised, placebo-controlled, phase 2a trial. Lancet HIV 2017;4(8):e331–40.

[65] Ledgerwood J, Coates E, Yamshchikov G, Saunders J, Holman L, Enama M, et al. Safety, pharmacokinetics and neutralization of the broadly neutralizing HIV-1 human monoclonal antibody VRC01 in healthy adults. Clin Exp Immunol 2015;182(3):289–301.

[66] Hua CK, Ackerman ME. Increasing the clinical potential and applications of anti-HIV antibodies. Front Immunol 2017;8:1655.

[67] Puri A, Sivaraman A, Zhang W, Clark MR, Banga AK. Expanding the domain of drug delivery for HIV prevention: exploration of the transdermal route. Crit Rev Ther Drug Carrier Syst 2017;34(6).

[68] Gunawardana M, Remedios-Chan M, Miller CS, Fanter R, Yang F, Marzinke MA, et al. Pharmacokinetics of long-acting tenofovir alafenamide (GS-7340) subdermal implant for HIV prophylaxis. Antimicrob Agents Chemother 2015;59(7):3913–9.

Notes on harm reduction and the opioid epidemic in the United States

12

Don C. Des Jarlais, PhD [1], Jonathan Feelemyer[2], Hayley Berg[2], David C. Perlman, MD [3]

[1]*Professor of Epidemiology, Social and Behavioral Sciences, College of Global Public Health, New York University, New York, NY, United States;* [2]*College of Global Public Health, New York University, New York, NY, United States;* [3]*Professor of Medicine, Icahn School of Medicine at Mount Sinai Chief, Infectious Diseases, Mount Sinai Beth Israel New York, NY, United States*

Introduction

All societies that have had access to psychoactive drugs have used them. There are multiple positive aspects of psychoactive drug use, from creating positive mood states, to stress and pain relief, to increasing social bonding, to simple preservation of health (for much of human history it was safer to drink locally available wine or beer than locally available water). Psychoactive drug use also has many negative aspects, from impairing psychological and social functioning, to disinhibition and release of aggression, to inebriation and accidents, to causing infections and fatal diseases, and to fatal overdose. The potential positive and negative consequences of psychoactive drug use have led to many different social mechanisms for regulating access to and use of psychoactive drugs, from incorporating drug use into religious rituals, to informal social norms, and to civil and criminal laws.

The "Harm Reduction" framework is the most recently developed framework for regulating psychoactive drug use, and we would argue, the most appropriate framework for use in large, complex societies in which patterns of drug use, and the individual and societal adverse consequences of use can change very rapidly.

Much of harm reduction theory and practice was developed in Western Europe and Australia [1–3], but as this book focuses on the current opioid epidemic in the United States, this chapter will also focus on harm reduction in the United States. There are three aspects of the US situation that have greatly influenced the course of harm reduction in this country. First is the sheer size of the psychoactive drug use in the United States. Recent estimates are that there are 6.2 million persons in the United States with illicit drug use disorders [4]. The large size of the US drug using population creates the potential for enormous profits to be a made from importing or manufacturing illicit drugs, and from diverting drugs from medical sources. With this large demand, eliminating supply is simply not possible. Second is the great extent to which interracial and interethnic conflict has been incorporated into drug policies in the United States. A full examination of the relationships between

The Opioid Epidemic and Infectious Diseases. https://doi.org/10.1016/B978-0-323-68328-9.00012-6

drug use and racial/ethnic conflicts in the United States is beyond the scope of this chapter, but we would note several aspects of US culture that have been of great importance to drug use and drug policies in the country. Many of the original European colonists belonged to religious groups who held extremely negative views of drug use, considering drugs to be products of the devil and drug use to be inherently sinful [5]. Slavery in the United States was developed in part to create very large-scale production of a psychoactive drug (nicotine in tobacco) [6]. Prohibition of alcohol in the United States in 1918 was a product of cultural conflict between rural/small city dominated by Protestants and urban areas dominated by Catholic immigrants. The bars and saloons portrayed as dens of evil that ruined family life were in particular associated with German immigrants, and Prohibition was passed at the end of World War I. Third, the United States is a federal system, with state and local governments having great but not complete authority in the area of public health. Thus, state and local governments have often implemented harm reduction programs despite intense opposition at the federal level (for example, implementation of needle/syringe exchange programs). Many states, however, are dependent upon the federal government for the funding of their public health programs, so that opposition to harm reduction at the federal level can also be quite effective.

What harm reduction is not

There have been several attempts to define and characterize harm reduction with many common elements but without a definitive consensus [7,8]. This is not surprising given the rapid development of the framework over the last several decades. We believe that, as a starting point for understanding the current state of harm reduction in the United States, with respect to policy and direct services, it is helpful to begin with consideration of what harm reduction is not. In our assessment, there is probably more agreement on what harm reduction is not rather than on what harm reduction is (at any given historical moment).

First, harm reduction is clearly not an ethnocentric condemnation of people who use certain types of drugs. This is specifically relevant in the context of illicit versus licit drugs. Legality typically creates a framework for moral judgment about a person based on the psychoactive drugs they choose to consume (for example, the use of alcohol or cigarettes vs. heroin in the United States). Harm reduction does not make this global distinction, but rather considers individual drugs and individual routes of administration in terms of the potential harms to be addressed. As noted above, there are long traditions of drug use in many different cultures. Drug use that is new to a dominant cultural group and associated with minority groups within the society has often been moralistically condemned, with heavy criminal penalties imposed on active use and possession. Examples include the use of opium by Chinese immigrants [9,10], use of marijuana by Mexicans [11], and, more recently, use of crack cocaine by African-Americans all in the United States [12]. The imposition of extremely heavy penalties for possession of drugs as well as quality of life crimes often associated with dependence (panhandling, etc.) was often in the name of fear of more serious crimes associated with drug use and which incorporated overt racism. This has led to mass incarceration in the United States which has widely been condemned as racist and stands, in some ways, in opposition to how the United States has treated the recent opioid epidemic which has largely affected white, working class individuals.

A second point is the desired outcomes of substance use treatment. Harm reduction does not insist that abstinence is the only acceptable outcome for the treatment of substance use disorders. Harm reduction includes the use of psychoactive medications during treatment. Medication-assisted treatment (MAT), particularly methadone and buprenorphine, and the use of psychiatric medications are not only acceptable components of the harm reduction approach to treatment of substance use disorders but can lead to important improvements in physical and mental health and overall quality of life [13].

Third, harm reduction is not confined to illicit drugs. Indeed, addressing licit drug use is an increasingly important aspect of harm reduction. In recent years, with the increase in the number of people who are becoming addicted to prescription opioids, harm reduction organizations have had to expand their services and outreach methods to work with communities where the primary drug problem has become the misuse of prescription opioids.

Fourth, harm reduction does not include unlimited commercial exploitation of psychoactive drugs. With their ability to generate dependence, both licit and illicit psychoactive drugs can be extremely profitable. Harm reduction recognizes the need for limitations on the distribution and marketing of drugs. In the United States, harm reduction organizations have been some of the biggest proponents for reform of prescribing practices for opioids and stricter regulation on how pharmaceutical companies market their drugs to healthcare providers and patients [14].

Finally, harm reduction does not expect to create a perfect world. It is not a vision of a drug-free world, in which no one uses psychoactive drugs, nor it is a vision in which everyone who uses drugs does so in a harm-free manner. Harm reduction necessarily involves trade-offs between different forms and quantities of individual and societal harms associated with the many varieties of psychoactive drug use.

Positive principles of harm reduction

The harm reduction perspective emphasizes the need to base policy on research, rather than on stereotypes of drug users, both illicit and licit users. There have been hundreds of studies of the major harm reduction interventions—MAT for opioid use disorders, syringe services programs (distribution of new syringes, cookers, cotton, smoking pipes, and other drug use paraphernalia) to reduce transmission of HIV, and antiretroviral treatment for HIV infection—and there is a strong scientific consensus that they can be very effective [15,16]. The current status of the research is that the benefits of harm reduction programs are sufficiently well established that it would be unethical to withhold these programs from a "control group" in future research. It is important to note, however, that harm reduction programs are not likely to be effective if they are poorly implemented. The programs need to treat people who use drugs with dignity and respect, and they need to be implemented on a large, public health scale.

The research has also shown that harm reduction programs do not lead to increases in illicit drug use. Indeed the US opioid epidemic, with its large increases in people who use drugs (PWUD), has been particularly severe in the areas of the county that historically have had the *least* amount of harm reduction services, such as Appalachia [17].

Harm reduction incorporates a human rights approach to health. Health and healthcare are seen as basic human rights, and that all persons receiving health-related services should be treated with dignity and respect. Harm reduction aims to preserve the importance of individual rights while providing adequate treatment for persons with psychoactive drug use problems. Most importantly, harm reduction has led to a growing recognition that adverse consequences of nonmedical drug use (such as HIV transmission) can be reduced without increasing illicit drug use. It thus acts as a wholistic view of "health" and what it means to have a substance use disorder.

Harm reduction is a collaborative process, involving persons who use drugs in both policy formulation and in implementing programs (such as peer harm reduction programs). Peers can assist in providing comprehensive and accurate information on how to use drugs safely, while delivering harm reduction supplies to drug users. Peers are also often nonjudgmental, an important aspect of fostering relationships with drug users, who are often stigmatized. Further, within harm reduction, people who use drugs are seen as members of the community, and the health of the community as a whole depends upon maintaining the health of persons who use drugs.

Finally, harm reduction is constantly evolving. Patterns of drug use and the individual and societal harms change continually and often rapidly; one of the most recent changes in drug use patterns has been the recent increase in opiate and fentanyl use in the United States [18]. Some problems associated with drug use have been reduced to minimal levels, but other problems require continuous efforts and new problems can rapidly arise. For example, combined prevention (including needle/syringe exchange programs, MAT, and antiretroviral treatment for HIV positive persons) has effectively ended the HIV epidemic among persons who inject drugs (PWID) in New York City [19]. However, HCV incidence among PWID is still unacceptably high in New York City, approximately 19.5/100 for those injecting for 6 years or less, which will likely end up being one of the next drivers of change in harm reduction theory [20].

As noted throughout this book, the current opioid epidemic in the United States is the latest public health crisis associated with psychoactive drug use. Before considering how harm reduction may be applied to this current public health crisis, it will be useful to consider the back and forth between drug use epidemics, harm-increasing responses to the epidemics, and resistance to harm reduction responses to the epidemics over the last century. The following historical timeline includes both "Harm-Increasing" (HI) events and "Harm Reducing" (HR) events, and a few "To Be Determined (TBD)" events. The TBD events are events that in our assessment have not yet reached a final equilibrium for increasing versus decreasing harm. The psychedelic revolution of the 1960s included a massive increase in drug use, which included positive experiences for many users, severely negative experiences for some users, and clearly inequitable law enforcement/incarceration for racial/minority groups in the United States. Societal assessment of psychedelic drugs, including marijuana, has continued, however, with increasing valuation of the possible medical uses and nonmedical uses of these drugs. The development of electronic cigarettes not only has the potential for reducing the severe harms associated with conventional cigarette use and of assisting some cigarette users to stop but also has the potential to create nicotine addiction in many youth. The eventual harms/positives balance for these developments many depend upon the societal mechanisms for regulating their use more than the intrinsic properties of the drugs themselves.

Historical timeline of harm reducing and harm-increasing events in the United States

- **Late 1800s to early 1900s**: Gradual transition of opioid use from medical prescription to illicit activities. (HI)
- **January 23, 1912**: The International Opium Convention is held at the Hague, becoming the first international drug control treaty signed into law. (HI)
- **Late 1910s to early 1920s**: Morphine maintenance clinics in multiple US cities. Shreveport, LA best known of these clinics. (HR)
- **1914**: Harrison Act outlawing narcotic drugs. (HR)
- **1914**: Cocaine made illegal. (HI)
- **1918**: Prohibition begins. Great increase in organized crime. (HI)
- **1930**: Creation of the federal Bureau of Narcotics, headed by Harry Anslinger. (HI)
- **1933**: Prohibition ends. Some criminal organizations move into distribution of heroin and cocaine. (HR, but some HI)
- **1945**: With end of World War II, increased importation of heroin into the United States, through the French Connection. (HI)
- **1964**: Surgeon General's report on the health risks of smoking. (HR)
- **Mid 1960s**: Development of methadone maintenance treatment for heroin addiction. (HR)
- **Late 1960 through 1970s**: Psychedelic drug revolution, including increased use of marijuana. (TBS)
- **1970s and 1980s**: Increased use of heroin and cocaine. (HI)
- **Early 1970s**: Original "War on Drugs," but including large expansion of methadone maintenance treatment programs. (HI, but some HR)

- **Late 1970s**: Rapid transmission of HIV among PWID in the northeast United States. (HI)
- **1980**: Mothers Against Drunk Driving founded. Currently has chapters in all US states. (HR)
- **1981**: AIDS outbreak first observed among PWID. (HI)
- **Mid-1980s**: Outreach HIV education programs implemented for PWID. (HR)
- **Mid-1980 and 1990s**: Crack cocaine epidemic, violence associated with distribution of crack, increased "War on Drugs" with severe penalties for possession and sale of crack. Spread of HIV through unsafe sex associated with crack use. (HI)
- **1988**: First syringe exchange in United States in Tacoma, WA. Founding of North American Syringe Exchange Network. (HR)
- **Late 1980s to present**: Continued expansion of syringe exchange programs in the United States, currently there are approximately 400 syringe exchange programs in the country. (HR)
- **1988**: Initial ban on use of federal funds for supporting syringe exchange operations. (HI)
- **1989–93**: US National Commission on AIDS advocates for legal access to sterile injection equipment and increased treatment for substance use disorders. Inclusion of PWUD as a protected class in the Americans with Disabilities Act. (HR)
- **Early to late 1990s**: Accumulation of evidence supporting effectiveness of syringe exchange programs. Increase in numbers of programs in the United States. (HR)
- **1996**: Development of combined antiretroviral treatments for HIV infection. (HR)
- **2000 onward**: Implementation of public health scale "combined prevention and care" (syringe service programs, leading to "ending HIV epidemics" in many high-income settings). (HR)
- **2000 onward**: Increase bans on smoking in public places. (HR)
- **2002**: FDA approval of buprenorphine for the treatment of addiction. (HR)
- **2000 onward**: Opioid epidemic in United States, with overprescription of opioid analgesics, with transitions to injecting and to heroin use. Syringe exchange programs and MAT expand but with local resistance in many areas. (HI)
- **Mid-2000s**: Development and commercialization of electronic cigarettes, widespread use by teens in mid-2010s. (TBD)
- **January 2001**: Distribution of naloxone for reversing opioid overdoses at Chicago Recovery Alliance for all staff, volunteers, and participants, gradually spreading in United States. (HR)
- **2011**: Discovery of direct acting antiretrovirals (DAAs) for the treatment of hepatitis C virus infection.
- **2012 onward**: Medical marijuana and recreational marijuana laws adopted in many states. (HR)

- **2013–16**: HIV outbreak among PWID in Scott County, IN. (HI)
- **January 2016**: Lifting of ban on use of federal funds to support syringe exchange programs, though federal funds cannot be used for purchase of syringes. (HR)
- **2016 onward**: Widespread distribution of fentanyl in illicit drug distribution. (HR)
- **2016 onward**: Consideration of and planning for safer injection facilities, but federal opposition has prevented implementation. (HR)
- **2017**: Declaration of opioid epidemic as a public health emergency. (HR)
- **2019**: "First Step" Act to reform drug laws—reduce criminal penalties for drug possession. (HR)

This historical timeline clearly demonstrates that the history of drug use and harm reduction in the United States has not been a simple or linear process. Events that have increased drug use harms have alternated with events that have promoted harm reduction. Harm reducing activities have often followed harm-increasing events, though often with considerable time between the harm augmentation event and a harm reduction response. We do believe, however, that the overall trend is toward increased harm reduction as a result of greater scientific understanding of drug use disorders and which interventions actually reduce drug-related harms, as well as the growing acceptance of health as a human right.

Harm reduction and the current opioid epidemic

The conceptual analyses of what harm reduction is not and what harm reduction is can provide an overall framework for applying harm reduction to the current opioid epidemic. The historical timeline lists development of specific harm reduction interventions for which there are strong evidence bases and should be utilized in addressing the current epidemic. We would note the following interventions are likely to have the greatest positive impact within the United States:

1. Outreach to persons who use drugs to provide factual information about hazards of specific forms of drug use, to develop trusting communications between health workers and persons who use drugs, and to provide information on how to obtain services for drug-related problems
2. Syringe service programs, that include syringe exchange and the most other health and social services as feasible
3. MAT for opioid use disorders
4. Distribution of naloxone to reverse opioid overdose
5. Safer injection facilities to prevent fatal drug overdoses and transmission of HIV and HCV, and to provide referrals to substance use treatment when these become practical in the United States [21]
   There is sufficient evidence to recommend against:

6. Incarceration of people for possession of small quantities of currently illicit drugs
   Finally, and perhaps most importantly, we would recommend:
7. Community education to reduce stigmatization of drug use

The current opioid epidemic in the United States is a severe and multifaceted challenge to public health. Harm reduction provides multiple tools for addressing this epidemic, but the epidemic is likely to change over time, creating a need for vigilance and a likely need for developing new harm reduction interventions.

Tips for clinicians

In this chapter, we have discussed harm reduction as a set of public policies and public health interventions that recognize the innate desires of human beings to use various psychoactive drugs and that medical and social science can be used to minimize the individual and societal harms often associated with psychoactive drug use. Harm reduction can also be a critical component of healthcare provide/patient relationships. We thus would like to conclude this chapter with suggested guidance for infectious disease healthcare providers when working with persons who use drugs:

1. Open, nonstigmatizing conversations about drug use so as to better understand individual health risks and offer appropriate, patient-centered interventions. Understand that not all individuals are ready for abstinence, but that any harm reduction can improve health outcomes.
2. Encourage use of sterile syringes if persons inject drugs. Prescribe syringes, if individuals live in a state where laws require prescriptions and permit prescribing of syringes. Discuss the importance of not sharing cookers, cotton, pipes, and other drug using paraphernalia, in addition to syringes to prevent acquisition of infectious diseases, particularly HCV.
3. Provide buprenorphine treatment so that you can treat both infectious diseases and opioid use disorders in same setting. Refer and link patients to other buprenorphine providers or methadone if not available in your clinical setting.
4. Know local community-based organizations, such as syringe exchange programs, that aid in drug user health and refer and link patients to these groups.
5. Offer PrEP to PWID, particularly if PWID are concurrently having nonprotected sex.
6. Treat HCV-positive sexual and drug using partners together, to prevent reinfection of the social unit.
7. Prescribe Naloxone to prevent opioid overdose.
8. Believe in the right to life even for people who use drugs.

References

[1] Hartgers C, Buning EC, van Santen GW, Verster AD, Coutinho RA. The impact of the needle and syringe-exchange programme in Amsterdam on injecting risk behavior. AIDS 1989;3:571—6.

[2] Tsai R, Goh EH, Webeck P, Mullins J. Prevention of human immunodeficiency virus infection among intravenous drug users in New South Wales, Australia: the needles and syringes distribution programme through retail pharmacies. Asia Pac J Public Health 1988;2(4):245—51.

[3] Wodak A. HIV infection and injecting drug use in Australia: responding to a crisis. J Drug Issues 1992;22(3):549—62.

[4] Lipari RN, Van Horn SL. Trends in substance use disorders among adults aged 18 or older. CBHSQ Rep. 2017 Substance Abuse and Mental Health Services Administration. Bethesda Md.

[5] Crocq M-A. Historical and cultural aspects of man's relationship with addictive drugs. Dialogues Clin Neurosci 2007;9(4):355—61.

[6] Meshnick A. A morbid disconnect: the battle over slave health in the early American tobacco industry. 2017.

[7] Single EJ. Defining harm reduction. Drug Alcohol Rev 1995;14(3):287—90.

[8] Lenton S, Single EJ. The definition of harm reduction. Drug Alcohol Rev 1998;17(2):213—9.

[9] Ahmad DL. Opium smoking, anti-Chinese attitudes, and the American medical community, 1850—1890. Am Ninet Century Hist 2000;1(2):53—68.

[10] Musto D. Opium, cocaine, and marijuana in American history. Sci Am 1991;265:40—7.

[11] Bonnie RJ, Whitebread C. The forbidden fruit and the tree of knowledge: an inquiry into the legal history of American marijuana prohibition. Va Law Rev 1970;56:971.

[12] Cornish JW, O'Brien C. Crack cocaine abuse: an epidemic with many public health consequences. Annu Rev Public Health 1996;17(1):259—73.

[13] Feelemyer JP, Jarlais DC, Arasteh K, Phillips BW, Hagan H. Changes in quality of life (WHOQOL-BREF) and addiction severity index (ASI) among participants in opioid substitution treatment (OST) in low and middle income countries: an international systematic review. Drug Alcohol Depend 2013;134:251—8.

[14] Burris S. Where next for opioids and the law? Despair, harm reduction, lawsuits, and regulatory reform. Public Health Rep 2018;133(1):29—33.

[15] World Health Organization, UNAIDS, UNODC. Technical guide for countries to set targets for universal access to HIV prevention, treatment and care for injecting drug users Geneva. 2012. Available from:http://www.unodc.org/documents/hiv-aids/WHO%20UNODC%20UNAIDS%20%20IDU%20Universal%20Access%20Target%20Setting%20Guide%20-%20FINAL%20-%20Feb%2009.pdf.

[16] Des Jarlais DC, Friedman SR, Ward TP. Harm reduction: a public health response to the AIDS epidemic among injecting drug users. Annu Rev Public Health 1993;14:413—50.

[17] National Institute on Drug Abuse. Opioid summaries by state. Bethesda MD: NIH; 2018.

[18] New York City Department of Health and Mental Hygiene. Increase in drug overdoses deaths linked to increased presence of fentanyl in New York City (Advisory #47). 2016.

[19] Des Jarlais DC, Arasteh K, McKnight C, Feelemyer J, Campbell AN, Tross S, et al. Consistent estimates of very low HIV incidence among people who inject drugs: New York city, 2005—2014. Am J Public Health 2016;106(3):503—8.

[20] Jordan AE, Des Jarlais DC, Arasteh K, McKnight C, Nash D, Perlman DC. Incidence and prevalence of hepatitis c virus infection among persons who inject drugs in New York City: 2006–2013. Drug Alcohol Depend 2015;152:194–200.

[21] Gaeta JM, Racine M. New strategies are needed to stop overdose fatalities: the case for supervised injection facilities. Ann Intern Med 2018;168(9):664–5.

Modeling the impact of harm reduction for opioid use disorder on infectious disease prevention

13

Annick Bórquez, PhD, MSc [1], Javier A. Cepeda, PhD, MPH [1],
Natasha K. Martin, DPhil [2]

[1]*Assistant Professor, Division of Infectious Diseases and Global Public Health, University of California San Diego, La Jolla, CA, United States;* [2]*Associate Professor, Division of Infectious Diseases and Global Public Health, University of California San Diego, La Jolla, CA, United States*

Introduction

Opioid use disorder (OUD) can lead to injection drug use, which is an important risk factor for blood-borne viruses such as HIV and hepatitis C virus (HCV), among other infections. Indeed, the burden of blood-borne viruses among people who inject drugs (PWID) is high globally. A systematic review and meta-analysis [1] found that 17.8% (95% uncertainty interval [UI], 10.8−24.8) of PWID are living with HIV, 52.3% (95% UI, 42.4−62.1) are HCV-antibody positive, and 9.1% (95% UI, 5.1−13.2) are hepatitis B virus (HBV) surface antigen positive. This equates to an estimated 2.8 million (1.5−4.5 million) PWID living with HIV, 8.2 million (4.7−12.4 million) PWID living with HCV antibody, and 1.4 million (0.7−2.4 million) PWID living with chronic HBV infection [2]. Among PWID in the United States, an estimated 8.7% (95% UI, 6.8%−10.7%) are living with HIV, 53.1% (95% UI, 38.1%−68.0%) are HCV-antibody positive, and 4.8% (95% UI, 3.0%−7.2%) are HBV surface antigen positive [1].

Fortunately, there is good empirical evidence from systematic reviews and meta-analyses that harm reduction interventions such as opiate agonist therapy (OAT) and needle and syringe programs (NSPs) can prevent the acquisition of HIV and HCV among PWID, particularly if provided in combination [3−5].

Despite this, coverage of harm reduction is low in the United States and worldwide. A systematic review and meta-analysis [6] found that globally there are 33 [7−36] needle-syringes distributed via the NSP per PWID each year, and only 16 [7−10,37−47] OAT recipients per 100 PWID. These levels are far below the World Health Organization recommended levels of coverage, defined as >200 needle-syringes distributed per PWID and >40 OAT recipients per 100 PWID. In the United States, an estimated only 30 [7−35,38−47] needle-syringes were distributed per PWID per year, and there are only 19 [7−21,38−47] OAT recipients per 100

The Opioid Epidemic and Infectious Diseases. https://doi.org/10.1016/B978-0-323-68328-9.00013-8

PWID [6]. Indeed, only four countries (Australia, Austria, the Netherlands, and Norway) have achieved a high coverage of both NSP and OAT. As a result, only an estimated 1% of PWID live in countries with a high coverage of both NSP and OAT [6].

Mathematical or epidemic modeling has been used extensively to explore and understand infectious disease epidemics among PWID worldwide. In the United States specifically, several epidemic modeling studies have examined HIV and HCV epidemic dynamics among PWID in both urban [48,49] and rural settings [37,50]. Through these studies, modeling has been used to understand important drivers of the epidemic and to identify priorities for prevention.

Modeling can also be used as a "virtual laboratory" to evaluate the population impact of existing harm reduction strategies. Often the evaluation of the impact of existing interventions such as NSPs and OAT at a population level is difficult using epidemiologic data only. For example, natural epidemic expansion or decline could mask or inflate the impact of intervention scale-up, respectively, in the absence of a counterfactual theories, which can be generated through modeling. Additionally, the presence of multiple interventions often makes disentangling the individual impact of each intervention component difficult. Finally, changes in incidence could also be a result of background changes in terms of injecting drug use epidemiology (initiation, cessation, or risk) instead of intervention effect. As a result, modeling studies are useful tools to generate counterfactual theories of the likely epidemic in the absence of the intervention and to disentangle the impact of epidemiologic changes and interventions on the epidemic.

Additionally, modeling can be used for forecasting—to predict the population-level impact of interventions such as harm reduction on disease epidemics and infectious disease transmission. Indeed, modeling has been used extensively to estimate the potential impact of harm reduction interventions, both alone and in combination with other interventions such as HIV and HCV treatment on HIV and HCV incidence and mortality among PWID [38–44]. Modeling provides a virtual test laboratory in which different intervention scenarios can be investigated and compared in lieu of implementing large community randomized controlled trials or in preparation for these trials. This is particularly important, because depending on the epidemic stage, the structure of injecting networks, and the injecting practices in a specific population, small increases in intervention coverage might result in large reductions in incidence, whereas in different populations, much higher coverage levels might be required [45]. In general, these modeling studies have underscored the substantial population prevention benefits that harm reduction, particularly in combination with other treatment and prevention modalities, can play in terms of reducing HIV and HCV incidence among PWID.

There are a broad range of methodological approaches used to evaluate the impact of harm reduction on infectious disease epidemics. Traditional "static" models evaluating the impact of harm reduction, such as OAT, on drug use and overdose incorporate only individual health benefits, whereas more complex "dynamic" transmission models mechanistically simulate the impact of OAT on associated infectious disease incidence at a population level. These dynamic transmission models therefore incorporate both individual and population prevention benefits and can be either deterministic (compartmentalizing the population into different groups and infection states, assuming the behavior is heterogeneous within each compartment) or individual based (simulating each individual separately within each population). The selection of model type (e.g., deterministic vs. individual based) is often based on the research question and available data. Models evaluating the impact of NSPs provision have generally fallen into two categories: models that utilize relatively simple calculations of change in infection incidence over 1 year predicted by a change in the population proportion of contaminated syringes circulating among PWID (entitled "circulation theory" models) and dynamic transmission models that assess long-term impact and account for the entire future chain of infections averted. As stronger systematic review data emerges on the impact of harm reduction interventions on an individual's risk of HIV and HCV incidence, more robust evaluations can occur estimating the short- and long-term impact of harm reduction on related infectious disease epidemics.

This chapter reviews the real-world and modeling evidence surrounding the impact and cost-effectiveness of harm reduction for OUD in the prevention of infectious diseases, with a focus on analyses for the United States.

Empirical evidence for harm reduction on acquiring HIV and hepatitis C virus infections

Harm reduction interventions for people who use and inject drugs include medication-assisted treatment and NSPs. Medication-assisted treatment includes OAT, with drugs such as methadone and buprenorphine, and opioid antagonist treatment, with drugs such as naltrexone. It is well known that OAT is effective in reducing fatal overdose. Evidence from a global meta-analysis of 21 cohorts of nearly 140,000 patients who underwent OAT found that methadone reduced the risk of overdose by 79% (relative risk [RR] 0.21; 95% CI, 0.13–0.34) [46]. Only one cohort study was conducted among patients who used buprenorphine, but the magnitude of the effect on fatal overdose prevention was similar (approximately 70% reduction) [47]. Two global systematic reviews and meta-analyses have found strong evidence that OAT reduces an individual's risk of acquiring HIV by 54% (RR 0.46; 95% CI, 0.32–0.67) [5] and acquiring HCV by 49% (RR 0.51; 95% CI, 0.4–0.63) [3]. The results were consistent across geographic regions. For example, the effect estimates in North America were similar to the overall pooled effect, with OAT reducing an individual's risk of acquiring HIV by 62% (RR 0.38; 95% CI, 0.23–0.65) [5] and HCV by 43% (RR 0.57; 95% CI, 0.42–0.77) [3]. Evidence of the effectiveness of antagonist treatments such as naltrexone on reducing HIV and HCV acquisition risk is mixed, and therefore will not be discussed here.

NSPs provide sterile needles, syringes, injecting equipment, education, and other prevention and support services. There is evidence that NSPs not only reduce injecting risk behaviors but also prevent the acquisition of HIV and HCV. A systematic review found that exposure to NSPs reduces an individual's risk of acquiring HIV by 44% (RR 0.6; 95% CI, 0.43−1.01) across all studies with high heterogeneity, and 0.42 (95% CI, 0.22−0.81) across six higher quality studies [4]. A Cochrane review [3] found weaker evidence for NSPs in reducing HCV, with the overall finding that high coverage of NSPs reduces an individual's risk of acquiring HCV by 23% (RR 0.77; 95% CI, 0.38−1.54) compared to no or low NSPs coverage, and combined OAT and NSPs results in a 76% reduction in HCV acquisition risk (RR 0.24; 95% CI, 0.09−0.62). However, there was high heterogeneity across studies regarding the impact of NSPs on HCV infection and the effect varied by region [3]. For example, high NSPs coverage in Europe was associated with a 56% reduction in HCV acquisition (RR = 0.44; 95% CI, 0.23−0.8) with low heterogeneity, whereas no effect was found for North America (RR = 1.58; 95% CI, 0.57−4.42), which had high heterogeneity [3]. There are several potential explanations for this geographic difference in the observed NSPs effect. First, while consistent measures of NSPs exposure through individual-level coverage estimates were available from Europe (measured by receiving one or more sterile syringes for each injection), measures in North American studies varied and focused more on the frequency of attendance at NSP instead of coverage. These inconsistencies in measurement contributed to the difference in heterogeneity between the studies, and these exposure measurement differences combined with differences in study design and injecting patterns may account for a lack of observed effect in North America. Additionally, the lack of federal funding for NSPs during the period the studies were performed has resulted in lower coverage of NSPs among PWID in the United States compared with the European sites, which may mask the intervention effect. Finally, the higher proportion of PWID injecting stimulants in the US studies could contribute to lower impact. Residual confounding may be important, especially in North America, where people who attend NSPs also report higher injection risk behaviors and factors associated with injecting/sexual risk (such as sex work and homelessness) so that adjustment for these factors may attenuate any positive association between HIV or HCV transmission and NSPs attendance.

Supervised injection facilities (SIFs), along with supervised drug consumption rooms more generally, are facilities that provide safer environments for drug use. These sites provide a place for hygienic consumption of drugs under the supervision of trained staff. The primary aim is to reduce unsterile drug use practices, prevent drug-related overdose deaths, and facilitate connections with drug use treatment and health and social services. Typically, SIFs provide sterile injecting equipment, counseling, emergency overdose care, and referral to the aforementioned services. The first SIF was established in 1986 in Switzerland, with subsequent expansion across Europe. Ten countries currently allow legal operation of SIFs (Australia, Canada, Denmark, France, Germany, Luxembourg, the Netherlands, Norway, Spain, and Switzerland). In the United States, the legal status of SIFs was unclear until

October 2019, when a District Judge ruled that "the ultimate goal of Safehouse's proposed operation is to reduce drug use, not facilitate it, and accordingly, §856(a) does not prohibit Safehouse's proposed conduct". Documentation of an unsanctioned SIFs in the United States operating since 2014 has been reported [7]. A review of reviews [8] indicated that there was "tentative evidence" to support the effectiveness of SIFs in reducing injecting risk behavior and improving injecting hygiene. Although encouraging, authors generally conclude that the evidence to evaluate any impact on HIV and HCV incidence is insufficient and further studies are needed in this area.

In summary, there is strong evidence that OAT reduces overdose, as well as an individual's risk of acquiring HIV and HCV infection. There is good but weaker evidence that high-coverage NSPs reduce the acquisition of HIV and HCV globally; however, there is high heterogeneity and evidence for stronger effect of high NSP coverage in Europe, but no effect in North America. In combination, there is strong evidence that the receipt of both OAT and high-coverage NSP prevents acquisition of HCV. There is tentative evidence that SIFs reduce injecting risk, but the evidence is insufficient and more studies are needed to evaluate the impact on HIV and HCV incidence.

Modeling the impact of harm reduction on HIV epidemics among people who inject drugs in the United States
Modeling opiate agonist therapy for HIV prevention

For more than 50 years, methadone treatment, a form of OAT, has been prescribed to treat patients with OUD in the United States [9] and was readily available prior to the emergence of HIV in the early 1980s. In the United States, early work by Zaric et al. [10] in 2000 used a dynamic transmission model to investigate the impact of a 10% relative increase in methadone coverage in two settings with low (5%) and high (20%) HIV prevalence resembling Los Angeles and New York City, respectively, and found that it would result in 34 and 264 HIV infections averted over 10 years, respectively, in each setting. This analysis assumed a relatively high (94%) reduction in HIV risk on OAT. While updated estimates of methadone effectiveness from global systematic reviews have become available since [5], this modeling study contributes valuable information to policy makers because it found that 36% and 28% of HIV infections averted in the low- and high-prevalence settings, respectively, would be among the general population, thus showing the benefits of methadone scale-up would go beyond the PWID population [10]. This information can be a key argument when advocating for the expansion of harm reduction services.

Modeling needle and syringe programs for HIV prevention

Initial studies evaluating the impact of NSPs on HIV epidemics utilized ecologic analyses, comparing HIV prevalence across sites with and without NSPs provision.

A 1997 ecologic analysis by Hurley and colleagues [11] used data from 81 cities across Europe, Asia, and North America, finding that HIV prevalence increased by an average of 5.9% per year in cities without NSPs (n = 52). By contrast, HIV prevalence decreased by an average of 5.8% per year in the cities with NSPs (n = 20). One particularly striking example was evident from New York City, where the introduction of NSPs occurred alongside a concomitant marked decrease of HIV incidence among PWID [12,13]. Nevertheless, ecologic studies are limited because changes in HIV incidence or prevalence could be due to other factors such as background changes in mortality and epidemiology, so disentangling the impact of NSP is difficult.

Numerous early studies utilized a simplified mathematic framework developed by Kaplan [14] called the needle circulation theory to evaluate the potential impact of NSPs in the United States and the associated cost-effectiveness (described in the section Modeling the impact of harm reduction among incarcerated populations on infectious diseases). Kaplan's analysis uses population estimates of the number of injecting events per year and the number of sterile syringes distributed per year by NSPs to generate estimates of the proportion of contaminated syringes circulating in a population. It is then assumed that the more syringes distributed via NSPs, the shorter the time a syringe is in circulation, which lowers the proportion of circulating contaminated syringes and subsequently reduces the associated injecting-related disease incidence. This hypothesis was supported by programmatic data indicating the mean circulation time, as well as the prevalence of HIV within syringes exchanged at a syringe exchange in New Haven, Connecticut, which was reduced across the 20 months of operations from 1990 to 1992 [15]. With this framework, Kaplan used programmatic data on the number of clients reached and syringes distributed to evaluate the impact of the New Haven SEP, estimating it reduced new HIV infections among attendants by 33% in 1 year [14]. Additionally, the analysis found that the SEP distributed 168 syringes per PWID per year and contacted 200 PWID, predicting that this distribution averted 1.62 HIV infections per year [16]. Interestingly, this model predicted that an optimal resource allocation of more syringes among fewer PWID (761 syringes per PWID per year among 165 PWID) could avert 2.5 HIV infections per year [16]. Another analysis by Laufer et al. [17] of NSPs in New York utilized a circulation theory as well as estimates of HIV incidence inside and outside NSPs in New York City to estimate the impact of seven NSPs located in New York City and Rochester, New York, in 1992. Using these estimates, these SEPs were predicted to decrease HIV incidence among clients by 60%, resulting in 87–92 HIV infections averted per year.

The predicted impact of NSPs varies substantially by epidemiologic setting and assumptions about intervention efficacy, but it generally indicates the marked impact on averting HIV with NSPs scale-up. For example, Lurie and colleagues [18], using a mixture of circulation theory and dynamic models, simulated four hypothetical cities with different epidemiologic characteristics and predicted that NSPs implementation could result in reductions in HIV incidence among PWID between 17% and 70%. A subsequent analysis by Lurie et al. [19] estimated the HIV infections associated with a lack of comprehensive NSPs in the United States. They estimated that 4394–9666 HIV infections could have been averted between 1987 and 1995 with a scale-up similar to that achieved in Australia [19]. An analysis by Nguyen et al. [20], also based on a circulation theory, estimated that a national investment of an additional $10 or $50 million for NSPs providing a minimal set of services would avert 194 or 816 new HIV infections among PWID over a year in the United States. Finally, an analysis by Geodel et al. used an individual-based dynamic transmission model to examine the impact of barriers to NSPs implementation in a rural US county similar to Scott County, Indiana, after the introduction of a single HIV infection. Using data from Scott County, they simulated the impact of an NSP with 55% attendance among PWID and reductions in self-reported syringe sharing from 34% to 2% among those attending the NSP. Using these assumptions, their analysis found that there would be on average 124 infections within 5 years if no NSP was implemented, whereas reactive implementation of an NSP beginning operations 10 months after the first infection (as occurred in Scott County) would prevent 76 infections. On the other hand, if NSPs were preexisting before the HIV infection introduction, they would avert 105 infections. Importantly, the proactive (preexisting NSP) scenario would result in lower prevalence among both PWID and the broader population, indicating the important community benefit of NSPs (Fig. 13.1). Gonsalves et al. [50] carried out a similar analysis of the Scott County outbreak using a deterministic model, also finding that the outbreak could have been reduced to ten or fewer infections through early intervention.

Despite these analyses, there remains uncertainty in how the expansion of NSPs translates to changes in individual-level syringe distribution coverage, syringe sharing, and the resulting HIV transmission. An analysis from Australia by Kwon et al. [21] used data on the dose-response relationship between individual-level syringe distribution coverage and individual self-reported syringe sharing, indicating that in the absence of NSPs the syringe sharing rate would have been 20%–45%, which reduced to <20% with the expansion of NSP in the early 1990s to achieve a coverage of roughly 50 needle-syringes distributed through NSPs per capita per year. However, subsequent increases in the number of needle-syringes distributed through NSPs per capita to above 150 did not substantially reduce sharing further. These data are important in quantifying the benefits of NSP provision and coverage, which may not be linear. Unfortunately, no equivalent data are available for the United States, although the relationship is likely to be similar. Using these data, Kwon estimated that NSPs in Australia reduced the incidence of HIV among PWID by 34%–70% from 2000 to 2010, a dramatic impact with a comprehensive national program.

Modeling combination opioid agonist therapy and needle and syringe program for HIV prevention

In an analysis, Bernard et al. [41] utilized dynamic transmission modeling to investigate the potential impact of scaled-up combination HIV prevention portfolios

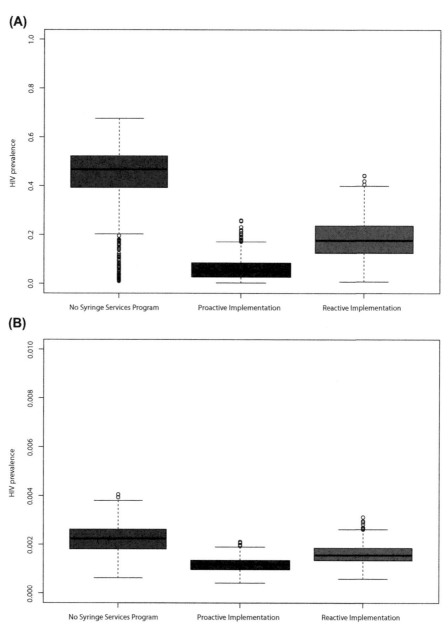

FIGURE 13.1 Modeled projections of HIV prevalence among **(A)** people who inject drugs and **(B)** people who do not inject drugs in a rural county in the United States at the end of a 5-year period following the introduction of a single infection with various syringe services program implementation scenarios.

including harm reduction on reducing HIV among PWID in the United States. They explored the impact of combinations of OAT, NSP, HIV testing and treatment, and HIV preexposure prophylaxis on HIV among PWID. Bernard and colleagues [41] found that scaling up OAT or NSP to 50% coverage among PWID could reduce HIV prevalence by a relative 16%–17% at 20 years, which would avert 22,000 or 35,000 HIV infections among PWID over 20 years, respectively. A combination of scaled-up OAT, NSP, HIV test and treat, and HIV preexposure prophylaxis interventions at high coverage (50% of eligible population) would avert 62,000 (95% confidence interval [CI], 37,000–92,000) over 20 years [41].

Using a model of HIV transmission among PWID in New York City, Marshall et al. [22,44] also investigated the impact of HIV prevention packages incorporating harm reduction. They examined the impact of a 50% relative increase in HIV testing, OAT coverage, NSPs impact on syringe sharing, and treatment as prevention coverage, implemented alone, in combination with another intervention (dual prevention strategy), or as a combination of all interventions (combination prevention), on HIV incidence among PWID. They found that, if implemented in isolation, increased OAT coverage resulted in a 26.3% (95% CI: 11.3%, 41.3%) relative reduction in HIV incidence by 2040 and increased NSPs access resulted in a 34.3% (95% CI: 19.4%, 49.2%) reduction but that neither of these individual strategies reduced HIV incidence to <1 per 1000 person-years by 2030 [44]. However, joint OAT and NSPs scale-up could result in an HIV incidence among PWID of <1 per 1000 person-years by 2040 [44]. Furthermore, the full combination prevention strategy resulted in a 62.4% (95% CI: 52.6%, 72.2%) reduction in incidence in 2040 compared to the status quo [44]. The combination prevention strategies all had higher impact on incidence compared with scenarios in which interventions were implemented alone, highlighting the epidemiologic benefits of a comprehensive combined intervention approach.

These US analyses are consistent with other global modeling studies that have concluded that scaled-up combination prevention including harm reduction could have a substantial impact on both individual acquisition of HIV and population-level transmission among PWID in a wide range of countries and epidemiologic settings [23–26,42,43].

Additionally, several international studies have evaluated the substantial impact that *existing* combination harm reduction programs have had on HIV epidemics among PWID. For example, two modeling studies have explored the relative impact that scaled-up harm reduction and antiretroviral therapy (ART) efforts could have

Scenarios examined were when a syringe services program was never implemented (*purple*), when a syringe services program was implemented after 10 incident HIV infections are diagnosed (*blue*), and when a syringe services program was existing at initialization (*red*). Boxes show 25%–75% centile; whiskers, 2.5 and 97.5 centiles.

Courtesy of William Goedel and Brandon Marshall.

had on the HIV epidemic among PWID in Vancouver [27,28]. In Vancouver, substantial declines in HIV and HCV incidence among PWID between 1996 and 2013 occurred alongside the expansion of both ART and harm reduction interventions [29]. In one study, Fraser et al. [27] used dynamic coinfection modeling and found that the large declines in HCV incidence observed (84% relative decline from 1996 to 2007) required substantial declines in injecting risk (by nearly 60%), which likely accounted for the majority of the observed decline in HIV incidence. As such, the authors conclude that the observed declines in HIV incidence should be seen as a success for intensive harm reduction interventions, whereas ART may have played a smaller role. In a separate analysis, Nosyk et al. [28] also used modeling to retrospectively investigate the impact and contribution of harm reduction and ART interventions on HIV incidence in British Columbia, Canada. They estimated that their implementation averted 3204 (2402–4589) HIV infections between 1996 and 2013 [28]. To estimate the maximum impact of harm reduction versus ART interventions, they implemented hypothetical scenarios in which ART had no impact on injecting transmission and in which the coverage of harm reduction had remained constant at 1996 levels. Under such extreme assumptions, 77% (62%–95%) and 44% (10%–67%) of HIV infections averted would be attributable to harm reduction and ART interventions, respectively [28]. They concluded that even if ART effectiveness on injecting transmission was as high as that for sexual transmission, harm reduction interventions would still have played a key role in lowering HIV incidence.

Modeling supervised injection facilities for HIV prevention

Several analyses have evaluated the population impact of SIFs on HIV among PWID in North America. Although only one government-sanctioned SIF has been functioning in North America for several years (Insite in Vancouver), interest has grown substantially in response to the overdose crisis and a few new SIFs have emerged. Several groups have investigated the effectiveness of Insite in reducing HIV incidence, with estimates varying from 4 to 119 HIV infections per year [30–34]. Analyses with lower estimates, such as those by Pinkerton et al. [31,32], did not consider behavior change in terms of sharing rates, whereas other studies incorporated data indicating lower rates of sharing among Insite attendants [30,34]. Additionally, higher estimates of infections averted tended to incorporate dynamic models that include the full chain of onward infections averted [34]. Other analyses evaluated the potential impact of opening SIFs in Toronto, Ottawa, and Montreal in Canada [35,36]. These analyses estimated that opening one to three SIFs would avert 2–3 HIV infections per facility in Toronto, 6–10 HIV infections per facility in Ottawa, and 11 HIV infections per facility in Montreal over 20 years [35,36]. The impact of opening fourth and fifth facilities on HIV incidence would be considerably less. In the United States, Irwin et al. [51,52] carried out similar analyses to estimate the potential impact of an SIF on HIV incidence in San Francisco and Baltimore, predicting that a single SIF could avert 3.3 and 3.7 HIV infections per year, respectively. Overall, these studies provide important evidence that SIFs can avert HIV infections, but the predicted impact depends on the epidemic setting, assumptions of intervention impact, and the model type.

Modeling hepatitis C virus infection and harm reduction in the United States

Modeling opioid agonist therapy and needle and syringe programs for hepatitis C virus infection prevention

Early theoretic analyses by Pollack et al. [53,54] evaluated the impact of NSPs on steady-state HCV prevalence among PWID in general settings with and without NSPs. These analyses compared methodological approaches and by utilizing dynamic modeling indicated that short-term incidence analyses overstate NSPs effectiveness in preventing HCV and recommended using longer-time time horizons with dynamic approaches [53,54]. More recent analyses evaluating the impact of existing harm reduction interventions on HCV infection incorporated updated effect estimates for NSPs on HCV incidence or observed empirical relationships between syringe coverage and sharing behavior, combined with transmission epidemic modeling. As detailed earlier, Kwon et al. [21,40] utilized observed relationships between individual-level syringe coverage and syringe sharing behavior in Australia and a dynamic transmission model to estimate that NSPs reduced the incidence of HCV infection among PWID by 15%−43% (19,000−77,000 cases) during 2000−10.

Another UK study evaluating the impact of the existing harm reduction provision by Vickerman et al. used surveillance data to estimate the proportion of PWID on OAT and the proportion receiving high-coverage NSPs (defined as receiving one or more sterile syringes for each injection) combined with the effect estimates for these interventions from systematic reviews and a dynamic transmission model. They found that the existing high levels of harm reduction coverage (>50% of each) could have prevented very high prevalence of HCV infection (>65% chronic prevalence among PWID, compared with the 40% observed) [39]. Another study by Fraser et al. [55] evaluated the scale-up of harm reduction programs in Scotland associated with government-funded national strategies, which promoted the scale-up of OAT, NSPs, and some increases in HCV treatment from 2008. They used modeling to test whether observed decreases in HCV incidence after 2008 could be attributed to this intervention scale-up and found that scaling up of all interventions averted 1492 (95% credible interval [CrI], 657−2646) infections over 7 years, with the majority due to the scale-up of OAT and NSPs (1016 infections, 95% CrI, 308−1996) [55].

No recent studies have evaluated the population impact of *existing* harm reduction provision on HCV infection in the United States, partly because coverage is very low in many settings and additionally because focus has shifted toward how settings can achieve incidence reductions of 80%−90% by 2030, in line with the goals of the World Health Organization [56] and US National Academies of Sciences, Engineering, and Medicine [57]. As such, analyses have tended to focus on the potential future impact of scaled-up levels of HCV treatment for both individual cure and population prevention benefit, such as analyses in Chicago, Illinois [58], and Hartford, Connecticut [59]. Furthermore, modeling analyses by Martin et al. [38] across several generalized HCV epidemic settings (20%, 40%, and 60% chronic HCV infection among PWID) indicated that scale-up of harm reduction alone could reduce HCV incidence by up to 40% within a decade, but that further reductions required a *combination* harm reduction and treatment strategy. Their analyses indicated that combination prevention strategies incorporating both treatment and harm reduction can be highly effective in achieving elimination targets and can reduce the numbers needed to treat.

This general work was supported by two recent US-focused studies that assessed what level of scaled-up combination intervention (harm reduction and HCV treatment) could achieve reductions of 90% in HCV incidence by 2030. The first work, by Fraser et al. [37], examined what is needed in Scott County, Indiana, a rural setting with a rapidly expanding HCV epidemic and increasing injecting drug use. They found that elimination can be achieved through scale-up of HCV treatment only, but that combination scale-up of harm reduction (NSP and OAT to 50% coverage among PWID) halves the treatment rate required. Importantly, they also found that harm reduction provision was essential for prevention of reinfection. If reinfections are not retreated, the epidemic will rebound due to reinfection unless harm reduction is present to sustain treatment impact (Fig. 13.2). This underscores the critical importance of harm reduction as a key component of HCV intervention strategies to prevent both primary infection and reinfection.

Fraser et al. [60] subsequently extended this modeling framework to evaluate how to achieve a 90% reduction in HCV incidence by 2030 among PWID in two US settings: one urban setting (San Francisco, California) and one rural setting (Perry County, Kentucky). They find that with existing harm reduction levels, HCV incidence will increase in Perry County (21.3 in 2017 to 22.6 per 100 person-years in 2030 [/100 person-years]) and decrease in San Francisco (12.9−11.9/100 person-years from 2017 to 2030) [60]. They also found that the scale-up of OAT and NSPs to 50% coverage among PWID reduces the treatment rate to achieve the incidence target in Perry County (from 13%/year to 5%/year); however, it has less impact on the treatment rate in San Francisco due to the existing high levels of coverage of NSPs [60].

These findings add to the growing body of evidence that dramatic reductions in HCV incidence among PWID (such 80%−90% reduction) can be achieved through the scale-up of combination harm reduction and treatment strategies in numerous global settings [38,61−63] and that harm reduction plays a key role in preventing both new infections and reinfections.

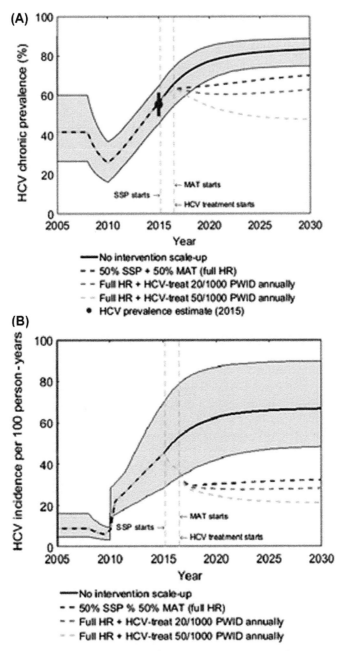

FIGURE 13.2 Modeled projections of hepatitis C virus (HCV) (A) chronic prevalence and (B) incidence among people who inject drugs (PWID) in Scott County, Indiana, over time with various combination intervention strategies.

Modeling supervised injection facilities for HCV prevention

Few studies have examined the impact of SIFs on HCV transmission. Bayoumi and Zaric [34] performed a dynamic economic evaluation of Vancouver's SIF and predicted 51 HCV new cases could be prevented across 10 years. A circulation theory analysis by Irwin et al. [52] estimated that opening a single SIF in Baltimore could avert 21 HCV infections per year. More studies are needed evaluating the potential impact of SIF on HCV transmission, particularly that incorporate dynamic models to assess the full chain of averted transmissions, and that are based on empirical estimates of the impact of SIF's access on HCV and HIV incidence.

Modeling the impact of harm reduction among the incarcerated population on infectious diseases

Owing to widespread policies criminalizing drug use, the concentration of PWID in incarcerated settings results in a high burden of HCV, HIV, and tuberculosis (TB) [64]. Several modeling studies have investigated the potential impact of harm reduction interventions targeting incarcerated populations on related infectious disease epidemics. Ndeffo-Mbah et al. [65] carried out a systematic review of studies modeling infectious disease transmission in incarcerated settings, identifying a wide range of studies that explore HIV, TB, HCV, HBV, and other sexually transmitted infections. Among these, several considered the provision of harm reduction interventions in this setting. Of the 14 studies included, Dolan et al. [64] investigated the impact of prison-based OAT followed by postrelease retention among PWID, considering two main general scenarios based on HIV prevalence among PWID: medium-risk (ranging from 5% to 20%) and high-risk (over 20%) communities. They estimated 100% OAT coverage among incarcerated PWID would reduce cumulative HIV incidence among PWID by 12% in a high-risk community and 28% in a medium-risk community over 5 years. Another study by Altice et al. [66] assessed the longer-term (20 year) impact of scale-up of OAT in prison. They found that in a setting with roughly 20% HIV prevalence among PWID in the general population, provision of 50% OAT coverage in prison with 12 months retention after

Median projections from 1000 model fits are shown, with 95% CrIs only shown for the no-intervention scale-up scenario. Full harm reduction (Full HR) is defined as 50% coverage of both SSP and MAT. HCV treatment started in mid-2016 with two scenarios being shown (20 or 50 per 1000 PWID being treated annually). Incidence is estimated among susceptible PWID. *MAT*, medication-assisted treatment; *SSP*, syringe services program.

release reduces HIV prevalence among PWID in the community by 28% and cumulative incidence by 20% across 15 years. Broadly speaking, these general results indicate that provision of OAT in prison could be an effective strategy for reducing HIV incidence among PWID in both short and long timeframes. Importantly, both studies note that additional impact is achieved by reducing incarceration rates among PWID, as incarceration was associated with increased syringe sharing in prison and the immediate period post release, and interruption of HIV ART.

In Scotland, national survey data indicate lower HCV incidence in prison than in the community (4.3 vs. 7.3 per 100 person-years), which is likely due to existing high levels of OAT. Indeed, after introducing prison OAT in Scotland (current coverage of 57% among PWID), evidence suggests reduction in HCV incidence among incarcerated PWID. Using an epidemic transmission model, Stone et al. [67] estimated that over the next 15 years, existing OAT and HCV treatment in prison could reduce disease incidence among all PWID by a relative 10.7% (95% CrI = 8.4%−13.3%). However, without prison OAT, HCV incidence would decrease by 3.1% (95% CrI = −28.5% to 18.0%), indicating the important role that prison OAT continues to play in HCV epidemics [67]. Another study by the same group indicated that scaled-up prison OAT and removal of the elevated HCV transmission risk after release (possibly achievable through OAT provision on release) could decrease HCV incidence by 30%−90% in four illustrative global settings (Scotland-like, Australia-like, Ukraine-Like, and Thailand-like) [68].

It is unknown what impact scaled-up levels of harm reduction such as OAT and NSPs among incarcerated populations could have on the HCV epidemic among PWID in the United States. One study [69] indicated that universal opt-out HCV testing and treatment in United States prisons for 1 year could prevent 800 new HCV infections in prison and 7200 infections outside prison over 30 years, underscoring the substantial community benefit of prison-based intervention strategies. As such, it appears likely that provision of harm reduction interventions in prisons and jails would have beneficial population impact among both incarcerated populations and PWID in the community. Further research is needed in this area to predict and assess the impact of prison-based harm reduction interventions on HCV in the United States.

Overall, this work underscores the importance of both scale up of evidence-based harm reduction strategies in prison and public-health-oriented drug law reform, which could reduce incarceration of PWID and the transmission of associated infectious diseases [24].

Cost-effectiveness of harm reduction interventions in the United States
Cost-effectiveness background

As indicated earlier, the evidence supporting the benefits of harm reduction interventions in preventing acquisition of HIV and HCV is clear, with substantial modeling evidence to indicate substantial impact on population-level transmission with scaled-up harm reduction in a variety of settings. However, decision-makers often additionally require evidence on the economic implications of a given strategy. Economic evaluation is "the comparative analysis of alternative courses of action in terms of their costs and consequences [70]." By cost, we adopt the standard definition from theoretic economics in which we mean the opportunity cost, or the most valuable alternative not selected. This broad definition includes not just monetary costs but other foregone outcomes, such as loss of productivity. In this regard, perspective of the intervention cost is critical. Perspectives can range from institutional (e.g., hospital, insurance company) to societal, which encompass costs outside the payer's domain. For example, if an investigator adopts a societal perspective, the lost wages for someone who is incarcerated due to opioid use is a cost that might have been averted if he or she were enrolled in a OAT program.

Cost-effectiveness analyses evaluate the value of an intervention (the costs relative to the outcomes) compared to the next best alternative scenario. Health outcomes in cost-effectiveness analyses can be generated from mathematical models and quantified in terms of "number of HIV cases averted" or could be standardized using a health utility, such as the quality-adjusted life-year (QALY). Briefly, a QALY is a measure of quality of life, which is a function of duration of years of life multiplied by the utility of living in that year state on a scale from 0 (dead) to 1 (perfect health). For example, 1 year of life in a perfect health state would be 1 life year × 1 utility value = 1 QALY.

The incremental cost-effectiveness ratio (ICER) is the most frequently used metric to guide decision-making on whether an intervention is cost-effective. It is calculated as the difference in costs of scenarios divided by the differences in health benefits (e.g., QALYs) between the two scenarios (e.g., intervention vs. standard of care). The ICER is therefore presented as an incremental costs per health benefit gained (e.g., dollars per QALY gained). This ICER is assessed against a willingness-to-pay threshold, and interventions with ICERs falling below the threshold are considered cost-effective. Unlike other countries such as the United Kingdom, the United States does not have an official cost-effectiveness threshold; however, a common heuristic is that interventions with an ICER less than $50,000–$100,000 per QALY gained are considered cost-effective [71]. In this section, we describe the cost-effectiveness of harm reduction interventions on prevention of infectious diseases, with a focus on US-based economic evaluations.

Cost-effectiveness of harm reduction in the prevention of infectious diseases

Opioid agonist therapy

Several economic evaluations have found OAT a cost-effective intervention for opioid use disorder in the United States, particularly when incorporating societal costs such as reducing crime [72,73]; however, only a few analyses incorporate the potential additional benefit on infectious disease transmission. Zaric et al. [10]

used a dynamic HIV transmission model to estimate the cost-effectiveness of expanded OAT provision in prevalence settings similar to New York and Los Angeles. The authors adopted a healthcare perspective and estimated the ICER of expanded OAT capacity by 10% to be $8200 per QALY gained in a high HIV prevalence setting (e.g., New York: 40%) and $10,900 per QALY gained in a low HIV prevalence setting (e.g., Los Angeles: 5%) compared to no expansion. The reduction in costs was mostly due to the offset in costs of preventing new HIV infections who would have initiated ART.

A subsequent study evaluated the cost-effectiveness of buprenorphine versus methadone, as these are the two most common OAT alternatives [74]. Overall, the authors found that buprenorphine was cost-effective in both high and low HIV prevalence settings if it did not affect methadone recruitment (ICER: $10,800−$44,200). However, buprenorphine was not cost-effective using the $50,000 per QALY gained threshold in either setting if the buprenorphine cost exceeded $30 per dose (ICERs ranged between $66,700 and $84,700 per QALY gained). Current costs for buprenorphine are roughly $16 per dose [75], indicating that it is cost-effective compared with methadone.

Needle and syringe programs

The economic benefits of NSPs were demonstrated decades prior to 2015, when Congress lifted the ban on NSPs to receive federal funding (federal dollars still cannot be used to purchase sterile syringes). Numerous global studies have found that NSPs are cost-effective in a variety of settings [76]; here we focus on the studies evaluating the cost-effectiveness in the United States.

In 1995, Kaplan [16] published an economic evaluation of the existing NSP in New Haven, Connecticut, which consisted of a mobile van, drug treatment referral coordinator, and outreach staff supervisor. Using a circulation theory model, Kaplan estimated that the program cost $150,000 per year (in USD 1995) and averted 1.62 HIV infections per year at a cost of $92,593 per infection averted. However, if the program were optimized to exchange more syringes among fewer PWID, it could have averted 2.5 infections per year at a cost of $60,000 per infection averted. Kaplan also predicted that if the program budget were up to roughly double that of the New Haven program, more infections would be averted and the NSP could be cost-saving [16]. In an economic evaluation of NSPs in the state of New York, Laufer [17] used a circulation model parameterized with setting-specific data finding an overall ICER of $20,947 per HIV infection averted; however, the cost per infection averted varied between $11,648 and $129,008 across the sites. Importantly, after adopting a societal perspective, NSPs were estimated to be cost-saving after consideration of the costs from donated goods and in-kind services provided [17].

In addition to this evaluation of an existing program, numerous studies have evaluated the potential cost-effectiveness of scaled-up NSPs in preventing HIV among PWID in the United States. In 1993, Lurie et al. [18] assessed the potential cost-effectiveness of NSPs in the United States using an assortment of circulation theory and dynamic models. Lurie and colleagues found that NSPs were consistently cost-effective in preventing HIV across four theoretic United States settings compared to no intervention owing to the offset in HIV treatment costs. It should be noted that in several states, sterile syringes can be purchased at pharmacies, and if policies were changed to increase access to sterile syringes, both NSPs and pharmacies could be cost-effective in terms of averting new cases of HIV infection [77].

In the early 2000s, Pollack [53] was among the first to analyze the potential cost-effectiveness of NSPs for HCV prevention using United States data. Using a transmission model, the author concluded the cost-effectiveness of NSPs was highly sensitive to the prevalence of HCV among PWID, with a lower cost per infection averted in settings with lower HCV prevalence. Since then, empirical data on the efficacy of NSPs in preventing HCV transmission [3], and advances in HCV treatment resulting in high cure rates, has enabled more robust economic evaluations. More recently, within the context of the opioid crisis in the rural United States, an economic evaluation conducted in Perry County, Kentucky, found the potential scale-up of NSPs from 0% to 50% coverage among PWID to be very cost-effective in preventing HCV transmission ($2650 per QALY gained) [78].

These studies are consistent with studies in other countries indicating that existing NSPs are highly cost-effective or cost-saving in preventing HIV and HCV transmission. For example, Kwon et al. developed an HIV/HCV coinfection model parameterized with data from Australia, which unlike the United States, provided high coverage ($\sim$200 syringes exchanged per PWID per year) at the onset of the disease epidemics. Their model indicated that NSPs were very cost-effective and had a positive return on investment ($1.3−$5.5) for the dollars spent on NSPs [21]. Furthermore, an economic evaluation from the United Kingdom indicates that existing NSPs are cost-effective in preventing HCV infection in three sites, and cost-saving in some settings, with difference in cost-effectiveness likely due to the population size and HCV prevalence among PWID [63].

Supervised injection facilities
Economic evaluations of SIFs are more limited, given their relatively recent emergence compared with OAT and NSPs. As various local and state governments in the United States consider opening SIFs, cost-effectiveness analyses have been conducted in several settings in Canada, which shares similar HIV epidemic characteristics as PWID in the United States. Several studies have assessed the cost-effectiveness of Vancouver's SIF *Insite*, all of which conclude that it is cost-saving, but with inconsistent estimates on the number of infections averted primarily due to differences in assumptions on behavior change and model structure used [30−34]. Lastly, although not directly related to injection risks, a cost-benefit analysis of a supervised smoking facility in Vancouver was found to have saved the government approximately 2 million CAD (1.5 million in 2018 USD) because of the reduction in the number of HCV cases averted [79].

The abundance of economic and outcomes data from Vancouver has served as key inputs for hypothetical economic models of SIFs in other North American settings. Enns et al. [80] used a dynamic transmission model, which incorporated the impact of SIFs on HIV and HCV, found a potential SIF in Toronto and Ottawa only cost-effective, with some simulations suggesting it could be cost-saving. Jozaghi et al. [36] also incorporated HIV and HCV benefits using circulation theory and found a potential SIF in Montreal cost-saving. A subsequent analysis by Irwin et al. [51] using circulation theory indicated that a potential SIF in San Francisco would be cost-saving because of its impact on reducing HIV infection, HCV infection, overdose, and skin and soft tissue infections while also increasing the number of individuals on OAT. A similar analysis incorporating these numerous outcomes by Irwin and colleagues [52] also found a hypothetical SIF cost-saving in Baltimore, Maryland. Overall, it appears possible that SIFs are cost-saving when incorporating the numerous benefits of SIFs on HIV, HCV, and other infections.

Combination harm reduction interventions

Newer studies have evaluated the cost-effectiveness of harm reduction within the context of comprehensive combination HIV intervention packages for PWID. Bernard et al. [41] found that OAT, NSPs, and Test & Treat, implemented alone or in combination, could be cost-effective interventions to prevent HIV infection among PWID in the United States. Importantly, however, they found that when coverage expansions included combined investment with other programs and were compared to the next best intervention, the most cost-effective strategy was to first scale OAT coverage up to 50%, followed by scaling NSPs coverage to 50%, then scaling Test & Treat coverage to 50%, with each coverage expansion producing an ICER <US$50,000 per QALY gained relative to the next best portfolio (Fig. 13.3).

One study evaluated the cost-effectiveness of combination harm reduction (OAT + NSPs) plus HCV treatment on HCV epidemics among PWID in Kentucky. This study found that in rural Kentucky, which has a high HCV incidence, combination harm reduction and HCV test and treat was found to be cost-effective compared with scale-up of OAT and NSPs alone [81]. Given the emergence of curative direct-acting antivirals (DAAs), modeling the impact and cost-effectiveness of combination prevention and treatment interventions on HIV and HCV transmission among PWID remains an active area of investigation.

Cost-effectiveness of harm reduction sites as locations for infectious disease or overdose interventions among people who inject drugs

In addition to direct prevention benefits in terms of infectious disease transmission, harm reduction services provide key opportunities for the diagnosis of infectious diseases. Cipriano et al. [82]. found that frequent (every 3—6 months) HIV screening among OAT clients in the United States was cost—effective. This study, in the pre-DAA era, found that annual HCV screening was moderately cost-effective (ICER, $80,800/QALY gained). More recent studies in the DAA era have found that rapid on-site testing for HCV infection in substance use treatment programs in the United States is cost-effective (ICER, <$30,000/QALY gained) compared

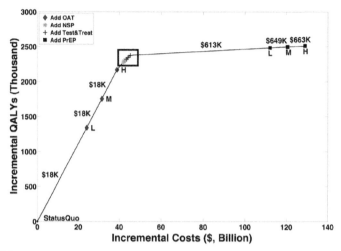

FIGURE 13.3

Cost-efficiency frontier of combinations of opiate agonist therapy (OAT), needle and syringe programs (NSPs), HIV test & treat, and HIV preexposure prophylaxis (PrEP) at status quo, low- (L), medium- (M), and high-coverage (H) levels on HIV prevention among PWID in the United States. QALYs, quality-adjusted life-years.

Reproduced from Bernard CL, Owens DK, Goldhaber-Fiebert JD, Brandeau ML. Estimation of the cost-effectiveness of HIV prevention portfolios for people who inject drugs in the United States: a model-based analysis. PLoS Med 2017;14(5):e1002312.

with referral for testing [83]. Combined rapid on-site HIV and HCV testing in substance use programs was cost-effective under a willingness-to-pay threshold of $100,000/QALY gained. An analysis by Schackman et al. [84] within the context of a randomized clinical trial examined the cost-effectiveness of and HCV screening and active linkage to care intervention at OAT sites in New York and San Francisco. They concluded the screening to linkage to care intervention to be cost-effective (ICER, <$25,000 per QALY gained).

Harm reduction sites can also play important role in providing overdose prevention interventions. Uyei et al. [85] developed a Markov state model to examine the cost-effectiveness of naloxone distribution at NSPs in the United States. They found that naloxone distribution through NSP is highly cost-effective (ICER, $323/QALY gained), and that naloxone distribution plus linkage to OAT from NSPs was cost-saving compared with NSPs alone [85].

Cost-effectiveness of harm reduction in the prevention of other infectious diseases

While the health benefits of harm reduction interventions are primarily focused on the prevention of blood-borne viruses such as HIV and HCV, PWID are nonetheless more likely to acquire other infectious diseases, such as TB, compared with the general population. As such, harm reduction interventions represent critical referral or screening sites to obtain treatment for comorbidities, which could otherwise go unaddressed. OAT programs have been shown to be important cost-effective sites to screen and treat TB. For example, Perlman et al. [86] evaluated the cost-effectiveness of a TB screening and directly observed therapy program at an NSP, parameterized mostly with data from New York City. Similarly in another study involving client data from five methadone sites in San Francisco, Snyder et al. [87] found that methadone treatment was highly cost-effective, and in certain circumstances cost-saving, because of the high proportion of patients who were successfully screened and completed preventative therapy.

Conclusion

There is strong global empirical evidence that OAT and NSPs (especially in combination with OAT) are effective in preventing HIV and HCV acquisition among PWID. Despite this, coverage of harm reduction is suboptimal and well below the recommended World Health Organization standards in the vast majority of countries worldwide, including the United States.

Modeling studies across numerous global settings have indicated that existing OAT and NSPs have likely prevented a substantial amount of HIV and HCV transmission among PWID. Studies focusing on the United States have indicated that scale-up of harm reduction could play an important role, both in isolation and in combination with other treatment and prevention interventions, in averting HIV and HCV infections in the future and that these interventions are cost-effective and potentially cost-saving.

Only a few modeling studies have assessed the potential impact of SIFs on infectious disease transmission in the United States, but these theoretic studies, based predominantly on data from Vancouver's SIF (Insite), indicate that US-based SIFs could be highly cost-effective in preventing HIV and HCV transmission. Empirical studies evaluating the impact of attendance at an SIF on an individual's risk of acquiring HIV, HCV, and other infections are warranted and will strengthen modeling studies of potential population impact.

To date, the vast majority of analyses have assessed the role of interventions in singular disease epidemics (e.g., HIV or HCV). Yet, OAT is known to prevent both HIV and HCV transmission, as well as reduce fatal overdose, reduce incarceration (which has been found to increase the risk of overdose, HIV infection, and HCV infection), and increase uptake and improve outcomes of HIV ART. More detailed studies are needed that incorporate these synergistic and interacting benefits on multiple infectious and noninfectious disease outcomes at a population level in different epidemic settings among PWID. Similarly, much of the evidence base has focused on evaluating the cost-effectiveness of individual harm reduction interventions on single health outcomes, which under reasonable assumptions indicate that harm reduction interventions are cost-effective and, in some instances, cost-saving, particularly when incorporating societal benefits such as OAT preventing reincarceration and associated criminal justice costs. Future economic evaluation should continue to broaden the scope of their analyses, evaluating combination harm reduction interventions, their synergies, and multiple health benefits. Continued work quantifying the additional societal benefits of these interventions in terms of work productivity, criminal justice costs, etc. will enable researchers to fully capture the health and economic benefits of harm reduction. Finally, as harm reduction services become more closely integrated with infectious disease treatment, economic and infectious disease modeling will become increasingly more important to ensure their sustainability.

In conclusion, there is an increasingly strong evidence base that harm reduction interventions such as OAT and NSPs for OUD reduce an individual's risk of acquiring HIV and HCV infections. Modeling studies have indicated that scale-up of these interventions can have multiple benefits on HIV and HCV epidemics among PWID and can serve as important sites for linkage to infectious disease testing and treatment. Scale-up of harm reduction for the incarcerated population while in custody and after release could have a substantial benefit in reducing HIV and HCV transmission both within criminal justice settings and in the broader community. Evidence for the impact of SIF on infectious disease transmission is limited, but these could be important components of the epidemic response. Additionally economic evaluations have indicated that scale-up of harm reduction interventions is cost-effective and potentially cost-saving. Scale-up of harm reduction, in addition to HCV and HIV treatment and naloxone, is urgently needed to address the opioid crisis and the related infectious disease epidemics in the United States.

References

[1] Degenhardt L, Peacock A, Colledge S, Leung J, Grebely J, Vickerman P, et al. Global prevalence of injecting drug use and sociodemographic characteristics and prevalence of HIV, HBV, and HCV in people who inject drugs: a multistage systematic review. Lancet Glob Health 2017;5(12):e1192−207.

[2] Vanhommerig JW, Thomas XV, van der Meer JT, Geskus RB, Bruisten SM, Molenkamp R, et al. Hepatitis C virus (HCV) antibody dynamics following acute HCV infection and reinfection among HIV-infected men who have sex with men. Clin Infect Dis December 15, 2014;59(12):1678−85. Epub 2014/09/05; PubMed PMID: 25186590.

[3] Platt L, Minozzi S, Reed J, Vickerman P, Hagan H, French C, et al. Needle syringe programmes and opioid substitution therapy for preventing hepatitis C transmission in people who inject drugs. Cochrane Database Syst Rev 2017 09/18;(9):CD012021. PubMed PMCID: PMC5621373.

[4] Aspinall EJ, Nambiar D, Goldberg DJ, Hickman M, Weir A, Van Velzen E, et al. Are needle and syringe programmes associated with a reduction in HIV transmission among people who inject drugs: a systematic review and meta-analysis. Int J Epidemiol 2014; 43(1):235−48.

[5] MacArthur GJ, Minozzi S, Martin N, Vickerman P, Deren S, Bruneau J, et al. Opiate substitution treatment and HIV transmission in people who inject drugs: systematic review and meta-analysis. BMJ 2012;345:e5945. PubMed PMID: 23038795.

[6] Larney S, Peacock A, Leung J, Colledge S, Hickman M, Vickerman P, et al. Global, regional, and country-level coverage of interventions to prevent and manage HIV and hepatitis C among people who inject drugs: a systematic review. Lancet Glob health 2017;5(12):e1208−20. PubMed PMID: 29074410.

[7] Kral AH, Davidson PJ. Addressing the nation's opioid epidemic: lessons from an unsanctioned supervised injection site in the U.S. Am J Prev Med 2017;53(6):919−22.

[8] MacArthur GJ, van Velzen E, Palmateer N, Kimber J, Pharris A, Hope V, et al. Interventions to prevent HIV and hepatitis C in people who inject drugs: a review of reviews to assess evidence of effectiveness. Int J Drug Policy January 2014;25(1):34−52. Epub 2013/08/27; PubMed PMID: 23973009.

[9] Joseph H, Stancliff S, Langrod J. Methadone maintenance treatment (MMT): a review of historical and clinical issues. Mt Sinai J Med Oct-Nov;67(5−6):347−64. Epub 2000/ 11/07; PubMed PMID: 11064485.

[10] Zaric GS, Barnett PG, Brandeau ML. HIV transmission and the cost-effectiveness of methadone maintenance. Am J Public Health July 2000;90(7):1100−11. Epub 2000/ 07/18; PubMed PMID: 10897189. Pubmed Central PMCID: PMC1446290.

[11] Hurley SF, Jolley DJ, Kaldor JM. Effectiveness of needle-exchange programmes for prevention of HIV infection. Lancet June 21, 1997;349(9068):1797−800. Epub 1997/ 06/21; PubMed PMID: 9269214.

[12] Des Jarlais DC, Marmor M, Paone D, Titus S, Shi Q, Perlis T, et al. HIV incidence among injecting drug users in New York City syringe-exchange programmes. Lancet October 12, 1996;348(9033):987−91. Epub 1996/10/12; PubMed PMID: 8855855.

[13] Des Jarlais DC, Perlis T, Arasteh K, Torian LV, Beatrice S, Milliken J, et al. HIV incidence among injection drug users in New York City, 1990 to 2002: use of serologic test algorithm to assess expansion of HIV prevention services. Am J Public Health 2005; 95(8):1439−44. PubMed PMID: 15985649.

[14] Kaplan EH, O'Keefe E. Let the needles do the talking! Evaluating the new haven needle exchange. Interfaces 1993;23(1):7−26.

[15] Kaplan EH, Heimer R. A circulation theory of needle exchange. AIDS 1994;8(5): 567−74. PubMed PMID: 8060540.

[16] Kaplan EH. Economic analysis of needle exchange. AIDS 1995;9(10):1113−20. PubMed PMID: 8519446.

[17] Laufer FN. Cost-effectiveness of syringe exchange as an HIV prevention strategy. J Acquir Immune Defic Syndr November 1, 2001;28(3):273−8. Epub 2001/11/06; PubMed PMID: 11694836.

[18] Berkeley: School of Public Health University of California. The Public Health Impact of Needle Exchange Programs in the United States and Abroad: Summary, Conclusions and Recommendations. 1993. https://harmreductionorg/wp-content/uploads/2012/01/ NEPReportSummary1993.pdf.

[19] Lurie P, Drucker E. An opportunity lost: HIV infections associated with lack of a national needle-exchange programme in the USA. Lancet March 1, 1997;349(9052): 604−8. Epub 1997/03/01; PubMed PMID: 9057732.

[20] Nguyen TQ, Weir BW, Des Jarlais DC, Pinkerton SD, Holtgrave DR. Syringe exchange in the United States: a national level economic evaluation of hypothetical increases in investment. AIDS Behav November 2014;18(11):2144−55. Epub 2014/05/16; PubMed PMID: 24824043. Pubmed Central PMCID: PMC4211599.

[21] Kwon JA, Anderson J, Kerr CC, Thein H-H, Zhang L, Iversen J, et al. Estimating the cost-effectiveness of needle-syringe programs in Australia. AIDS November 13, 2012;26(17):2201−10. https://doi.org/10.1097/QAD.0b013e3283578b5d. Epub 2012/08/24; PubMed PMID: 22914579.

[22] Marshall BDL, Paczkowski MM, Seemann L, Tempalski B, Pouget ER, Galea S, et al. A complex systems approach to evaluate HIV prevention in metropolitan areas: preliminary implications for combination intervention strategies. PLoS One 2012;7(9): e44833.

[23] Mabileau G, Scutelniciuc O, Tsereteli M, Konorazov I, Yelizaryeva A, Popovici S, et al. Intervention packages to reduce the impact of HIV and HCV infections among people who inject drugs in Eastern Europe and Central Asia: a modeling and cost-effectiveness study. Open Forum Infect Dis March 2018;5(3):ofy040. Epub 2018/03/30; PubMed PMID: 29594179. Pubmed Central PMCID: PMC5861407.

[24] Borquez A, Beletsky L, Nosyk B, Strathdee SA, Madrazo A, Abramovitz D, et al. The effect of public health-oriented drug law reform on HIV incidence in people who inject drugs in Tijuana, Mexico: an epidemic modelling study. Lancet Public Health 2018; 3(9):e429−37.

[25] Cepeda JA, Eritsyan K, Vickerman P, Lyubimova A, Shegay M, Odinokova V, et al. Potential impact of implementing and scaling up harm reduction and antiretroviral therapy on HIV prevalence and mortality and overdose deaths among people who inject drugs in two Russian cities: a modelling study. Lancet HIV 2018;5(10):e578−87.

[26] Rhodes T, Guise A, Ndimbii J, Strathdee S, Ngugi E, Platt L, et al. Is the promise of methadone Kenya's solution to managing HIV and addiction? A mixed-method mathematical modelling and qualitative study. BMJ Open March 6, 2015;5(3):e007198. Epub 2015/03/10; PubMed PMID: 25748417. Pubmed Central PMCID: PMC4360c822.

[27] Fraser H, Mukandavire C, Martin NK, Hickman M, Cohen MS, Miller WC, et al. HIV treatment as prevention among people who inject drugs - a re-evaluation of the evidence. Int J Epidemiol 2017;46(2):466−78. Epub 08/12; PubMed PMID: 27524816.

[28] Nosyk B, Zang X, Min JE, Krebs E, Lima VD, Milloy MJ, et al. Relative effects of antiretroviral therapy and harm reduction initiatives on HIV incidence in British Columbia, Canada, 1996-2013: a modelling study. Lancet HIV July 2017;4(7): e303−10. Epub 2017/04/04; PubMed PMID: 28366707. Pubmed Central PMCID: PMC5494273.

[29] Wood E, Kerr T, Marshall BDL, Li K, Zhang R, Hogg RS, et al. Longitudinal community plasma HIV-1 RNA concentrations and incidence of HIV-1 among injecting drug users: prospective cohort study. BMJ 2009;338:b1649−. PubMed PMID: 19406887.

[30] Andresen MA, Boyd N. A cost-benefit and cost-effectiveness analysis of Vancouver's supervised injection facility. Int J Drug Policy January 2010;21(1):70−6. Epub 2009/05/09; PubMed PMID: 19423324.

[31] Pinkerton SD. Is Vancouver Canada's supervised injection facility cost-saving? Addiction August 2010;105(8):1429−36. Epub 2010/07/27; PubMed PMID: 20653622.

[32] Pinkerton SD. How many HIV infections are prevented by Vancouver Canada's supervised injection facility? Int J Drug Policy May 2011;22(3):179−83. Epub 2011/04/01; PubMed PMID: 21450450.

[33] Andresen MA, Jozaghi E. The point of diminishing returns: an examination of expanding Vancouver's insite. Urban Stud 2012;49(16):3531−44.

[34] Bayoumi AM, Zaric GS. The cost-effectiveness of Vancouver's supervised injection facility. CMAJ 2008;179(11):1143–51.

[35] Bayoumi AM, Strike C. Report of the Toronto and Ottawa supervised consumption assessment study. 2012.

[36] Jozaghi E, Reid AA, Andresen MA. A cost-benefit/cost-effectiveness analysis of proposed supervised injection facilities in Montreal, Canada. Subst Abuse Treat Prev Policy July 9, 2013;8:25. Epub 2013/07/11; PubMed PMID: 23837814. Pubmed Central PMCID: PMC3710233.

[37] Fraser H, Zibbell J, Hoerger T, Hariri S, Vellozzi C, Martin NK, et al. Scaling-up HCV prevention and treatment interventions in rural United States—model projections for tackling an increasing epidemic. Addiction 2018;113(1):173–82.

[38] Martin N, Hickman M, Hutchinson S, Goldberg D, Vickerman P. Combination interventions to prevent HCV transmission among people who inject drugs: modelling the impact of antiviral treatment, needle and syringe programmes, and opiate substitution therapy. Clin Infect Dis 2013;57(Suppl. 2):S39–45.

[39] Vickerman P, Martin N, Turner K, Hickman M. Can needle and syringe programmes and opiate substitution therapy achieve substantial reductions in hepatitis C virus prevalence? Model projections for different epidemic settings. Addiction 2012. https://doi.org/10.1111/j.1360-0443.2012.03932.x.

[40] Kwon JA, Iversen J, Maher L, Law MG, Wilson DP. The impact of needle and syringe programs on HIV and HCV transmissions in injecting drug users in Australia: a model-based analysis. J Acquir Immune Defic Syndr August 1, 2009;51(4):462–9. Epub 2009/04/24; PubMed PMID: 19387355.

[41] Bernard CL, Owens DK, Goldhaber-Fiebert JD, Brandeau ML. Estimation of the cost-effectiveness of HIV prevention portfolios for people who inject drugs in the United States: a model-based analysis. PLoS Med 2017;14(5):e1002312.

[42] Alistar SS, Owens DK, Brandeau ML. Effectiveness and cost effectiveness of expanding harm reduction and antiretroviral therapy in a mixed HIV epidemic: a modeling analysis for Ukraine. PLoS Med 2011;8(3):e1000423.

[43] Vickerman P, Platt L, Jolley E, Rhodes T, Kazatchkine MD, Latypov A. Controlling HIV among people who inject drugs in Eastern Europe and Central Asia: insights from modeling. Int J Drug Policy November 2014;25(6):1163–73. Epub 2014/12/03; PubMed PMID: 25449056.

[44] Marshall BD, Friedman SR, Monteiro JF, Paczkowski M, Tempalski B, Pouget ER, et al. Prevention and treatment produced large decreases in HIV incidence in a model of people who inject drugs. Health Aff March 2014;33(3):401–9. Epub 2014/03/05; PubMed PMID: 24590937. Pubmed Central PMCID: PMC4469974.

[45] Garnett GP, Cousens S, Hallett TB, Steketee R, Walker N. Mathematical models in the evaluation of health programmes. Lancet August 6, 2011;378(9790):515–25. Epub 2011/04/13; PubMed PMID: 21481448.

[46] Sordo L, Barrio G, Bravo MJ, Indave BI, Degenhardt L, Wiessing L, et al. Mortality risk during and after opioid substitution treatment: systematic review and meta-analysis of cohort studies. BMJ 2017;357:j1550.

[47] Kimber J, Larney S, Hickman M, Randall D, Degenhardt L. Mortality risk of opioid substitution therapy with methadone versus buprenorphine: a retrospective cohort study. Lancet Psychiatry October 2015;2(10):901–8. Epub 2015/09/20; PubMed PMID: 26384619.

[48] Escudero DJ, Lurie MN, Mayer KH, Weinreb C, King M, Galea S, et al. Acute HIV infection transmission among people who inject drugs in a mature epidemic setting. AIDS October 23, 2016;30(16):2537−44. PubMed PMID: 27490641. Pubmed Central PMCID: PMC5069170.

[49] Escudero DJ, Lurie MN, Mayer KH, King M, Galea S, Friedman SR, et al. The risk of HIV transmission at each step of the HIV care continuum among people who inject drugs: a modeling study. BMC Public Health 2017;17(1):614. PubMed PMID: 28738861.

[50] Gonsalves GS, Crawford FW. Dynamics of the HIV outbreak and response in Scott County, IN, USA, 2011-15: a modelling study. Lancet HIV October 2018;5(10): e569−77. Epub 2018/09/18; PubMed PMID: 30220531. Pubmed Central PMCID: PMC6192548.

[51] Irwin A, Jozaghi E, Bluthenthal RN, Kral AH. A cost-benefit analysis of a potential supervised injection facility in San Francisco, California, USA. J Drug Issues 2016;47(2): 164−84.

[52] Irwin A, Jozaghi E, Weir BW, Allen ST, Lindsay A, Sherman SG. Mitigating the heroin crisis in Baltimore, MD, USA: a cost-benefit analysis of a hypothetical supervised injection facility. Harm Reduct J May 12, 2017;14(1):29.

[53] Pollack HA. Cost-effectiveness of harm reduction in preventing hepatitis C among injection drug users. Med Decis Making October 1, 2001;21(5):357−67.

[54] Pollack HA. Ignoring 'downstream infection' in the evaluation of harm reduction interventions for injection drug users. Eur J Epidemiol 2001;17(4):391−5.

[55] Fraser H, Mukandavire C, Martin NK, Goldberg D, Palmateer N, Munro A, et al. Modelling the impact of a national scale-up of interventions on hepatitis C virus transmission among people who inject drugs in Scotland. Addiction November 2018; 113(11):2118−31. Epub 2018/05/22; PubMed PMID: 29781207.

[56] World Health Organization. Global health sector strategy on viral hepatitis 2016−2021, towards ending viral hepatitis. 2016.

[57] National Academies of Sciences Engineering and Medicine. Eliminating the public health problem of hepatitis B and C in the United States: phase one report. 2016.

[58] Echevarria D, Gutfraind A, Boodram B, Major M, Del Valle S, Cotler SJ, et al. Mathematical modeling of hepatitis C prevalence reduction with antiviral treatment scale-up in persons who inject drugs in Metropolitan Chicago. PLoS One 2015;10(8):e0135901. PubMed PMID: 26295805.

[59] Zelenev A, Li J, Mazhnaya A, Basu S, Altice FL. Hepatitis C virus treatment as prevention in an extended network of people who inject drugs in the USA: a modelling study. Lancet Infect Dis 2018;18(2):215−24.

[60] Fraser H, Vellozzi C, Hoerger T, Evans J, Kral A, Havens J, et al. Scaling-up hepatitis C prevention and treatment interventions for achieving elimination in the United States − a rural and urban comparison. Am J Epidemiol 2019 ;188(8):1539−1551.

[61] Gountas I, Sypsa V, Anagnostou O, Martin N, Vickerman P, Kafetzopoulos E, et al. Treatment and primary prevention in people who inject drugs for chronic hepatitis C infection: is elimination possible in a high prevalence setting? Addiction 2017; 112(7):1290−9. https://doi.org/10.1111/add.13764.

[62] Fraser H, Martin NK, Brummer-Korvenkontio H, Carrieri P, Dalgard O, Dillon J, et al. Model projections on the impact of HCV treatment in the prevention of HCV transmission among people who inject drugs in Europe. J Hepatol 2018;68(3):402−11.

[63] Platt L, Sweeney S, Ward Z, Guinness L, Hickman M, Hope V, et al. Assessing the impact and cost-effectiveness of needle and syringe provision and opioid substitution therapy on hepatitis C transmission among people who inject drugs in the UK: an analysis of pooled data sets and economic modelling. Southampton UK: Queen's Printer and Controller of HMSO; 2017. This work was produced by Platt et al. under the terms of a commissioning contract issued by the Secretary of State for Health. This issue may be freely reproduced for the purposes of private research and study and extracts (or indeed, the full report) may be included in professional journals provided that suitable acknowledgement is made and the reproduction is not associated with any form of advertising. Applications for commercial reproduction should be addressed to: NIHR Journals Library, National Institute for Health Research, Evaluation, Trials and Studies Coordinating Centre, Alpha House, University of Southampton Science Park, Southampton SO16 7NS, UK; Sep 2017.

[64] Dolan K, Wirtz AL, Moazen B, Ndeffo-mbah M, Galvani A, Kinner SA, et al. Global burden of HIV, viral hepatitis, and tuberculosis in prisoners and detainees. Lancet 2016; 388(10049):1089−102.

[65] Ndeffo-Mbah ML, Vigliotti VS, Skrip LA, Dolan K, Galvani AP. Dynamic models of infectious disease transmission in prisons and the general population. Epidemiol Rev June 1, 2018;40(1):40−57. Epub 2018/03/23; PubMed PMID: 29566137. Pubmed Central PMCID: PMC5982711.

[66] Altice FL, Azbel L, Stone J, Brooks-Pollock E, Smyrnov P, Dvoriak S, et al. The perfect storm: incarceration and the high-risk environment perpetuating transmission of HIV, hepatitis C virus, and tuberculosis in Eastern Europe and Central Asia. Lancet 2016; 388(10050):1228−48. Epub 07/14; PubMed PMID: 27427455.

[67] Stone J, Martin NK, Hickman M, Hutchinson SJ, Aspinall E, Taylor A, et al. Modelling the impact of incarceration and prison-based hepatitis C virus (HCV) treatment on HCV transmission among people who inject drugs in Scotland. Addiction 2017;112(7): 1302−14. PubMed PMCID: PMC5461206.

[68] Csete J, Kamarulzaman A, Kazatchkine M, Altice F, Balicki M, Buxton J, et al. Public health and international drug policy. Lancet 2016;387(10026):1427−80.

[69] He T, Li K, Roberts MS, Spaulding AC, Ayer T, Grefenstette JJ, et al. Prevention of hepatitis C by screening and treatment in U.S. prisons. Ann Intern Med 2016;164(2): 84−92. Epub 11/24; PubMed PMID: 26595252.

[70] Drummond M, Sculpher M, Torrance G, O'Brien CB, Stoddart S. Methods for the economic evaluation of health care programmes. Press OU; 2005.

[71] Neumann PJ, Cohen JT, Weinstein MC. Updating cost-effectiveness-the curious resilience of the $50,000-per-QALY threshold. N Engl J Med August 28, 2014;371(9): 796−7. Epub 2014/08/28; PubMed PMID: 25162885.

[72] Barnett PG. The cost-effectiveness of methadone maintenance as a health care intervention. Addiction April 1999;94(4):479−88. Epub 1999/12/22; PubMed PMID: 10605844.

[73] Basu A, Paltiel AD, Pollack HA. Social costs of robbery and the cost-effectiveness of substance abuse treatment. Health Econ August 2008;17(8):927−46. Epub 2007/11/10; PubMed PMID: 17992708. Pubmed Central PMCID: PMC3512566.

[74] Barnett PG, Zaric GS, Brandeau ML. The cost-effectiveness of buprenorphine maintenance therapy for opiate addiction in the United States. Addiction September 2001; 96(9):1267−78. Epub 2001/10/24; PubMed PMID: 11672491.

[75] NIDA. How Much Does Opioid Treatment Cost?. 2018. https://wwwdrugabusegov/publications/research-reports/medications-to-treat-opioid-addiction/how-much-does-opioid-treatment-cost.

[76] Wilson DP, Donald B, Shattock AJ, Wilson D, Fraser-Hurt N. The cost-effectiveness of harm reduction. Int J Drug Policy February 2015;26(Suppl. 1):S5–11. Epub 2015/03/03; PubMed PMID: 25727260.

[77] Holtgrave DR, Pinkerton SD, Jones TS, Lurie P, Vlahov D. Cost and cost-effectiveness of increasing access to sterile syringes and needles as an HIV prevention intervention in the United States. J Acquir Immune Defic Syndr Hum Retrovirol 1998;18(Suppl. 1): S133–8. Epub 1998/07/15; PubMed PMID: 9663636.

[78] Fraser H, Barbosa C, Young A, Havens J, E T, Ward Z, et al. Cost-effectiveness of scaling-up syringe service provision among people who inject drugs in Perry County, Kentucky. In: International symposium on hepatitis care in substance users (INHSU) 2018, Lisbon, Portugal September 19–21, 2018 oral presentation; 2018.

[79] Jozaghi E. A cost-benefit/cost-effectiveness analysis of an unsanctioned supervised smoking facility in the Downtown Eastside of Vancouver, Canada. Harm Reduct J November 13, 2014;11(1):30. Epub 2014/11/15; PubMed PMID: 25395278. Pubmed Central PMCID: PMC4251950.

[80] Enns EA, Zaric GS, Strike CJ, Jairam JA, Kolla G, Bayoumi AM. Potential cost-effectiveness of supervised injection facilities in Toronto and Ottawa, Canada. Addiction 2016;111(3):475–89.

[81] Fraser H, Barbosa C, Vellozzi C, Hoerger T, Evans J, Hariri S, et al. Cost-effectiveness of scaling-up HCV prevention, testing and treatment interventions among people who inject drugs in the US. In: International symposium on hepatitis care in substance users (INHSU) 2017 oral presentation; 2017.

[82] Cipriano LE, Zaric GS, Holodniy M, Bendavid E, Owens DK, Brandeau ML. Cost effectiveness of screening strategies for early identification of HIV and HCV infection in injection drug users. PLoS One 2012;7(9):e45176. Epub 2012/10/03; PubMed PMID: 23028828. Pubmed Central PMCID: PMC3445468.

[83] Schackman BR, Leff JA, Barter DM, DiLorenzo MA, Feaster DJ, Metsch LR, et al. Cost-effectiveness of rapid hepatitis C virus (HCV) testing and simultaneous rapid HCV and HIV testing in substance abuse treatment programs. Addiction 2015; 110(1):129–43. PubMed PMID: 25291977.

[84] Schackman BR, Gutkind S, Morgan JR, Leff JA, Behrends CN, Delucchi KL, et al. Cost-effectiveness of hepatitis C screening and treatment linkage intervention in US methadone maintenance treatment programs. Drug Alcohol Depend April 1, 2018;185:411–20. Epub 2018/02/27; PubMed PMID: 29477574. Pubmed Central PMCID: PMC5889754.

[85] Uyei J, Fiellin DA, Buchelli M, Rodriguez-Santana R, Braithwaite RS. Effects of naloxone distribution alone or in combination with addiction treatment with or without pre-exposure prophylaxis for HIV prevention in people who inject drugs: a cost-effectiveness modelling study. Lancet Public Health March 2017;2(3):e133–40. Epub 2017/12/19; PubMed PMID: 29253386.

[86] Perlman DC, Gourevitch MN, Trinh C, Salomon N, Horn L, Des Jarlais DC. Cost-effectiveness of tuberculosis screening and observed preventive therapy for active drug injectors at a syringe-exchange program. J Urban Health September 2001;78(3):550–67. Epub 2001/09/21; PubMed PMID: 11564856. Pubmed Central PMCID: PMC3455907.

[87] Snyder DC, Paz EA, Mohle-Boetani JC, Fallstad R, Black RL, Chin DP. Tuberculosis prevention in methadone maintenance clinics. Effectiveness and cost-effectiveness. Am J Respir Crit Care Med July 1999;160(1):178–85. Epub 1999/07/03; PubMed PMID: 10390397.

Index